A Falling House of Cards

The Victorian Government and the Pandemic Hotel Quarantine Disaster

Dr Carl A. Gibson

A Falling House of Cards

All illustrations are the property of Executive Impact Consulting Pty Ltd, unless otherwise noted.

National Library of Australia Cataloguing-in-Publication data is available upon request.
ISBN: 978-0-6450000-8-5

Composition and book design by Executive Impact Publishing an imprint of Executive Impact Consulting Pty Ltd.

The material contains case studies and anecdotal commentary. The material presented in this book comprises discussion based upon factual information derived from the Coate Inquiry (including the two reports, witness statements and transcripts), as well as plausible inferences and suppositions where verifiable information is not available. This by necessity means that some assertions in this book may prove to be incorrect as and when further information is made available in the public domain. The author apologises in advance for any situations where this may occur in the future. Further, this book makes no claim as to the culpability or otherwise of persons and organisations named in this in book. The author has endeavoured to provide information to allow the reader to reach their own conclusions.

Contents

Foreword

Early January 2020, and my family and friends had thought that I had lost the plot. I was warning them to get ready, to make sure that they had sufficient food, water, and batteries for a couple of weeks. I was urging them to get prepared for what could be a few weeks of serious disruptions, maybe even civil unrest. They probably thought that my love of horror movies and TV series had finally sent me over the edge, here I was predicting the early stages of the zombie apocalypse. From my perspective, I was reading epidemiological reports and speaking with infectious disease experts, former colleagues from an earlier career, and I was beginning to get very worried about the information coming out of China.

To be honest, I had been waiting for *the* pandemic for several decades. Although I had spent more recent time at senior levels in the public and private sectors, my original career was in infectious virus diseases. I worked in both research and leading field investigations into emerging diseases, working with some of the world's most iconic research institutions. One of my scientific mentors was fanatical about the 1918 influenza pandemic ('Spanish Lady) and its origins. He spent a number of years trying to isolate the virus from frozen corpses, individuals that had died during *that* pandemic, and had been buried within the Arctic Circle. His passion 'infected' me and the prospect of a new emerging disease became my driving force for many years.

Since the 1990's working in Australia, I had ensured that each of my employers had plans in place in readiness for the pandemic that almost every virologist believed was overdue. With each emerging disease outbreak (bird flu, SARS, MERS, swine flu, etc.), I of course wondered if this could be the big one, monitoring the situation but not becoming overly concerned. But the picture that I was beginning to build in early 2020 was causing a mental itch that I could not relieve. Something about this one felt different, but I could not honestly say why I was more worried about this outbreak. That this outbreak had occurred in China might have been part of my intuitive response. Historically, China had been a hotspot for emerging respiratory diseases[1,2]. Its cultural traditions that

---

[1] Including the emergence of SARS in 2002, H2N2 influenza in 1957; H3N2 influenza in 1968; H5N1 influenza in 1996 and H7N9 influenza in 2013 (Kaina, 2021; Honigsbaum, 2020). It has also been postulated that the 1918 H1N1 influenza pandemic may also have originated in China, although Kansas and France have also been suggested (Worobey et al, 2019; 2014; Oxford and Gill, 2019; Vergano, 2014; Kilbourne, 2006; Barry, 2004).

[2] Growing populations, land use changes, continuing encroachment and exposure of human populations to potentially infected wildlife (through urban expansion, wet markets, tourism

exposed vulnerable individuals to new zoonotic pathogens from captured wildlife in crowded markets along with indifferent food handling standards, provided a perfect recipe for an outbreak[3].

Its population size and population density, the mass movement of people during holiday periods, along with its global air connections and traffic volumes would provide for ready widespread transmission. Whilst the Chinese Communist Party's historical lack of transparency about internal crises, would help to ensure that any emerging respiratory disease within China would spread rapidly to the rest of the world.

Dr Carl A. Gibson
Queensland, October 2023.

---

etc.), with remnant wildlife populations acting as reservoirs of novel pathogens, combined with the supply of wild animal originated traditional medicines, poor sanitation and food handling practices all come together to create a 'perfect storm' (Rulli et al, 2021; Emanuel and Moore, 2020; Kuchipudi, 2020; Mitchel et al, 2020; Liu, 2017). Whilst other SE Asian countries may also be regarded as hotspots for emerging diseases, China's prominence may also be because of its more extensive surveillance capabilities ensuring that such emerging diseases are detected more readily. However, it appears that this heightened surveillance is then countered by labyrinthine and secretive bureaucracies which hinder a rapid effective response as was seen in the 2003 SARS pandemic (Huang, 2004).

3 Despite the presence of potential 'hotzone' wet markets, through 2021 there was increasing evidence for a laboratory source for the COVID-19 Pandemic. This seems more and more likely as previously undisclosed emails emerge indicating beliefs of a possible lab origin for the disease, held by scientists that publicly tried to discredit such hypotheses and shut down any debate (Achenbach, 2023; Devine , 2023; Knapton, 2022; Gorman and Zimmer, 2021; Wade 2021).

Prologue

On 27th March 2020 a decision was made somewhere in the Victorian Government that would result in what has since been termed as the worst public policy and administration failure in Australia's history, and is ranked in the world's ten worst industrial accidents of the last 100 years (Gottliebsen, 2020b). This was a decision that returned Victorians to enforced isolation; imposed the severest restrictions on human rights[4], liberty, and freedom of speech ever seen in a democratic nation; caused mass unemployment and economic chaos; isolated Victoria from the rest of Australia; set the economic and societal recovery of the whole of the Australia back months; and most tragically of all caused over 800 otherwise preventable deaths. This single public health failure represented 99% of Victoria's known COVID cases during 2020 (Taylor, 2020a), and as of 4 January 2021 was still responsible for over 70% of the cases and over 90% of the deaths nationally (Albrechsten, 2021). To put the extent of the quarantine failures into perspective, Victoria had responsibility for only 11.9% of the total travellers coming into hotel quarantine in Australia[5] (compared with NSW taking 53.4%), with only Tasmania, South Australia and the Northern Territory taking lower numbers (Grout et al, 2021).

This decision by the Victorian Government was to establish hotel quarantine[6] for travellers entering Australia from overseas, using private security guards to provide front line containment. A different model than was adopted by other states and territories, which instead deployed police and Australian Defence Force personnel at the quarantine hotels. Hotel quarantine was part of the Australian Government's response to the growing global COVID-19 (SARS-CoV-2) pandemic, a part that was tasked to the various state and territory governments.

---

[4] In September 2021, Melbourne, the Victorian state capital took on the mantel as the most lock-downed place on earth (Burgess, 2021; Stewart, 2021). Melbourne residents being subjected to over 8 months of what amounted to home detention, allowed out of the home for two hours a days for essential activities within 5km of home (in 6 lockdowns over the pandemic period). Compounding which, visitors to the home were banned, including close family members. The only way in which a child (say a teenager at university) could legally be allowed to visit their parents was for them to have been employed as a construction worker to do work in the home.

[5] Up to the 31st of January 2021.

[6] This was known as 'Operation Soteria', named (ironically as it turned out) after the ancient Greek goddess of safety and salvation, deliverance, and preservation from harm.

The failed Victorian Hotel Quarantine Program is estimated to have cost in excess of $195 million[7] (blowing out the original budget of $80 million), with tens of millions of dollars going to outsourced providers, with little in the way of robust procurement or effective contract management. Questions still have to be answered on what value for money the Government received from consultancy advice on the Program that it purchased from Boston Consulting Group ($393,000), PwC ($304,000), Deloitte ($200,000), and from KPMG for broader pandemic advice (a staggering $3.5 million)[8]. The government's increased dependency on external consultants should have come as no surprise, since under Daniel Andrews' time as Premier, consultancy costs have exploded by more than 300%, with $175million being spent in the 2020-2021 financial year alone (Towell and Crock, 2021).

Although this decision by the Victorian Government appears to be the primary driver of the subsequent failures that resulted in this catastrophe, it was not an isolated decision. There were a range of other decisions, beliefs, assumptions, cultures, ideologies, and vulnerabilities within the Victorian Government and its bureaucracy that played major causal roles in the disaster that was to come. However, the dire situation that Victoria faced in the first half of 2020 was not really just because a pandemic occurred. This was a disaster of the Victorian Government's own failing that had been building since it was first elected. A continuing degradation in governance and capability created inherent problems within government and its bureaucracy that coalesced in March 2020 to provide a perfect storm for the disaster that was to unfold.

---

[7] Varga and Snowden, 2020.
[8] Consultancy.com.au, 2020.

1
The start of the pandemic

Wuhan, 2019

Sometime in early to mid-November 2019 (Ma, 2020), a novel respiratory disease emerged in Wuhan, a city of over 11 million people in central China. Through November the number of infections steadily increased in the community, with up to 5 new cases occurring daily in the early stages. However, the Chinese government continued to deny human-to-human transmission was occurring for many weeks, even though a localised epidemic of a contagious disease was emerging. One of the earliest confirmed hospitalisations occurred on 16 November 2019, a 65 year old worker from the city's large wet market (the Hunan Wholesale Seafood Market)[9]. Within a few days of this there were over 60 identified cases, a number of which were also either workers from the wet market or their close family members. This naturally focussed attention on the wet market as a potential source of the outbreak, something that will be discussed later.

Less than a week later multiple hospitals and other health facilities in Wuhan started to report clusters of patients with a strange pneumonia similar to SARS and MERS[10] , and hospital workers treating sick patients were themselves becoming infected, clear evidence of human-to-human transmission (Hu et al, 2021). On 31 December 2019, the health authorities in Wuhan notified the World Health Organisation (WHO)[11] about this novel disease (Wu and McGoogan, 2020). Although the WHO announced the emergence of this new disease on 9 January 2020, human-to-human transmission continued to be denied until it was publicly acknowledged on 21 January 2020.

Even then the WHO continued to downplay the potential seriousness of the outbreak, despite evidence of the disease's spread beyond China's borders. By 23 January 2020, the whole city of Wuhan was placed into quarantine lockdown, but it was not until over a week later on 31 January that the WHO finally declared a global emergency (AJMC Staff, 2021), and not until 11 March

---

[9] 'Seafood Market' is a little misleading, as the market also sold large number of live mammals, birds, and reptiles for slaughtering for food.

[10] Previous human coronavirus diseases occurring in 2003 (SARS – severe acute respiratory syndrome) and 2012 (MERS – Middle East respiratory syndrome).

[11] World Health Organisation

2020 that they declared a pandemic. The inaction and slow responsiveness of the WHO has been widely criticised (Feldwisch-Drentrup, 2020), with suggestions that China's increasing influence and control over the WHO, and a compromised Director General promoted the economic and political interests of China ahead of the Agency's public health priorities (Calbert and Abuthnot, 2021). The WHO's slowness and ineffectiveness allowed a local epidemic to grow into a pandemic. This was not the first time that the WHO had been implicated in creating health disasters through incompetence and inaction[12]. Nor was it the only government organisation to make the pandemic worse by sacrificing good science for politics, ideology, misinformation, and secrecy.

The focus on the wet market

There has been considerable scientific, political, and public interest in the origins of the pandemic, and different theories have received highly polarised partisan support. There has been a consistently promoted belief that the SARS-CoV-2 virus had emerged in the wet market as a result of transfer from freshly butchered meat or from the sale of live animals such as bats or pangolins. However, the plausibility of the wet food market as the 'ground zero' for COVID-19 was subsequently challenged by a variety of different evidence. Over the course of 2020 it become increasingly plausible that this was part of deliberate campaign of misdirection by Chinese officials seeking to cover up the nature of the emerging pandemic (Sparrow, 2021; Markson 2021b Editorial Board, 2020; Yuan, 2020). In the early stages of the pandemic, various interests (including some gullible mainstream media) promoted the narrative of infected bats and pangolins being sold in the wet market as the source of the pandemic.

However, it later transpired that these animals were not present in the market when the COVID-19 outbreak started in Wuhan, and no evidence could be found that these animals had been in the market in the months before the outbreak. Despite the growing number of disconnects between the 'official' narrative and the growing evidence, the media and certain western institutions continued for months with the natural origin theory for SARS-CoV-2 (the

[12] The WHO (World Health Organisation) has been widely condemned for its failure to deliver on its core responsibilities (including slow responses to emergencies) on multiple occasions, including: Ebola in West Africa; Cholera in Haiti; Zika virus in the Americas, 2009 H1N1 pandemic; tuberculosis, HIV and AIDS in the 1990's, (Kamradt-Scott, 2018; Castro, 2017, Huang, 2016; Wibulpolprasert and Chowdhury, 2016; Colen, 2015; Condon and Shina, 2008).

scientific name for the virus causing COVID-1)[13], even going so far as to attack any dissenters to this unproven hypothesis as conspiracy theorists.

Whilst the official line of bats and pangolins as the prime suspects was eventually discounted[14], further widespread testing and epidemiological studies failed to find any of the other types of animals that were at the market to be the potential source of the outbreak in Wuhan (Shi, 2021). Beyond finding the suspect animal source of the pandemic, the wet market itself increasingly looked less and less likely to be the ground zero. The known epidemiology of the early stages of the outbreak did not support the market as the primary emergence site. Although many of the known human-to-human transmissions occurring from about the 8 December 2019 were clustered within and close to the wet market (Chen et al, 2020b; Li, 2020), the earliest infections in November had no epidemiological connection with the wet market (Shi, 2021). Genetic analysis (Graham and Baric, 2020) also supports human infection prior to the wet market outbreak, again strongly implicating some other location in Wuhan as the source of the outbreak. This naturally led to speculation about the possible involvement of the nearby Wuhan Institute of Virology (WIV) being ground zero for this unique viral disease.

Much of the renewed interest in the Wuhan laboratory's possible role as the pandemic's origin then started to focus on the conduct of 'gain of function' research into bat coronaviruses. It is now widely accepted that this type of genetic manipulation research was part of the WIV research program. Convincing evidence presented to US Congressional committees strongly support the WIV as the source of SARS-CoV-2 and the start of the COVID-19 pandemic. Increasingly popular suspicions circled around the possibility that either an already human-adapted wild virus was present in the laboratory, or that Chinese scientists had intentionally or accidently genetically engineered a bat coronavirus to increase its ability to infect humans (McCaul, 2020). Whatever the origins of the virus, it began to look increasingly plausible that the WIV was ground zero for the pandemic.

---

[13] The virus responsible for the 2003 SARS pandemic was named SARS-CoV-1.

[14] The SARS-CoV-2 virus does not have genetic markers indicating that it could have naturally passed through intermediate hosts such palm civets or pangolins (Macdonald, 2021).

The Focus on the Wuhan Institute of Virology

For most of 2020, there were stringent denials from the Chinese government, the WHO, and from numbers of western scientists that the pandemic could have resulted from a laboratory escape. Many media outlets and various 'experts' claimed that any suggestions about the involvement of the WIV was 'racist propaganda' or the realm of conspiracy theorists (Barclay, 2020; Beusekorn, 2020, Calisher, 2020; Cohen, 2020; Daszak, 2020). However, the situation was not that clear cut. Some of those scientists leading these denials about the WIV's involvement had significant potential conflicts of interest, having been involved in virology research with or directly funding the Wuhan laboratory (Dilanian et al, 2021; Dunleavy, 2021; Editorial Board, 2021; Wernau, 2021). Even the WHO was implicated in hindering its own investigations into the pandemics origins through behind the scenes deals with the Chinese government in the lead up to its 2020 report (Calbert and Arbuthnott, 2021).

However, as the pandemic continued, the laboratory leak theory continued to gather credible support (Thacker, 2021a). Increasing amounts of evidence showed that the WIV was in fact involved in coronavirus research, that it was undertaking research on bat viruses including bat coronaviruses closely related to SARS-CoV-2, that it did hold live bats within the facility[15], that it was undertaking gain of function research (McCaul, 2021; Markson, 2021a), and that earlier independent reports had criticised manifestly unsafe laboratory practices. All of which increased the plausibility for a laboratory leak to have occurred (Glasgow, 2021).

China's refusal to allow access for a new investigation into the pandemic's origins, along with their punishment of countries calling for further investigations[16], only added fuel to the possibility of the WIV's involvement as the source of the pandemic. Dr Anthony Fauci[17] was originally unsupportive of the lab leak theory in public statements during 2020. It later emerged that Fauci may have had serious conflicts of interest in that he provided funding for

---

[15] Despite earlier denials.

[16] Chinese state-controlled media have also been reporting a named Swiss scientist's claims that the US government is pressuring the WHO to undertake a second investigation into the Wuhan laboratory (WIV). However, in light of the Swiss Government's finding that a scientist of that name does not actually exist (Tang, 2021b), it appears to be more disinformation from the ruling Chinese Communist Party.

[17] Head of the US National Institute of Allergy and Infectious Diseases and advisor to the US President.

coronavirus work at the Wuhan laboratory (Markson and Mendes, 2021), with allegations that some of this funding was for gain of function research banned in the USA, and that he had mislead Congress about activities at the WIV (Browne, 2021).

With continuing investigations releasing some of his emails, Fauci began to claim he was never dismissive of the source being the Wuhan laboratory (Fink, 2021), despite his apparent central involvement in the laboratory leak theory denials and secretly commissioning papers rejecting a possible laboratory origin. Even the Director General of the WHO has backtracked on his original position and now accepts that a leak from the WIV is a possibility that should be investigated (Tang, 2021a). A possibility that is further strengthened by US intelligence reports indicating that three of the WIV workers became ill with a COVID-19 like illness and sought hospital treatment in November 2019 (Dilanian, 2021), well before the apparent wet market outbreak.

A more recent WHO investigation (SAGO, 2022) has provided some initial reporting that because information has not been provided by China, it is not yet possible to identify the origins of the virus. The WHO points out that although some of the early cases were linked to the Huahan Seafood Market, other cases came from other markets, whilst yet other cases had no exposure to any markets. There has also been no evidence provided about the extent of mild disease or asymptomatic cases during the early stages of the Wuhan outbreak. One compelling conclusion is that the outbreak at the Seafood market was an 'amplification' event (where the virus significantly increased in transmission in the human population) rather than an actual seeding event (where the virus was first introduced or 'spilled over' into humans), and that genetic studies suggest that there were several seeding events into the human population.

Some earlier epidemiological evidence and molecular analysis of the SARS-CoV-2 genetic makeup suggests a natural origin rather than laboratory genetic engineering of the virus (Holmes et al, 2021), although this has been disputed, including by some virologists. The closest related viruses found to date in bats has a 96.8% common genomic sequence to SARS-CoV-2. In virological terms that is a substantial difference, but is *suggestive* of an originating relationship, the virus responsible for SARS (in 2003) showed a similar percentage of common genome with the most closely related bat viruses (Chen et al, 2001). Although with SARS the potential intermediate hosts were quickly found after that pandemic. However, the WHO concluded that the relationship is not sufficiently strong to identify the original source of the virus. This means that although a bat and natural transmission was more likely than a gain of function research origin, it does not yet rule out the possibility that this was not due to deliberate manipulation. Further, this still means that an accidental laboratory leak of a bat virus is still a strong possible origin for the COVID-19 pandemic.

This most recent WHO report is also critical of the increasingly discredited January to February 2021 WHO investigation[18] (Australian Government, 2021; Beaumont, 2021; Pezenik, 2021) that disregarded the data about 76,000 patients with respiratory illness in the months prior to the official date of the pandemic commencing in Wuhan. The WHO report raised the real possibility that a significant number of these patients may have COVID-19 but were excluded because they were asymptomatic or had mild symptoms that did not fit the stringent criteria adopted by the earlier WHO team.

Even if the virus was not manipulated deliberately, this does not rule out the possibility that the origin of the pandemic was a result of an accidental exposure or escape of the virus. It is entirely plausible that a researcher could have been exposed to infected bat samples or virus samples in the laboratory, or exposed in the field when collecting those samples. This is an entirely realistic scenario since scientists from the Wuhan had collected samples from horseshoe bats (known to be reservoirs of the closest naturally occurring viruses to SARS-CoV-2). That the closest population of these bats to Wuhan (and from where the scientists collected their samples) is some 1500km from the city (Cheriyedath, 2021) even more discounts the possibility of a natural route of transmission to humans, and makes the laboratory route of a naturally occurring virus even more likely.

---

[18] The initial investigation was widely criticised because of its superficial examination of the issues, obstruction by the Chinese officials into exploring key issues, and alleged conflicts of interest of some of those that were members of the WHO investigation team. This included scientists with apparent ties to the Chinese Government and People's Liberation Army (Markson, 2021c), and an individual scientist that had had provided funding into the study of bat coronaviruses at the Wuhan Institute of Virology (Pascault, 2021). A similar probe by a taskforce, put together by the medical Journal – The Lancet, was dissolved in the face of alleged conflicts of interest and deep divisions about a laboratory versus natural origin for SARS-CoV-2. There were also criticisms about the appointment of Dr Peter Dasak as the initial Chair of the taskforce, the same scientist with alleged conflicts of interest that was a member of the original WHO investigation team. Although he was removed as Chair, other members refused to allow Dasak to be removed from membership of the Taskforce. It was later revealed that the new Chair and three other members of the Taskforce were co-investigators with Dasak on a virus research project funded through the organisation run by Dasak (Cohen, 2021). None of these apparent conflicts of interest were declared. Peter Dasak was later exposed as the person that orchestrated a letter to The Lancet signed by a number of well-known scientists that decried any suggestion of the Wuhan laboratory's involvement in the origins of the pandemic, and labelled it as a conspiracy theory (Thacker, 2021b).

The US National Intelligence Council issued a report (NIC, 2019) putting forward both a laboratory accident and a natural origin as the most plausible origins of the COVID-19 pandemic.

What is more worrying than the probability of a deliberately engineered virus or a laboratory accident as the origin for COVID-19, has been the reaction of much of the political elite and mainstream media to the possibility of such a deliberate act or accident occurring. For months, the growing evidence of potential laboratory involvement was dismissed, derided, or allegedly covered up by senior health officials (Chellaney, 2022). Obfuscation and misdirection by politicians and bureaucrats occurred not only in China, but in other countries where vested interests prevailed. Whilst proponents for looking at the 'lab leak' theory were labelled as conspiracy theorists, bullied into silence, or were 'cancelled'. A compliant media unquestioningly accepted the official line. These very same tactics became familiar against critics of the Victorian Government during 2020, that is before the Coate Inquiry revealed at least part of the truth.

The Situation in Australia

The imposition of bans and restrictions

In the face of a burgeoning potential pandemic, Australia commenced the screening of international arrivals on 23 January 2020, with the first four in-country cases of COVID-19 reported on 25 January (Doherty, 2020; Hunt and Murphy, 2020) in travellers arriving from China (Dunstan, 2021). One of these, Australia's first case, was an infected traveller from Wuhan arriving in Melbourne on 19 January (Hunt, 2020). On 31 January, Australia introduced a ban on travellers entering the country directly from China, with further bans being imposed shortly after on travellers from Italy, Iran, and South Korea. Some three weeks later, on 20 March 2020, this ban was extended to prevent the entry of all non-citizens and non-residents into the country (Worthington and Snape, 2020), along with increasing restrictions on gatherings, business operations, and social distancing requirements. Following which travel bans were further extended to prevent Australian citizens and residents from leaving the country from 25th March, 2020 (Meixner, 2020).

The overriding aim of travel bans was not to fully prevent an emerging infectious disease such as COVID-19 from entering the country, but rather to delay widespread community transmission (Everett et al, 2020). The Australian Government's early response was very successful in limiting the number of infected cases entering the country, with new case rates beginning to plateau at about 50 per day by mid-March, with daily case numbers dropping in New South Wales and Sydney. By the 19 March 2020, Australia had recorded a total of 700 cases of COVID-19, and the first wave appeared to be running out of steam, then the Ruby Princess cruise liner arrived in Sydney.

The Ruby Princess Debacle

It has long been known that close contact environments provide a high risk situation for the transmission of contagious diseases. Large cruise ships have frequently provided such an environment for significant outbreaks of respiratory diseases (including influenza and Legionnaires disease), gastrointestinal disorders (Including Norwalk, hepatitis A and cyclosporiasis) and chickenpox (Tardievel et al, 2020; Zhang et al, 2016; Kak, 2015; Minooee and Rickman, 1999). It should therefore have been no surprise that a cruise ship presented an exceptionally high risk environment for the transmission of COVID-19.

Indeed, as early as February 2020, the 'hot zone' potential of cruise ships was highlighted by an outbreak of COVID-19 on the Diamond Princess operated by Princess Cruises (owned by Carnival Corp.). The vessel, with 3700 people on board was being held in quarantine at the port of Yokohama in Japan from the 3 February 2020, after previously visiting Hong Kong. Over the next 14 days, despite various infection control measures, including cabin isolation, the disease spread rapidly through passengers and then crew (Nakazawa et al, 2020). Outside of the pandemic raging through China, that one cruise ship came to hold the most cases of COVID-19 of anywhere in the world at that time (Baraniuk, 2020). About the same time another Carnival Corp. cruise ship (the Zaandam) was trying, without success, to find a port anywhere along the west coast of South America that would allow it dock (Campbell, 2020).

Yet another Carnival Corp. ship (The Grand Princess) experienced a serious outbreak commencing in mid-February starting with passengers on a cruise out of San Francisco, which infected crew and continuing passengers on a second cruise departing immediately after the end of the first cruise. The US Government's response was immediate, following confirmation of positive cases on board. The Grand Princess was directed to an isolated non-commercial facility and all passengers were transported to US military bases for mandatory 14 day quarantine (Walker, 2020). Carnival Corp. was not alone, with multiple other cruise ships experiencing some level of COVID-19 transmission on aboard during the early stages of the pandemic (Campbell, 2020). It would have been expected that the crew and operators of Princess Cruises' should therefore have been aware that their vessels could become hot spots for COVID-19. Australian Border Force and New South Wales health bureaucrats should also have had a heightened awareness that incoming cruise vessels carried a greatly elevated risk of carrying passengers infected with COVID-19.

Then another of the Diamond Princess' sister ships, the Ruby Princess arrived in Sydney the following month on 9 March 2020. The cruise ship's arrival in Sydney came at the end of a ten day cruise around New Zealand, with 2600 passengers plus crew onboard. Well before this arrival, it was known that there had been a massive increase in world-wide cases of COVID-19, with its presence confirmed in 114 countries (Walker, 2020). New Zealand had identified its first imported cases in February 2020, including at least one probable infected person arriving from the Diamond Princess in Japan. Local transmission of COVID-19 being confirmed in early March (Ministry of Health, 2020).

During an earlier voyage from Sydney in late February, travelling around New Zealand, some 22 passengers became ill with an unidentified acute respiratory illness, which was assessed by NSW Health as being "low risk", allowing all passengers to disembark without screening or restrictions. The following day the Ruby Princess took on 2,995 new passengers and set off on another voyage around New Zealand, visiting five different ports. This included taking onboard a crew member that had recently arrived from Italy, where surging numbers of COVID-19 were occurring. As the cruise proceeded, an exponentially increasing number of cases of an unknown acute respiratory disease were identified by the ship's doctor. This information was provided to NSW Health.

By the 7 March, 170 passengers were known to have a respiratory illness, with 18 being described with 'influenza-like' signs and symptoms. Following a series of back and forth communications between the Ruby Princess and NSW Health, the vessel was rated as "medium risk" and was allowed to dock in Sydney on 9 March. When a health screening team arrived on board later that morning, they were confronted by 360 apparently unwell passengers gathered together in the enclosed space of the ship's dining room, none wearing face masks or practising social distancing. Screening (based on signs and symptoms) identified 240 symptomatic individuals. However, based upon the screening and two earlier positive influenza test results, the medical officer in charge decided that COVID-19 was not present on board the ship. Apart from six passengers with high fever, all other passengers were allowed to disembark, without any form of control or restriction put in place. The six suspect individuals were tested but returned negative COVID-19 results and were subsequently allowed to disembark, and new passengers and crew were allowed to board the Ruby Princess the next day for a new cruise.

As a result of poor procedures (including a flawed risk assessment), miscommunication amongst officials, inadequate capabilities and negligence, a large number of cruise passengers with active COVID-19 infections were allowed to disembark, catch public transport and taxis, and then board aircraft to travel throughout Australia, and internationally. The infected passengers from the Ruby Princess introduced a significant surge of new cases into Australia, directly accounting for 10% of known infections, and through subsequent community transmission being responsible for the majority of the following exponential spike in cases (Probyn, 2020; Thiessen, 2020, Walker, 2020). Coincidently on 9 March, Melbourne recorded its first local transmission of COVID-19, a schoolteacher who had apparently been infected by their partner (ABC News, 2020a), recently arrived from the USA.

The well-publicised disaster on the Diamond Princess, and the experiences of other sister ships should have raised some high-risk warnings and provided some powerful lessons for managing the Ruby Princess' arrival. Unfortunately, for Australia it appears that these risks were ignored in NSW. Even with the widespread publicity from the Ruby Princess debacle and the epidemiological knowledge that was gained about the spread into the community, it appears that this wealth of lessons was not learned sufficiently by the Victorian Government.

Despite the large upsurge in cases resulting from the Ruby Princess, the various measures that had been put in place by the National Cabinet[19] and individually by the various jurisdictions, was able to substantially contain the first wave of infection to less than 500 new cases per day at its peak on 27th March. Following the introduction of mandatory quarantine for all incoming travellers on the 27th March, case numbers rapidly declined through April, to no known new locally acquired cases by mid-April 2020 (PAEC, 2021; Price et al, 2020). The combined efforts of Commonwealth, state and territory governments had apparently effectively contained a major pandemic first wave, avoiding the public health crises that were emerging in many other countries.

---

[19] The National Cabinet was formed on the 13 March 2020 to provide some national consistency across the Commonwealth, states, and territories.

This first wave of COVD-19 resulted in about 3,000 cases in NSW, 1,500 in Victoria and about 2,500 across the rest of Australia, with 103 deaths occurring nationally.

Victoria: a mounting crisis

As numbers of international cases mounted in early March 2020, with almost every news broadcast showing scenes of infected patients in China and Europe and increasing morbidity and mortality rates, health professionals in Victoria began to realise the seriousness of the impending global pandemic (van Diemen, 2020).

In the face of mounting cases, the Victorian Government started to impose the first of its restrictions. On 13 March 2020, the crowds waiting for the opening of the Melbourne Grand Prix were suddenly told that the event had been closed down, followed later that day by further cancellation announcements for attendance at AFL (Australian Football League) fixtures, Melbourne Food and Wine Festival, and the Melbourne International Comedy Festival. This was followed three days later by a declaration of emergency for Victoria (Dunstan, 2021). On 22 March 2020, the Premier announced the early end of the school term and other shutdowns. The immediate aftermath of this announcement saw widespread panic buying in the supermarkets, one of the first casualties of which was supermarket shelves emptied of toilet paper and flour.

National coordination

On the 27 March 2020, the National Cabinet agreed to allow small numbers of overseas travellers (mainly returning Australian nationals) to enter Australia through designated ports of entry and subject to strict quarantine requirements. Australia has had a long history of imposing mandatory quarantine (for specific notifiable diseases), from before federation, and most states had operated remote quarantine stations from the 1850's until the 1980's. The decision to move to a nationally agreed compulsory detention and quarantine of incoming passengers appears to have been originally based upon a paper written by Victoria's Chief Health Officer (Dr Brett Sutton). The

Australian Health Protection Principal Committee[20] made the recommendation which was accepted subsequently by the National Cabinet.

The National Cabinet's decision seems to have been driven by the combined fear of significantly increasing COVID-19 cases present in Australia at that time (3,162 cases on the 27 March 2020), and the fear of what National Cabinet appears to have been told where a significant number of infected people deliberately refusing to self-isolate[21]. This advice seems to have been based upon the misinformation that there was extensive deliberate non-compliance with the self-isolation requirements that had been in place up to then (for example for infected passengers and close contacts from the Ruby Princess). However, it was revealed during the Coate Inquiry that this information was incorrect. In fact, most of the small number of non-compliance cases that did occur where due to confusion created by inadequate provision and dissemination of government information to those required to self-isolate.

Mandatory quarantine, in late March, therefore appeared to be a blunt instrument which was used to deal with government incompetence rather than a necessary measure to deal with a 'make believe' wilfully rule breaking public. In Victoria's case this fear was further heightened by the knowledge that the state's ailing public health and hospital systems were in imminent danger of being overrun by potentially growing numbers of COVID-19 cases. This decision to concentrate uninfected and infected travellers together into poorly ventilated hotels along with inadequate and inexperienced staff would prove to be an absolute recipe for disaster. Whilst home-based isolation would certainly have reduced this risk, this would have required a resourced and competent public health system to provide monitoring and oversight. This was something that Victoria's chronic under-resourcing could simply not have managed. So mandatory detention replaced more pragmatic public health measures.

---

[20] Provided by the AHPPC (Australian Health Protection Principal Committee), which is the peak government body comprising the Commonwealth's State and Territory Chief Medical/Health Officers.

[21] Coate, 2020a p. 16.

Victoria does it Dan's way?

On the same day as the National Cabinet decision on 27th March 2020, Premier Daniel Andrews conducted a media briefing announcing the set-up of the Hotel Quarantine Program, *with the use of private security*. The following day, the Program got underway as hotels were stood up as quarantine facilities. On Sunday 29th March the first international travellers arrived at Melbourne Airport, and were then transported to various hotels in the CBD to start their 14 days of mandated quarantine.

This was a major decision for any government and should have required the establishment of a well-rehearsed strategic and operational approach employing highly skilled and experienced decision-makers. In Victoria this obviously did not happen. Decisions involving millions of dollars should have gone through a contestable process and scrutiny within the Victorian Cabinet (that has been a major role for Cabinet in democratic governments for hundreds of years, continuing even in times of war). However, in Victoria, the state government's Cabinet was effectively excluded from the decision-making and oversight, and instead key decisions affecting the lives of millions of Victorians seem to have been made somewhere between the Premier and his close advisors, and a few senior bureaucrats. Most of these were 'orphan decisions' for which no Labor Minister or senior public servant has ever accepted accountability or responsibility.

Where, under other Premiers (both Labor and Liberal), decisions were made subject to contestable advice from independent and highly skilled public servants, under Daniel Andrews governance and decision making in the Victorian Government had changed dramatically. It certainly appeared that his political advisers were fulfilling this function, with all of the power centralised in Andrews' Private Office and the Department of Premier and Cabinet (DPC). Against precedent, this "army" of 400 political advisers across government came under the control of Andrews' Chief of Staff, further alienating democratic processes and the involvement of what should have been an independent skilled public service. Accompanied by a tripling of the size of DPC in just six years, from the start of the pandemic, the Premier wielded more direct personal control over government than any other leader in Australia's history. Where once senior public servants were appointed for their experience and evidence of previous high performance, the Labor government in Victoria seemed to have increasingly based its appointments on ideological conformity and the closeness of the relationship to Dan Andrews himself (Le Grand and Sakkal, 2021). As a result, many of the checks and balances of necessary good governance simply disappeared.

That Dan Andrews should be driving strategy with little recourse to other Ministers or Cabinet scrutiny should have come as no surprise. Since taking power as Premier, Andrews had progressively removed a lot of the decision-making and authority from Ministers and government departments and consolidated it within his own domain. Andrews seems not to have learned that such an approach could lead to disaster.

More recently, the 'Victorian Government's' decision to break another election promise and suddenly cancel the Commonwealth Games, seems to have been a unilateral Dan Andrews' decision. A decision that was apparently done in secret, not only excluding Cabinet but also allegedly not involving the Deputy Premier Jacinta Allan, who was also the Minister responsible for the Games (and who succeeded as Premier on Andrews' resignation). It is now apparent that an external law firm was engaged to work on the cancellation, in the month prior to the public announcement. In fact, the lawyers started work on the cancellation less than 24 hours after Jacinta Allan had told the Public Accounts and Estimates Committee of Parliament that "tremendous progress" was being made on preparations for the Games (Kolovos, 2023; Eddie, 2023). Jacinta Allan claiming that she had only been told about the lawyers on the day that they had been engaged. It also emerged that the Secretary of the Department of Premier and Cabinet (and close confidant of the Dan Andrews) had travelled to London to inform the Commonwealth Games Federation of the cancellation three days before Cabinet met to make the decision about the cancellation. These revelations also raised serious concerns that Dan Andrews had also mislead the media and the public about the justification for cancelling the Games, as well as allegations that the government tried to obstruct the Liberal led Senate Inquiry into the cancellation (Rollason and Wong, 2023).

With so many of the decisions around hotel quarantine and the pandemic response seemingly made by political supporters under Andrews' control rather than from independent experts, is it any surprise that Victoria's pandemic response was so disastrous and so draconian?

The early illusion of success

The early stages of the Hotel Quarantine Program were marked by hubris and proclamations of success. This was an expression of an incredible level of flawed confidence in capability that ran contrary to any understanding of risk and reality about running a quarantine program for a known highly infectious disease. Certainly, by late March there was a wealth of information in the public domain, in specialist literature, and covered extensively by the media showing how readily the SARS-CoV-2 virus could be transmitted, especially in densely populated environments. The well-publicised experiences of the Diamond Princess cruise ship in Japan, and the Ruby Princess in Sydney had created a high level of awareness about the infectious nature of asymptomatic individuals, and the ease of transmission even when people were isolated in cabins and rooms.

There was even a growing understanding of the role that staff working in 'isolation facilities' could play in transmission from infected individuals placed into isolation. This was not some special esoteric knowledge locked away in the ivory towers of academia, it was very much public knowledge. These experiences showed what extreme risk exposures incoming travellers and quarantine attempts could present if not managed in appropriate facilities and with trained staff.

The Coate Inquiry concluded that at the time of setting up the Hotel Quarantine Program, that it had been well established that the SARS-CoV-2 virus could be transmitted by aerosols, droplets, contaminated surfaces, including by close contact, by airborne transmission (when aerosols were created by certain procedures)[22], and by asymptomatic super spreaders[23]. Risk factors that seem to have been frequently ignored in the operation of the quarantine hotels.

By 27th March, with the commencement of the hotel quarantine scheme, Ministers and officials should have been on high alert that they were facing a series of wicked problems[24]. Problems that required a very different approach

[22] Coate, 2020a p. 14.

[23] Where between 17 to 20% of infected people could be asymptomatic (Coate 2020a) p.15)

[24] Wicked problems are issues or situations that are characterised by extreme levels of complexity and novelty, and by a multitude of interconnections with other factors and problems. Wicked problems are very difficult if not impossible to fully understand by just simply trying to 'dissect the problem'. Understanding a wicked problem takes time and needs to be looked at from multiple perspectives, with a very robust approach to surfacing and challenging assumptions. Wicked problems are also extremely difficult to solve. There is usually no single solution that will solve a wicked problem, and as solutions are implemented,

to the familiar routine, but often barely adequate, day-to-day processes of government.

This understanding, if it ever existed at senior levels of the bureaucracy, did not appear to percolate down to any effective management of the Program, or affect changes in behaviour of some frontline workers in the quarantine hotels. Within the Victorian Government the extreme risks associated with quarantine and isolation appears to have been unrecognised, rejected, or deliberately ignored in both assigning initial responsibilities and then in the management of the Program.

In standing up the Hotel Quarantine Program on 27 March 2020 and in the subsequent days and weeks, decisions were made to use inadequate facilities, to use inappropriate, unskilled and under-resourced workforces, to put inexperienced and sub-optimal leadership in place, to give key responsibilities to individuals for roles that they were clearly untrained and unsuited, to allocate tasks to departments that they were wholly incapable of managing competently, to not develop plans, procedures and technical instructions, and to not train frontline staff in even the most basic of requirements. These decisions were often based on a complete ignorance of the assumptions on which they were based (many of which were false assumptions), to ignore manifest risks, and to fail to put in place adequate risk mitigations, especially when these ran counter to the prevailing ideology.

The Coate Inquiry revealed that the Victorian Government went through the first few months of the pandemic with ineffectual responses and inadequate preparedness. Although the hotel quarantine idea was initially promoted by Victoria nationally, it had no pre-existing quarantine plan of its own in place. Post second wave, Victoria's defence for this negligence came across as rather childish in nature, along the lines of *'it wasn't just us, the Commonwealth didn't have preplanning either'*. Accordingly, the Coate Inquiry report thought it was 'unfair' to blame Victoria, just because the Commonwealth had not specifically told the Victorian Government that it had to undertake some basic common-sense preparation. In fact, in the aftermath of the 2009 influenza pandemic the Commonwealth had recommended that the States review their policies on

---

further wicked problems often arise or become apparent. Attempted solutions to wicked problems are also usually irreversible, the consequences of errors can therefore be catastrophic and irrecoverable. Familiar routine approaches for problem-solving and decision-making are therefore highly likely to fail disastrously in the face of wicked problems. Successful resolution of a wicked problem requires a radically different approach, with an informed leadership and decision-makers that are experienced in complex problem-solving under high uncertainty.

quarantine and isolation (DHA, 2011). A recommendation that Victoria *decided not to implement*[25].

Victoria: from success to catastrophe

The Department of Jobs, Precincts and Regions (DJPR) was given the responsibility to set up the Hotel Quarantine Program. Who made this decision has still not been made public, although it appears to have involved a phone call from the Secretary of Premier and Cabinet to the DJPR Secretary on 27 March 2020[26]. To some Ministers and bureaucrats, this may have seemed to be an obvious decision. After all the Program has the word 'hotels' in its title, and DJPR had previously organised trade fairs and trade delegations, and that had involved sourcing some hotel rooms. Just the sort of limited expertise required to design and manage a disease quarantine program in a global health emergency.

As one arm of the Victorian Government (DJPR) went about organising the Hotel Quarantine Program, another arm of government, Emergency Management Victoria (EMV) started to set up the State Control Centre. In ignorance of what DJPR had been tasked to do, EMV established 'Health' as the control agency (as required under Victoria's Emergency Management Manual and emergency management arrangements at the time). A political process had already started to subvert the state's tried and tested emergency management capabilities. Even following the 27th March State Control Centre meeting which brought the various agencies together (but to which the Chief Health Officer and his team appear not to have been invited), there was still confusion about roles and responsibilities. This lack of clarity led to ongoing disputes between DHHS[27] and DJPR about which agency was in overall control of the Program[28]. This situation was a major contributor to the disaster that was to ensue.

From the start of the Hotel Quarantine Program, the Victorian Government and its bureaucracy seemed to have been in a celebratory mood. The Program was obviously an 'outstanding success', with more time being spent on self-congratulatory promotion than was given to understanding what was actually happening on the frontline within the hotels. This hubris appears to have been reinforced by a complete failure to understand the multitude of risks that had

---

[25] Coate, 2020a, p. 15.
[26] Coate, 2020a, p. 17.
[27] Department of Health and Human Services.
[28] Coate, 2020a, p. 18.

been created, in large part, through naivety and ignorance. From all of the available evidence, it appears that an emerging and highly complex disease crisis was approached with all of the understanding and care that would have gone into organising the average office Christmas party (but even work social events usually require a risk assessment!). The Coate Inquiry concluded that no thought was put into the suitability of hotels for housing quarantined individuals, no thought into how cleaning would be undertaken, no thought into how catering would be provided to 'detainees', nor how security would actually be managed[29].

The waning of the first wave

As restrictions placed on the Victorian public continued through April and May, community transmissions started to lessen dropping to single digit daily case numbers by early June 2020. Even as this first wave of COVID-19 declined, Victoria was struggling to manage even these few remaining cases (Henderson, 2021), the early warning signs of a fragile and fractured heath system becoming increasingly apparent.

With the overconfidence that typified much of the Hotel Quarantine Program, control measures started to relax and during April 2020 individuals detained at the hotels were allowed to go outside of the hotel for fresh air, with a private security guard escort. The opportunity for contact between staff and potentially infected people in quarantine increased as security guards handled traveller's luggage, took 'care packages' and special food deliveries to hotel rooms, and went shopping for special items, including children's toys, for those in isolation.

During May 2020 it looked as though Victoria, and more broadly Australia, had flattened the curve. On 26 May 2020, a duty manager at one of the quarantine hotels became infected and tested positive, with five security guards and their families being infected subsequently. This seems not to have raised too much concern about the effectiveness of the Program, and by 6 June Victoria believed it had no new cases in the community. As a result, the government, with increasing confidence, started to ease the restrictions with remote learning finishing, and schools reopening three days later, and on the 11 June, the Victorian Government allowed the mass gathering at a Black Lives Matter protest to occur.

---

[29] Coate, 2020a, p. 18.

However, apparently unknow by those in charge of the Program, multiple containment breaches were occurring in two of the quarantine hotels. Despite a very small number of the thousands of incoming travellers being placed into Quarantine being infected with the virus (just over 1%), the virus was already infecting security guards at the Rydges and Stamford Plaza hotels, and was being actively transmitted into the Victorian community. This community transmission increased through the rest of May and into June, with the government making no public admission about the source of this burgeoning outbreak. With a Victorian system close to collapse, Premier Daniel Andrews had to ask the Commonwealth for flights into Melbourne to be diverted to other States for two weeks and temporarily closed down the quarantine Program. Unfortunately, it appears the Victorian Government again did not appreciate the seriousness of the situation they were being faced with, and those two weeks in June eventually turned into five months before Victoria's Program could recommence operation in October 2022[30].

It is now known that this series of breaches at the two quarantine hotels occurring during May and June 2020, were ultimately responsible for 99% of the second wave cases[31]. However, it appears that government bureaucrats and Ministers were unaware about what was happening in the quarantine hotels.

A volte-face

Whilst infection control failures and quarantine breaches were occurring, with community transmission increasing in the second week of June 2020, and despite the obvious degree of contagion risk and mounting criticism, the Victorian Government permitted (some would say encouraged) the Black Lives Matter protest in Melbourne to go ahead. At the time the government and mainstream media played down the significance of the *potential* for widespread community transmission at such events. A number of commentators with apparent left-leaning views even justified the holding of protests in breach of COVID restrictions because the black lives issues outweighed the safety and lives of the whole of the Victorian community (Albrechtson, 2021). Whilst Premier Daniel Andrews said it would not be possible to stop the protests, the government in NSW had a very different view and through the Supreme Court imposed bans on the event proposed for Sydney (Ward and Rabe, 2020).

---

[30] Coate, 2020b, p. 9.

[31] Coate, 2020a, p. 14.

Less than a week later, on 11 June, one of the protestors proved to have been infected with the COVID-19 virus, with at least 5 other protestors testing positive subsequently. Despite some claims to the contrary, no reliable evidence has been presented that indicates the BLM protestor contributed in any significant way to the expansion of the second wave. Subsequent research into other massed protests internationally also suggested that such protests did not appear to be significant amplifying or super-spreader events (Neyman and Dalsey, 2020). However, at the time of the protest there was a clear and present risk of significant transmission occurring. A far greater disease risk than was presented by many of the individuals that were fined or arrested by Victoria Polices for being more than 5km from their homes or for sitting alone in a park drinking coffee during the lockdowns.

Premier Daniel Andrews received criticism for his mixed messaging, first telling the public that BLM protestors would not be fined if they attended the event, then later stating that people should not attend (Edsall, 2020; SBS 2020), although the protest was still allowed to proceed. After the protests were held, government and police action were limited to the fining of only three of the protestors for breaching restrictions.

The Victorian Government and Victoria police however showed a marked volte face when a series of later protests against government lockdowns and vaccine mandates occurred. Attendance at protests was criminalised and mass arrests and fines occurred (O'Sullivan, 2020). The protests were severely condemned by Labor Government Ministers, and the use of force against protestors by Victoria Police was unprecedented in modern Australian history. The use of baton rounds, tear gas grenades, the firing of cs gas pellets and dye pellets from weapons eerily resembling assault rifles, and the use of snatch squads to make mass arrests of protestors became a common sight on the streets of Melbourne. Whilst the protests were illegal for breaching the CHO's directives (as should the BLM protest have been), and presented a tangible risk of increasing community transmission, community outrage mounted at what was perceived as unwarranted police brutality.

That some members of the protests acted violently is obvious, police were placed into dangerous situations, ultimately because of government decisions, that should not have occurred and some police officers were injured. That is never acceptable, the police have a difficult enough job in general policing as it is. I know first-hand the challenges and dangers of policing violent protests. I spent over a decade on the front line as a sworn officer in London in the UK, at protests so violent that they make the Melbourne lockdown protests look like a children's tea party. Yet I can honestly say that I never witnessed any unwarranted or disproportionate use of force by London's Metropolitan Police at these events, whatever the provocation.

However, as more video footage emerged of the Melbourne protests, it became apparent that police were not just targeting violent individuals but were using exceptionally heavy-handed tactics on peaceful individuals. Certainly, VicPol's reputation took a battering with events such as charging and throwing to the ground a woman in her seventies who was walking away at the time, and then whilst she was on the ground spraying her in the face with capsicum foam. This and other scenes of police use of high levels force, including using pepper spray on journalists, as well as arresting and handcuffing other journalists (Flower, 2021a) looked to be specifically targeting the media. At least one journalist was removed by VICPOL's Protective Services Officers prior to a press briefing, allegedly on instructions from the Premier's Private Office (Yemini, 2021).

However, despite the apparent overuse of force by police, what was more disturbing was the government's reaction. Whilst Labor MPs were quick to condemn the protestors, there was absolute silence about even the *possibility* that VicPol *might* have used excessive force in some cases[32]. In fact, the Victorian Government's answer to the mounting protests was to *criminalise the organising of protests* (VEOHRC, 2020) which resulted in Victoria Police mounting "an over-zealous" response (Koob, 2021), including an early morning arrest and handcuffing of an obviously pregnant woman in her own home and still wearing her pyjamas (Schelle, 2021). Some of the reported tactics of VicPol at antigovernment protests have drawn comparisons from many observers about their similarity to the tactics used by the Chinese Communist Party to crush dissent during the Hong Kong pro-democracy protests. The Executive Director of the Institute of Public Affairs called out the Victorian Government for creating a "police state" (Roskam, 2020a, 2020b).

Most Victorian police members that I have had the privilege of knowing and working with over many years have had the highest levels of personal integrity and have been unreservedly dedicated to serving the people of Victoria. Increasing instances of political interference of the police over the last decade have only resulted in an increasing distrust of VicPol by the general public. Concerns about the insidious and destructive nature of interference by the government in police operational matters has created a great deal of concern,

---

[32] That at least some of these alleged cases represented actual unlawful police brutality was confirmed by a Victorian Police officer being charged for "recklessly causing injury" in January 2021, when he allegedly assaulted a member of the public at Melbourne's Flinders Street Station, during protests in the CBD (ABC News, 2022).

including significant criticism and allegations from former senior police officers such as former Chief Commissioners Kel Glare and Sir Ken Lay (Le Grand and Cooper, 2019; Lewis, 2019; Varga, 2019; Houston and Preiss, 2018; Minear, 2018; Smith, 2018; Smith 2016; Munro, 2011; Op Ed, 2011).

Such interference in the policing of Victoria by the government has been a great disservice to a great institution and a betrayal of those sworn officers, men and women that put their lives and their mental health on the line every day.

Reality bites back

Then, just when it looked like the Victorian Government's lockdowns and other civil restrictions had actually worked, daily case numbers suddenly and without apparent explanation started to balloon through June 2020. As the rest of Australia emerged from the first wave and life started to return to some degree of normality, something very wrong was happening in Victoria. Clusters of community infection began to emerge in working-class suburbs with high immigrant populations, like Truganina, Flemington, Hallam, and Sunshine West. The kinds of community where many of the quarantine hotel security guards lived. The second wave developed rapidly, and the government soon lost control of what was described as a "public health bushfire" (Briggs, 2020).

Towards the end of June 2020 further mandatory restrictions were introduced to try to curb the increases in community transmission, including bans on family gatherings. It was not for some weeks after the onset of the second wave, on 30 June, that Premier Dan Andrews finally admitted that much of the recent explosion in cases was a result of breaches at the quarantine hotels. As the extent of the second wave became apparent at the end of June, international flights to Melbourne were suspended until 7 December 2020. Reinstatement of international travel was eventually allowed under what was claimed to be a fully revised and reset hotel quarantine program. Premier Daniel Andrews made public claims that this new revamped Program was now the leading approach nationally for hotel quarantine. These were claims that apparently ignored health and safety breaches that had resulted in WorkSafe Victoria issuing improvement notices days before Andrews made his statements to the media (Murray, 2021). There were calls (that were of course ignored) from one of Australia's leading infectious disease experts (Professor Lindsay Grayson) to close down the Program again, because the Victorian Government could not be trusted to manage the Program[33] properly and that it was putting the rest of the country at risk (Dow et al, 2021; Trioli, 2021). Subsequent waves, deaths, and recurring lockdown after lockdown readily demonstrated that this new Hotel Quarantine Program was anything but "gold standard", as the Premier had asserted.

With numbers still climbing, 'progressive lockdowns' were reintroduced on 2 July 2020, and extended on 9 July. With the 2nd wave still not under control, a full metropolitan Melbourne lockdown was instituted on 2 August, with further restrictions for businesses. These restrictions were then further extended to include regional Victoria on 6 August.

Infected individuals from Victoria eventually spread the disease across the border into NSW and Queensland. However, this was not to be the end of breaches from the quarantine hotels, or of further new pandemic waves and lockdowns in Victoria.

Victoria, alone, had started its second wave of infection and community transmission.

The effectiveness of Victoria's control measures

The Victorian Government implemented a whole range of measures in response to the both the first and second waves. Including completely changing its advice on several occasions. Victorian Government advice through the first wave and into the second wave was that face masks provided no protection against COVID-19 (contrary to advice being provided by the US Centers for Disease Control at the time). We now know that this advice appears to have been less based on scientific evidence and was more to do with concerns about the lack of planning that led to shortages of masks for health and emergency services workers. By the 23 July 2020, the government had changed its mind and introduced the mandatory wearing of facemasks, perhaps in response to increased availability of supplies.

---

[33] Professor Grayson also stated that the basic premise of the Hotel Quarantine Program was seriously flawed, that these so called 'cold hotels' would contain asymptomatic infected individuals and were always potentially hot hotels. In other words that the establishment of 'hot' and 'cold' hotels was effectively scientific nonsense. He also believed that Victorian bureaucrats just did not understand the basic concepts of infection control and quarantine management. Infection control in quarantine hotels was 'sloppy' compared to the way that hospitals were managing the same risks.

The original aim of these measures was, according to Premier Daniel Andrews, to *"flatten the curve so our health system is not overwhelmed"* (Andrews 2020d). However, it is now apparent that many of these measures did little to flatten the curve at the time. Modelling of the effectiveness of the initial July lockdowns of Melbourne and the Mitchel Shire indicates that these measures were not successful in reducing the rate of infection (McQuire, 2020). Even the subsequent introduction of mandatory facemasks, provided little effect in bringing the outbreak under control. It was only the massive limitations on freedom of movement and association, beyond anything seen in any western democracy, introduced from 6 August 2020 for four months, that started to materially reduce the rates of spread.

It seems at some stage that the Victorian Government's intent changed from 'flattening the curve' to trying to eliminate the virus, something that persisted over the six lockdowns. Perhaps because the government realised how fragile its health system was, and that even flattening the curve of the pandemic would still result in the fractured health system being overwhelmed.

There is still a great deal of debate about whether lockdowns were necessary. It could be argued that, although a very blunt instrument, the long term neglect of Victoria's health system, left the Government with little alternative but to shut Victorians into their homes for months on end. That even relatively small numbers of COVID-19 cases would have overwhelmed Victorian's hospitals, triple zero system, and ambulance services soon became obvious over subsequent waves (and Victoria realistically only experienced tiny outbreaks in it pandemic waves compared to what was occurring overseas).

Ostensibly, these lockdowns were supposed to provide a breathing space for the government to get the health system in order. However, two years of breathing space later, what did the government actually achieve? Especially when the health system, continuing well in 2022, experienced regular breakdowns in emergency call taking, delayed or non-attendance of ambulances for critical emergencies, hours-long waits for ambulances on hospital ramps before patients were examined, never before seen levels of 'code browns'[34] as hospitals failed, at least 15 patients dying because of a lack of ambulance and medical attention. On top of which, significant mental health and morale problems manifesting in doctors, nurses, and paramedics, all

[34] A code brown is a transition to a critical hospital emergency response to deal with a sudden surge in incoming patients, usually as a result of a major external incident. The code browns declared during the pandemic were the first health system wide emergencies declared in Victoria's history.

combined to bring Victoria's health system close to total collapse (Dow, 2022a; Dow et al, 2022; Tsirtsakis, 2022; Baxdale, 2021; Tomazin et al, 2021) even in what turned out to be the absence of predicted large numbers of COVID patients.

A number of different research studies have since been published about the effectiveness of lockdowns for controlling pandemic waves, but opinion remains contentious. One of the reasons for contention is that many commentators do not adequately distinguish between the outcomes of initial lockdowns and those of subsequent later lockdowns[35]. This is further complicated by the absence of any standard understanding of what comprises a 'lockdown', which results in the term being applied very differently by different researchers. Many of the studies reviewed for this book regarded a 'lockdown' as any non-pharmaceutical intervention, which included restrictions on international travel, limiting massed gatherings (such as theatres and sporting events), and closing down educational facilities. Accordingly, looking at the impact of such a broad range of measures would generally produce more evidence for the effectiveness of lockdowns, rather than the relatively limited success revealed by applying the definition of a lockdown simply detaining citizens involuntarily in their homes for 23 hours every day for months on end.

Available evidence seems to show that lockdown interventions in the *very early stages of a pandemic* can be very effective (Alfanzo and Ercolano, 2020; Caristisa et al, 2020; Kharroubi and Saleh, 2020). Such as stay at home orders that are mobilised early in the pandemic and are *of short duration* (Joshi and Musalem, 2021; Mégarbane et al, 2020; Wang et al, 2020). However, it also needs to be borne in mind that many of the studies promoting the success of lockdowns "over-estimated the benefits and under-estimated the costs" (Allen, 2021). Research shows that for Canada, lockdowns may be the greatest peacetime policy failure in the country's history[36].

Furthermore, the effectiveness of lockdowns in later stages of the pandemic appeared to be less convincing, declining by up to a third after the first four

---

[35] The issue is further complicated because there is no standard understanding of what comprises a lockdown. Many of the studies reviewed for this book regarded a 'lock down' as any non-pharmaceutical intervention and including restrictions on international travel, limiting massed gatherings (such as theatres and sporting events), and closing down educational facilities. Accordingly, looking at the impact of such a broad range of measures would generally appear to be more effective than if the definition of a lockdown was restricted to the model were citizens were involuntarily detained in their homes for 23 hours every day for months on end.

[36] Allen, 2021.

weeks and continuing to decline as the length of a lockdown increased (Joshi and Musalem, 2021). Internationally published studies have shown that some types of restrictions, those that reduce super spreader exposures such as closing down businesses with high rates of cases along with universities and schools, did achieve lower infection rates and reduced the number of deaths (Kleczkowksi, 2022).

However, jurisdiction-wide and repeated community lockdowns (stay at home orders) had only marginal or little effects (Fuss et al, 2022; Goldstein et al, 2021; Herby et al, 2022; Sharov, 2020; Brauner et al, 2020). It is certainly plausible that success of any restrictions has had more to do with people already voluntarily limiting their movements (out of fear of infection) rather than government enforcing mandatory compliance (Spiliopolos, 2021). Full lockdowns may flatten the curve by spreading out the infections over a longer time period when implemented early (which could give the health system time to uplift capability before large cases numbers occur), but can then extend the duration of the pandemic (Oraby et al, 2021). Whilst it has also been shown that the effectiveness of lockdowns diminishes when applied to subsequent pandemic waves (Dainton and Hay, 2021).

The case has been made that "less disruptive and costly"[37] interventions can be as effective as the onerous burden of whole lockdowns (Kryola, 2021; Haug et al, 2020). Adam Kleczkowski summarised his review of lockdowns with: *"full and particularly repeated – lockdowns can be seen as a failure of other more gradual public health policies"*.

Overall, it appears that assumptions about the effectiveness of lockdowns, that were made during the first two years or so of the pandemic, are not borne out by the evidence. With recent research suggesting that highly restrictive lockdowns were no more effective than lesser interventions, including restrictions on massed gatherings and voluntary measures, such as social distancing (Spiliopoulos, 2022; Bendavid et al, 2021; Bjørnskov, 2021; Bonardi 2020). There is also compelling evidence that restrictive prolonged lockdowns may have had manifestly overall poor health outcomes, resulting in the loss of 20 times more life years than they save (Yanovskiy and Socol, 2022). With this research recommending that any future lockdowns must be accompanied by a robust cost-benefit analysis, something that was apparently not conducted or was ignored in the Victorian Government's decision-making.
The disastrous long term health and wellbeing effects of over zealous and onerous restrictions is becoming more evident, with health costs of lockdowns

---

[37] Haug et al, 2021.

far exceeding the benefits (for example, the avoidance of additional COVID 19 cases) by at least 5 to 10 times (Ellis, 2022; Bennett et al, 2021; Joffe, 2021; Dayaratna and Vanderplas, 2020; Swainston, 2020).

That the early lockdowns eventually provided a temporary respite is acknowledged[38]. Some lives were undoubtedly saved until COVID-19 vaccination became available months later. However, this was achieved at an immeasurable cost to Victorian citizens' financial security and long term health and wellbeing. It is absolutely certain that over coming years Victoria will see a large number of premature deaths, just because of cancelled and delayed health services (such as cancer screening) an issue that was occurring in other highly locked down jurisdictions (COVIDSurgCollaborative, 2021). To which must be added what is likely to be further significant numbers of early deaths due to the stress, social isolation, and family breakups that predominated during the lockdowns (Butterworth et al, 2022; Fontanesi et al, 2020; Greyling et al, 2020). It is also believed that there were significant increases in (often unreported) child abuse during lockdowns (Garstang et al, 2020). Many scientific and medical experts now recognise that the number of otherwise preventable deaths and long term adverse health effects of the lockdowns will far exceed those due to COVID-19 infection.

The picture for Victoria is grim, and the Victorian Government's decisions have had far reaching consequences for every Australian. Victorian Government debt due to COVID stood at $82 billion up to September 2021 (Towell, 2021), and has continued to balloon since then. Calculating economic cost of the Victorian lockdowns carries a lot of uncertainty, but estimates of costs to the taxpayer of $300 to $400 million per day (Sky News, 2020a), and about $1billion of economic impacts for each week that the State was locked down is not unreasonable (Cockburn, 2021). Modelling of the impacts of lockdowns, including relative loss of lives, shows that lockdowns have had a disproportionally adverse effect compared with what would have been alternative strategies (Foster, 2021; 2020a). I agree wholeheartedly with Professor Gigi Foster's statement on lockdowns, made to Victoria's Public Accounts and Estimates Committee: *"...unemployment, business collapse, education neglect, health neglect and loneliness. The virus does not do these things; government directives do these things..."* (Foster, 2020b)

Just because the lockdowns have had such awful impacts and because their effectiveness has been highly contentious, the Victorian public have an absolute

---

[38] Research indicates that lockdowns, in their early days, can be very effective at reducing community transmission. However, this effectiveness declines significantly overtime (Fritz et al, 2023).

right to know on what basis decisions were made that have so severely impacted upon their lives. At the time the Victorian Government made decisions about each of the lockdowns, a wealth of information was freely available about the relative merits and the potential for harm from various mitigation strategies against COVID.

Was the Victorian Government completely ignorant about this available information? Or did the government decide to ignore information that was not aligned to its ideology? Did the government receive flawed medical advice, or was valid advice provided by health experts that was then wilfully disregarded by the government?

Victoria's Chief Medical Officer (Dr Brett Sutton) has acknowledged the "terrible, terrible consequences" of the lockdowns, whilst also claiming that they were a "necessity" (9News Staff, 2021). However, there has been a strong resistance to providing the public with exactly why this was a "necessity". Premier Daniel Andrews and other Ministers adopted a veil of secrecy over their decisions. The Victoria Government consistently refused to disclose what medical advice they used to make their decisions about lockdowns, actively blocking the Freedom of Information requests for disclosure (Staley, 2021). After being ordered by the Office of the Victorian Information Commissioner in October 2021 (Piovesan, 2021) to release 176 documents from the Department of Health, the Victorian Government was still refusing to release key information in June 2022. The Department of Premier and Cabinet launching an appeal to the Victorian Civil and Administrative Tribunal in a bid to keep certain health advice secret (Wu, 2022).

The tragedy of the second wave

The tragedy of the second wave was not just that millions of Victorians lost their freedom and many of them lost their jobs. It was not just a tragedy because of the massive mental health problems created by lockdowns, the full extent of which we may never really understand. It was not just a tragedy because 801 people died with COVID-19. It was a tragedy because all of this was avoidable, but for bungling decision-making by the Victorian Government. This tragedy of government failure was made more poignant by the nature of the second wave, where the vast majority of those that died were some of Victoria's most vulnerable people, 655 of whom were aged care residents[39] . They died

[39] Representing 95% of all aged care deaths that occurred throughout Australia during the second wave.

ultimately because of government and bureaucratic incompetence. Nor did this tragedy simply cease with the end of the second wave. Subsequent lockdowns continued to claim more collateral damage, more victims.

In the aftermath of the tragedy, the Commonwealth and Victorian Government played the blame game with both trying to avoid accountability for what had happened (Clun, 2020). The Australian Government had responsibility for aged care facilities and was criticised for its lack of governance and oversight of some facilities where excessive fatalities occurred during the pandemic (Lucas, 2021; Lucas and Clun, 2020). The extent to which they fulfilled or failed in these responsibilities are important questions but lay outside the scope of this book. Despite the Commonwealth's direct role, the interactions with the Victorian Government introduced a number of critical errors that made major contributions to the tragedies that would unfold.

The situation at two Melbourne residential aged care facilities have received particular attention: 'St Basils' and 'Epping Gardens', where the large extent of the outbreaks and the facilities lack of preparedness for a pandemic have been highlighted (NARI, 2021). At St Basils 45 residents died (out of 94 infected and a total of 117 residents) and at Epping Gardens there were 38 deaths (out of 103 residents infected), along with large numbers of staff infected at both facilities. However, the high mortality rates do not convey the true extent of the horror faced by residents and staff. The trauma faced by residents, locked down and with no access to family, whilst friends were dying all around them, along with the despair felt by staff as they could do little to manage the spiralling situation until they were eventually placed into quarantine themselves. The aged care debacle was all the worse because it was entirely foreseeable[40].

An independent review (Gilbert and Lilly, 2020) determined that both facilities were substantially unprepared for the pandemic, with inadequate planning, a lack of exercising of emergency arrangements, inadequate infection control arrangements, ineffective leadership and management, inadequate clinical governance, and an over-reliance on external assistance (that the Victorian Government was unable to provide when it was actually required). This out-of-control situation was greatly exacerbated by Victoria's DHHS delays[41]. In particular, delays in providing information to the facilities about infected

[40] *"Homer Simpson could have foreseen the catastrophe in aged care coming with COVID-19"* Professor Joseph Ibrahim, Law and Ageing Research Unit, Monash University, quoted in Cousins, 2020.

[41] This included a six day delay before a testing team even attended the sites.

residents, because the State's laboratory testing and contact tracing systems were both overwhelmed and close to collapse. The Victorian Government then decided to replace existing skilled aged care staff with inexperienced and inadequate temporary agency workers. The handover process was described as chaotic, with inadequate and confusing communications from government and little time provided to induct the replacement workers and management before all of the existing facilities' staff were stood down and ordered off the premises. This was a decision, approved by Victoria's Chief Health Officer, that was described by independent doctors as "frankly dangerous" (Editorial Team, 2021).

The emerging situation was apparently made worse because the under-resourced and struggling hospital system was unable to accept the transfer of many of the infected residents. Several residents that were transported to hospitals by ambulance following emergency (triple 000) calls on the advice of a doctor, were refused admission by the hospital and sent back to the aged care facility. Concerns were also raised about agency staff working at multiple sites and potentially being a source for further transmission into unaffected facilities. Concerns that were apparently ignored by the government. During a subsequent wave over a year later, allegations were still being made that lessons from the second wave had still not been learnt and that staff were still working across multiple sites (Turner-Cohen, 2021). A situation that raised little apparent interest or action from the Victorian Government. Many of these problems were already present well before the pandemic. But were apparently ignored by the Victorian Government for years.

Systematic disarray

With a decayed health system, a hospital system on the brink of failure, a woefully under resourced public health team, a dysfunctional contact tracing system, and serious infighting, the Victorian Government had absolutely no hope of slowing down, let alone containing the second wave, without resorting to drastic measures. In the face of a failing system, it had only one choice, to impose another lockdown, to remove basic freedoms from millions of its own citizens. Yes, this was somewhat successful, but this success was quickly overturned by successive breaches, because fundamental and obvious problems in the various agencies had not been fixed.

The major reason for the imposition of lockdowns and other restrictions on people's liberty and human rights was to 'flatten the curve' to slow down the increase in numbers of COVID-19 numbers and hospitalisations. This was ostensibly to provide a window of time, 'breathing space', during which both the public health and hospital systems would be able to be prepared for any increase in demand arising from the pandemic.

These restrictions and lockdowns were essential for Victoria because its health system was already under critical stress long before the pandemic occurred. One only had to listen to doctors and nurses working in the Victorian Health system, over the last eight or so years increasingly complain about the problems they were facing, to realise that this was a health system on the edge of collapse. It would only require another stressor 'the straw that broke the camel's back', to tip the system over the edge.

The real fear in government was that any material increases in hospitalisations due to COVID-19 would break that 'camel's back'. They certainly had every right to hold that fear. The Victorian health system was massively underfunded and under resourced. An independent report published in 2022 showed just how far behind Victoria was compared to the rest of Australia in the lead into the pandemic (Productivity Commission, 2022; AAP, 2022; Credlin, 2022). Numbers for the financial year 2019/20 show that Victoria provided the least recurrent hospital funding per person of any of the other States and Territories. Victoria had the least number of hospital staff (per 1000 people) of any state or territory apart from South Australia and was also the second worse in Australia for the number of hospital beds. The Victorian health system also demonstrated deteriorating performance in hospital waiting times for emergencies and for non-urgent surgeries. Since the government was unable to address a chronically failing health system during years of routine operation, it would have been well outside of their abilities to fix these massive problems over a few months in the midst of a pandemic induced crisis.

In the face of lockdowns, the Premier promised $billions of additional funding for the health system which would fund 4,000 additional intensive care beds. Over two years later, only a handful of additional ICU beds were provided, with no transparency on what had happened to the beds or where the promised funding had gone.

One journalist's account of their experience in a Victorian public hospital towards the end of the second year of the pandemic is particularly harrowing. They described the health system as "chaotic", "beyond broken", and "third world", and that the system was broken before the pandemic occurred (9 News, 2022). Some off the record conversations with health staff have carried a similar theme, feelings of abandonment by the Andrews government and anger at Labor politicians making light of the crisis situation in the hospitals. These problems continued well into 2022, with overwhelmed ambulance and hospital systems, multiple avoidable deaths of patients due to delays in ambulance and medical aid. All happening with the Andrews government continuing to blame the pandemic, rather than the underlying reasons for the years of a failing health system.

A pandemic...... the big surprise

It is now a widely accepted conclusion (from the Coate Inquiry, and from many informed analysts and commentators) that the Victorian Government's management of the Hotel Quarantine Program and other significant aspects of the pandemic response was characterised by appalling and uninformed decision-making. Notwithstanding that those fragile governmental systems and a creaking bureaucracy were rapidly overwhelmed by the developing pandemic, did the Victorian Government even attempt to adequately manage the risk of a pandemic prior to January-February 2020?

Many supporters of the Andrews government have tried to defend its decisions and actions as 'reasonable' in what was an unwarranted and unforeseeable situation. Arguing that the government reacted as best as it could in the face of the unprecedented and unexpected pandemic. However, this is at best misdirection and is in a reality a specious argument.

The prospect of a pandemic resulting in significant disruption to civil society was entirely foreseeable, and almost all jurisdictions in the developed world had been preparing for such an eventuality for several decades. In the late 1990's and 2000's it was accepted practice across almost all Victorian Government agencies to have in place pandemic plans, many supported by detailed risk assessments. Throughout the first decade or so of this century the Australian Government, through the Emergency Management Australia Institute at Mt Macedon in Victoria, ran multiple training courses and planning workshops for managing disruptions, which included pandemic preparedness. Many senior managers from Victorian Government agencies, including health, justice, police, and infrastructure portfolios, as well as from the Department of Premier and Cabinet attended these capability development sessions.

Detailed pandemic plans were developed across government, and these plans continued to be updated well into the following decade. In the 2010's multiple different exercises were conducted in the Victorian public sector, even including a number of universities, that were looking at potential pandemic scenarios. The author of this book was involved in conducting several

workshops for different government agencies looking at continuity of government, quarantine, workforce, and supply chain issues under various pandemic scenarios.
A pandemic of some sort impacting upon Victoria was most certainly *not* unexpected, there had been substantial planning effort, over at least twenty years. Nor was a pandemic a merely theoretical exercise. A lot of thinking about pandemics was undertaken, based on learning from domestic and international experience of dealing with SARS, MERS, H1N1 influenza, Zika, Ebola, HIV, as well as specific experience in Victoria from a number of major veterinary disease outbreaks with human infection potential.

The various Victorian Governments of the 1990's and 2000's anticipated and were prepared for a pandemic. Their decision-making and public health arrangements were honed through training, exercising, and real-life exposure to large-scale disease outbreaks within Australia and overseas. The pandemic was not unprecedented, it was not unexpected, it was entirely foreseeable. However, the Victorian Government in 2020 was woefully unprepared for and incapable of managing the COVID-19 pandemic when it occurred.

How then could so many decisions and actions be undertaken in 2020 that seemed to completely ignore the experience, planning, and preparedness gained over the previous decades?

Why was the Victorian Government in 'panic' mode in late March 2020, when the Hotel Quarantine Program was being initiated, when it had two months of publicly available warnings about an emerging pandemic?

The Victorian Government also knew, well in advance of the WHO declaration of a pandemic, that a disease outbreak was occurring with the potential to become a disease of global significance. Why was the concept of quarantine seen as something novel and without precedence?

Even if we put the issue of a pandemic to the side for a moment, there are a several notifiable human diseases which have required mandatory quarantine under Australian law[42] since 1908, and now includes Lassa Fever, Marburg, Ebola, Crimean Congo haemorrhagic fever, highly pathogenic avian influenza in humans, SARS, cholera, smallpox, rabies, plague, and yellow fever (NDSS, 2010). Surely, someone, somewhere in the Victoria Government still had some understanding of setting up quarantine arrangements in 2020. Without the need to abrogate responsibility to groups whose only really experience was in

[42] Quarantine Act, 1908.

organising conferences and trade delegations, or in running the occasional routine tender?

On 11 February 2020, the World Health Organisation issued guidance on the management of quarantine requirements for international travellers (WHO, 2020), in line with the requirements of international law[43] (Plotkin, 2007; WHO, 2005). However, when the Victorian Government finally got around to developing a specific pandemic plan in mid-March 2020, it ignored the WHO requirements and guidance, and comprehensively failed to include quarantine considerations in its new pandemic plan (DHHS, 2020). This was despite the Australian Government's "Australian Health Management Plan for Pandemic Influenza" published in August 2019 specifically identifying the need to consider isolation and quarantine arrangements (DOH, 2019).

Why then was the Victorian Government so unprepared for the decisions and actions that had to be taken in late March, when the prospect of quarantine and community outbreaks had been 'on the table' for several months. Even the proposal for using CBD hotels as quarantine facilities was not something entirely new. The initial idea had originated within the Victorian Government weeks before the fateful decision on 27th March 2020.

Throughout the pandemic, the Victorian Government was only too quick to blame the complacency and noncompliance of its citizens as root causes of the various waves of disease that hit the State. It is a reasonable assumption that rapid spread of COVID-19 through the community would occur if infected individuals knowingly failed to isolate, broke quarantine, or deceptively crossed borders. Or if people with the signs and symptoms of COVID-19 did not get tested and did not voluntarily self-isolate, or enough people in the general population did not observe social distancing, hand washing, mask wearing etc., then small outbreaks would quickly turn into big outbreaks. From that perspective, then the Victorian Government may have had some limited justification for blaming a small number of its citizens (Carney, 2020). However, throughout history, attempts at controlling widescale infectious diseases (including attempts at quarantine) have faced these same problems, and have prepared for when breaches would eventually happen. Surely, the Victorian Government was not so naïve in its pandemic planning as to assume that for the first time in history such breaches would not occur.

---

[43] Which included binding International Health Regulations from 2005 that the Victorian Government had to comply with for preventing the international spread of disease.

The vast majority of Victorians did what was expected of them. That a minority would not comply ended up apparently playing such a major role in the transmission of the disease was because the government's arrangements were quite simply not up to the task expected of them. That complacency and non-compliance increased with each subsequent wave and resulting lockdown had less to do with a deliberately malfeasant population, and more to do with people's weariness and rejection of broken promises and continuing government incompetence. If the government did not expect noncompliance (and the growing 'lockdown fatigue), then they were simply not competent in their assessment of risk. If they did expect non-compliance and appreciate the risk this presented, but failed to manage this risk, then they were negligent.

2
An overview of the Victorian Hotel Quarantine Program

Introduction

There has been intense media and public interest into how Victoria, alone amongst all of the States and Territories, could so badly manage a hotel quarantine program. Mismanagement that resulted in the deaths of over 800 of its citizens. There has been much blame given to the decision to appoint private security guards to manage significant aspects of the Program, and compelling evidence presented at the Coate Inquiry, and subsequent media revelations, demonstrated how this decision contributed to the disaster that was to follow.

However, this book tries not to engage in counterfactuals, we make no attempt to say if certain aspects of the Program were managed differently, then a specific outcome would or would not have occurred. For example, it is just not possible to say that if private security guards were not used, and that if Victoria had adopted a nationally consistent approach, then this catastrophe would not have occurred. Unfortunately, there were a number of other severe chronic problems within the Victorian Government at this time that introduced fatal weaknesses into its attempts at controlling COVID-19 in the State. Even if police and ADF personnel had been deployed instead of private security, a serious quarantine failure would in all likelihood still have occurred, with a subsequent devastating community outbreak and mass fatalities. There were sufficient manifest latent failures within the Victorian Government's capabilities, systems, and decision-making that would have created the necessary conditions, irrespective of whoever provided front-line security, that almost guaranteed a failure of monumental proportions. However, the decision to appoint private security guards, and to appoint an unsuitable security provider introduced egregious and otherwise avoidable vulnerabilities. This made it a certainty that serious breaches would occur, and substantially elevated the potential for catastrophic outcomes to eventuate.

The extremely high level of risk associated with the Hotel Quarantine Program was obvious from the very start, and those factors that then contributed to the

Program's abject failure should have been foreseen[44]. However, the lack of sufficient public health and infectious disease control focus at the time, the absence of effective leadership, and too few competent bureaucrats meant that this failure was inevitable.

That quarantine breaches could occur was a clear high risk that should have been recognised and addressed. That the risk was apparently ignored or inadequately dealt with is an indictment on those involved in critical decisions. Victoria has not been alone in experiencing quarantine failures, and other Australian jurisdictions have experienced outbreaks from quarantine and transmission into the community. What distinguished the March 2020 outbreak in Victoria was the State's inability to quickly contain the community spread of the disease, the large number of fatalities that occurred, and the lengthy restrictions on societal and personal liberties that had to be enforced to contain an out-of-control situation. An out-of-control situation, which was not really because of COVID-19, but instead was caused by an already struggling public health system, ideology before outcomes, and an incapable bureaucracy. COVID-19 was just the 'straw that broke the camel's back. That the Hotel Quarantine Program's disastrous failure was the result of long-term leadership, institutional ,and cultural neglect is in itself deplorable. That the factors that contributed to this failure were absolutely foreseeable[45] and avoidable makes this disaster inexcusable.

The escape of the SARS-CoV-2 virus[46] from hotel quarantine into the community was a result of failed government decision-making at all levels, that placed multiple senior public servants into positions of power and control without the experience, knowledge, and capabilities to undertake the tasks expected of them. This occurred whilst some of the real expertise was apparently sidelined or excluded.

Once the virus was out and into the Victorian community, it spread rapidly because of antiquated, cumbersome, and slow contact tracing and testing systems. This was a result of flawed decisions made at the highest levels, months and even years before the pandemic emerged. The Victorian public health system was struggling long before the pandemic came onto Australia's shores. Leaked Victorian Government reports prepared in May 2019 provide evidence that Victoria's public health team was massively underfunded and was the worst resourced in Australia (Ilanbey and Baker, 2020). So much so that it

---

44 Coate 2021a, p.28.
45 Coate, 2020a, p. 28.
46 The scientific name for the virus causing the COVID-19 pandemic.

was claimed that even if staff numbers were suddenly doubled in Victoria, it would still be behind other jurisdictions.

In State's pandemic preparedness, in establishing and managing the hotel quarantine program, and in the subsequent response to the outbreak, there was little understanding of or attention paid to underlying vulnerabilities. There appears to have been an almost complete absence of anything resembling effective risk management. On what seems to be the rare occasion when risk assessment was undertaken, this was often either not communicated to, or was disregarded by key decision-makers within government.

The Victorian Government's Inquiry into the hotel quarantine failure (Coate, 2020a) found that no individual was to blame, but that the hotel quarantine failure resulted from multiple systemic failures. However, it must be remembered that outside of the rarefied contemplations of the Inquiry and out in the real world, systemic failures do not just occur on their own. These failures are always a result of multiple serious errors in decision-making that establish and perpetuate inadequate and failing systems. Someone, somewhere, made each of those flawed contributing decisions. Whilst the 'Final Report' of the Coate Inquiry did not seek to assign blame, a detailed reading of the evidence and transcripts provides significant clues as to how some of these decisions may have come about, and the culpability of some individuals in making those decisions.

In what should have been an Inquiry to uncover the truth about events, and to establish real lessons learned to prevent such a tragedy from occurring again, we instead saw the Premier, Ministers, and senior bureaucrats protecting themselves with an unprecedented army of barristers and supporting legal teams (Robins, 2020). The cost of this legal protection amounted to at least $12.3m of taxpayer money, almost twice the cost of conducting the Inquiry (Varga, 2021a). This was public money that could instead have been made available to what was quickly becoming an overwhelmed and grossly underfunded public health system. Instead, millions of dollars of taxpayer money were diverted away from protecting the health of Victorians to protecting the tenure of those in positions of power. The machinations of such an 'army' of lawyers have without doubt helped the obfuscations, avoidances, and blame shifting of many of those they represented, as well as successfully confusing and redirecting the attention of Counsel-assisting the Inquiry and the general public.

Allegations of mismanagement of the quarantine hotel system continued into 2021, along with further outbreaks, extensive lockdowns and the further suspension of civil rights. This was despite the formation of a new agency CQV[47] established to fix the hotel quarantine system's catastrophic problems. Through 2021, as further community outbreaks occurred, the new system repeatedly showed that whatever changes had been made, these were not up to the task. CQV continually struggled and was unable to cope adequately, even with relatively small numbers of positive cases and close contacts, in what was described as the continuing "Victorian hotel quarantine chaos" (Varga 2021c). There were even reports of growing tensions between CQV and the Victoria's public health team over process inadequacies.

These subsequent outbreaks, with the allegations of inadequate management and 'leaked secrets', make it appear the lessons about the need for good governance and transparent decision-making had still not been learned effectively.

Following the Inquiry, it was evident that one of the crucial issues in preventing breaches was ensuring that staff did not work across multiple quarantine hotels, that had However, the December 2020 'reboot' of the quarantine system still appeared not to have prevented the obviously dangerous practice of staff working across different high risk sites. Subsequent allegations in March 2021, about another contractor, Healthcare Australia[48], revealed apparent problems with staff shortages, failures to complete online training, "unfair rostering", delayed pharmaceuticals, movement of staff between hotels, and bullying and harassment. All of which was uncovered, not through any government oversight, but through a whistle-blower's revelations to the media. Perhaps even more worrying was the Victorian Government spokesperson's response to the allegations, in which they neither expressed concern about the continuing management failures with the quarantine program, or expressed any interest in further investigating the matters. Instead, just repeating the measures they *believed* were in place, in other words – '*nothing to worry about here, nothing to see here, move along now!*'.

In early October 2021, Melbourne became the world's most locked-down place in the world (Table 1). The Victorian Government's own knowledge of the gross inadequacies of the health system left them with little choice but to keep Victorians locked away in their own homes for months. With little overall

---

[47] COVID-19 Quarantine Victoria, established in November 2020.

[48] Coincidently, the CEO of Healthcare Australia resigned In February 2021 following the misadministration of COVID-19 vaccinations in aged care residences, four times the correct doses had been administered by a doctor that had not completed the mandatory training (Smethurst, 2021a).

improvement in capability over the first year of the pandemic, the inability to control even a small, limited outbreak of COVID-19 would result in lockdown after lockdown.

It is difficult to argue against lockdowns in the face of out-of-control community transmission and a health system in absolute disarray. Although lurching from one lockdown into the next does not appear to be especially competent management[49]. At the same time lockdowns are a blunt instrument that come with extreme economic losses and largely incalculable individual financial hardship, poor social and mental health outcomes, and long term serious adverse health impacts. Whist 'effective', it also needs to be remembered that an immediate recourse to harsh lockdowns in the face of relatively small numbers of cases, reflects a lack of the government's own confidence in its own capabilities and a reflection of an inadequate health system, rather than a balanced risk assessment and pragmatic approach. In other words, Victoria had to have lockdowns not just because there was a pandemic, but because the state's health systems were left to decline for far too long[50].

---

[49]Less than two weeks after leaving its fifth lockdown, Premier Daniel Andrews announced another snap seven day lockdown (Andrews, 2021), in response to a handful of cases of the delta variant of the virus. Just over a month later, the Victorian outbreak was growing at a faster rate than in NSW, despite Victoria's more draconian lockdown measures and entering the outbreak with higher vaccination rates (Fitzsimmons, 2021). As of early October 2021, this seven day lockdown was in its 54th day and still continuing, with case numbers higher than those for NSW (Paynter 2021b).

[50] Even with the knowledge of the potential to become a health crisis over a prolonged time, it appears that the Victorian Government still did not adequately drive long overdue improvements in the health system's capabilities and capacity. Despite Daniel Andrews announcing $1.3 billion funding for 4,000 new ICU beds in April 2020 (Andrews, 2020b), some eighteen months later only 50 new beds had appeared to provide a state-wide total of 500 ICU beds (O'Brien, 2021a), with the Health Department unable to explain where the bulk of the funds had gone.

Table 1: Melbourne lockdowns

Lockdown	Commenced	Ended	Days
First lockdown	16 March 2020: restrictions, 30 March 2020: stay at home lockdown	12 May 2020	43 days
Second lockdown	20 June 2020: increased restrictions 8 July: stay at home lockdown	27 October 2020	111 days
Third lockdown	12 February 2021: stay at home lockdown	15 February 2021	5 days
Fourth lockdown	27 May 2021: stay at home lockdown	10 June 2021	14 days
Fifth lockdown	15 July 2021: stay at home lockdown	27 July 2021	12 days
Sixth lockdown	5 August 2021: Stay at home lockdown	21 October 2021	78 days
	Total days in lockdown		**263 days**

In comparison: Perth spent 63 days in lockdown, Brisbane - 67 days, Greater Sydney - 159 days, whilst in other countries: Auckland – spent 183 days in lockdown, Paris - 113 days, London - 99 days, New York - 83 days, Quebec - 47 days, Moscow - 43 days, Delhi - 42 days, PNG -14 days.

An overview: from failure to catastrophe

The Victorian Government's frequently trotted out excuse was that the pandemic was unprecedented and that the need for quarantine was an issue that arose quickly and required great haste in putting in place a solution. This, however, appears far from the truth. The prospect of a future pandemic was well understood within all Australian jurisdictions, and under previous Victorian Governments there had been a great deal of focus on pandemic preparedness. Unfortunately, under the Andrews government, in the years leading up to 2020 there appears to have been general decline in commitment and effort directed towards both public health and pandemic capability. Yes, some limited pandemic planning for an influenza outbreak was still being undertaken in some organisations, and occasional emergency management exercises were being conducted (again focusing on influenza outbreaks). However, the quality and practicality of these efforts were becoming increasingly divorced from the reality of the actual changing infectious disease landscape and the reasonable efforts required to manage the public health risk (refer to SEA, 2021a for an overview).

The problem with hotels

Whist the Coate Inquiry considered the use of hotels for mass quarantine was unprecedented[51], this was not actually the case. There has been a long history of establishing quarantine facilities, including the use of hotels (BBC, 2020a). In numerous countries, for well over a hundred years, hotels have been used for quarantine of individuals infected with smallpox, diphtheria, influenza, bubonic plague, as well as for repatriated wounded in the First World War (James, 2021). Even in the early stages of the COVID-19 pandemic, and weeks before Victoria's 27 March 2020 decision to use hotel rooms for incoming travellers, emergency plans in several jurisdictions were considering their use. The hotel industry itself was offering rooms for individuals needing to self-isolate (Cowe et al, 2020), at least a week before the decision was made on the Hotel Quarantine Program.

This author can remember reviewing government pandemic plans at least 15 years ago where the use of hotels and university student campus accommodation was highlighted for use as mass casualty wards and for isolation purposes. Although this earlier pandemic planning was undertaken with some understanding of infectious disease control and the problems that these sort of facilities would present. An understanding that seems to have been missing in action March 2020.

There is a long standing history of the problems with infection control within hotels, and their unsuitability for containing the spread of infectious diseases. The role of hotels as foci for transmission of infectious diseases such as SARS, swine flu, typhoid, measles, and Legionnaires disease has been known for decades (Fung et al, 2020; CHP, 2019; Hung , 2018; Wong et al, 2015, Paull et al, 2012; Fernstrom and Goldblatt, 2013; Boone, 2007; Hollingsworth, 2007; Ali and Keil, 2006; Cheesborough et al, 2000; Fraser et al, 1977). Perhaps one of the best known case studies of so called 'superspreader[52]' events (and one that should be familiar to most people in infectious disease control) demonstrated how an hotel could play a major role in amplifying a disease outbreak. In the early stages of the 2003 SARS pandemic, a respiratory disease doctor, infected

[51] Coate, 2020a, p. 28.

[52] A 'superspreader' is a person, location, or event that results in the infection of an unusually large number of individuals.

with SARS, stayed for one night at the Metropole Hotel, in Kowloon, Hong Kong. During that one night stay, multiple other guests on the same floor were infected, these other guests then travelling and spreading SARS across the world. It was later estimated that about half of the world's SARS cases could be traced back to this single superspreader event (CDC, 2003a; Baric, 2007; Paull et al, 2012; Normile, 2013; Wong et al, 2015; Wick, 2022). One would reasonably assume that the wealth of information about hotels and the spread of infectious disease, including the repeated publication of the SARS superspreader event account over the following twenty years would be sufficient to raise some concerns within the Victorian Government. Even if key advisors and decision makers had completely missed reading the scientific literature, then surely they would have been alerted by the mainstream media repeating the Metropole Hotel story as part of their coverage of the emerging pandemic in February 2020 (CNBC, 2020).

These were critical issues about using hotels to house infected individuals, issues that seem to have been forgotten, ignored, or deliberately disregarded in the rush to the fatal decision of 27 March 2020.

Overview of the private security decision

A lot of the attention on the Victoria Government's mishandling of the Hotel Quarantine Program has been focused on one key decision, the decision to appoint outsourced private security providers to manage the arrangements at the quarantine hotels. This was a decision that set the Victorian response apart from other States and Territories, that instead used a more competent workforce in the form of police and ADF[53] personnel. This was the central decision that led to conditions where quarantine was breached on multiple occasions, allowing widespread community transmission of COVID-19, thereby creating Victoria's 'second wave'. This was not a decision taken in isolation, and it is highly probable that a sequence of other decisions, some completely unrelated to any management of the pandemic, contributed to and influenced the making of this one momentous decision.

Nor was the decision to appoint private security the final disastrous decision. A range of decisions and actions, taken after the announcement of the appointment of private security, exacerbated this dangerous situation, introducing further vulnerabilities and risks. This all eventually resulted in 801

[53] Australian Defence Force

deaths, and the denial of basic freedoms for 4.96 million people living within metropolitan Melbourne, and elsewhere in Victoria.

In hindsight it is easy to see that a number of significant decisions were made that were significantly flawed, and fault could be levied from the Premier and senior Ministers, to agency heads and other senior bureaucrats, as well as to the senior management of some private companies. Even the decisions and actions of some individual security guards are likely to have contributed to this catastrophe. However, blame is easy to assign with the benefit of hindsight, but few people (excluding psychopaths) go out of their way to deliberately make decisions that deliberately cause harm. The vast majority of people make decisions with the best of intentions and do so using the information that they have to hand at that moment in time.

The aim of this case study is to explore the conditions prevailing at the time that certain decisions were made. To try and understand what information was available, how situationally aware individuals may have been, what other factors could have influenced their perceptions and biases, their individual and group sensemaking, and ultimately their decision-making.

Tyche[54] or incompetence

The economic, social, and health outcomes of the hotel quarantine failure were 'bad' by any subjective or objective analysis. However, a bad outcome does not necessarily mean that it was the result of a bad decision, and ostensibly good decisions often result in bad outcomes[55]. This disjunction can particularly be the case when faced with situations of high uncertainty and high risk (Eckfeldt, 2017; Bezos, 2016; Ariely, 2010). Effective decision-making recognises the potential for bad outcomes from good decisions, and accordingly relies on 'reversibility', the ability to 'wind-back' a decision (or modify it) if the outcomes look to be undesirable.

---

[54] Tyche was the ancient Greek goddess of fortune, who would bring either good or bad luck, the latter often visited on those at the heights of hubris. Her Roman incarnation, Fortuna, behaved in a similar manner and was believed to visit ill-fortune on those public officials that were not virtuous.

[55] Conversely a bad decision can give rise to a good outcome, although this would be expected to be a much rarer event.

Inadequate decision-making

The majority of everyday decisions that all of us make are reversible. We may not have all of the information that we need or fully understand the situation, yet if we make the 'wrong' decision, we can change the decision (reversible) with reasonable ease. We make such reversible decisions in our personal lives (what to eat, what movies to see, what clothes to buy, event what places to visit on holiday, etc.) and in our professional lives (day-day-day operating decisions, who to allocate tasks to, who to employ, etc.). Even though some of these decisions will have adverse outcomes, we can either 'walk-back' that decision, manage the impacts (at some relatively low time and financial cost), or accept that we will achieve some if not all of the objectives we intended from that decision. Any harmful consequences from a reversible decision can be readily coped with (recoverable).

However, under conditions of high uncertainty and high complexity, the stakes are likely to be much higher, decisions can be difficult or impossible to turn back or alter (irreversible) and the consequences can be devastating and unrecoverable. Dealing with irreversible and unrecoverable decisions requires a very different approach, and skilled decision-makers know when and how to apply different decision-making approaches and put in place additional controls for such decisions. Dealing with irreversible decisions is discussed in more detail in Chapter 5.

It appears that many of those making key decisions related to the Hotel Quarantine Program were neither aware of the existence of irreversible decisions, nor were they sufficiently skilled to make them. From the evidence presented to the Inquiry it appears that there was no distinction in approach between what were simple routine (and reversible) decisions and those that were highly complex, unique, and irreversible decisions. From the limited evidence available it appears that decisions appear to have been made using similar simple routine approaches, irrespective of their complexity and irreversibility.

It is unlikely that we will ever know the extent to which the many decisions contributing to the hotel quarantine failure were 'good' or 'bad', although based upon the disastrous outcomes we can say that they were ineffective overall.

However, it appears that some key and ultimately disastrous decisions variously:

- Were not based upon an adequate consideration of all of the information available at the time (*ill-informed*).
- Did not seek to understand or deal with the effects of prevailing uncertainty (*poor management of risk*).
- Did not fully understand the historical or developing context (*inadequate or inappropriate situational awareness*).
- Had an insufficient appreciation of the significance of what was happening and how the developing situation could evolve (*inadequate sensemaking and anticipation*).
- Were often made by individuals or groups without the requisite skills, knowledge, and experience (*inadequate cognitive, emotional, and experiential competencies*).
- Were subject to unsurfaced and unchallenged assumptions (*low validity*).
- Were influenced or directed by a range of other external factors, often unrecognised or unacknowledged (*unmanaged bias and tacit coercion*).
- Where subject to high levels of uncertainty, ambiguity, error, and variability (*high noise*[56])

Being prepared

Ultimately, the effectiveness of the response to, and management of a crisis is dependent upon effective preparedness. A contention that has been repeatedly proven, both in the observance and in the omission on multiple occasions during the COVID-19 pandemic (Collins et al, 2020). Failures and inadequacies in public health preparedness and response have in many circumstances been attributed to chronic underfunding, insufficient expertise, and the politicisation of public health in many jurisdictions within Australia and overseas (Sheehan and Fox, 2020; Public Health Ontario, 2020; WHO, 2019; Katz et al, 2017; Watson et al, 2017; Bevington, 2014; Rokkas et al, 2014; WHO, 2014; MacIntyre, 2011; Weeramanthri et al, 2010).

The apparent gaps in public health capability and low levels of preparedness may also extend to other types of hazards and crises, (Sheehan and Fox, 2020;

[56] For a discussion on the effect of 'noise' in professional judgements see Kahneman and Sibony, 2021.

Westcott et al, 2019), and be especially low in a community context. Whilst there have been repeated warnings about such issues over many years, action has been frequently lacking (Ilanbey and Baker, 2020). For example, the Victorian Government's public health and wellbeing plan (Victorian Government, 2019) manages to avoid infectious diseases altogether[57], whilst focusing on climate change, healthy eating, exercise, and tobacco. It is well known that infectious disease funding within Australia has been subject to repeated cycles of "panic and neglect" (McNeill et al, 2020), rather than informed strategic planning.

Hence, it should come as no surprise that such long-term neglect of public health has resulted in a fractured and often incapable pandemic response within the state. Internal Victorian Government documents, predating the pandemic, show that even if public health funding had been doubled, the State would still have less public health officers than any other state in Australia (Faruqi, 2020).

One of the key questions that still remains, given the wide knowledge about such under funding and under resourcing (especially when compared to NSW and Queensland), is why leadership appeared to have done so little about it, especially in the face of several years of high workloads and then a growing pandemic (Ilanbey and Baker, 2020). Why such an inadequate investment in public health occurred has not yet been answered. Even at the height of the pandemic, the Victorian Government was still able to spend time and substantial resources on pursuing its identity politics agenda, whilst health capability appears to have been relatively neglected. Funding that could have been diverted to improving capabilities in quarantine hotels, upskilling public health expertise, improving hospital capacity, adequately resourcing the triple zero system, better resourcing Ambulance Victoria, etc. With widespread failures across the Victorian health system, there was still plenty of taxpayers' money being spent on what many would regard as pet vanity projects.

Within Australia, there have been repeated calls over the last three decades for a national public health and infectious diseases capability similar to the US Centers for Disease Control and Prevention (CDC) or its European equivalent (Kamradt-Scott and Roper, 2020). The lack of progress has had one primary cause, Federal and State politics, with NSW and Victoria in particular resisting an Australian national CDC. Conversely, good practice *requirements* for public

---

[57] To be fair, infectious disease is mentioned a single time in its 60 pages, although it is only in respect of the one of the effects of climate change. Pandemic does not rate a single mention.

health emergency management are well established within Australia and internationally (DoH[58], 2020; Public Health Ontario, 2020; CDC, 2019; NSW Health, 2015[59]; 2019; EMV[60], 2017; Vic Health, 2017; SA Health, 2015; US DHSS, 2007). However, during the COVID-19 pandemic, what *should have been done* appeared on many occasions to be different to the practical reality. This should have been unsurprising given that woeful mismanagement has been a feature of other public health emergencies in the past, including Zika, MERS, H1N1 influenza, and SARS (Kim et al, 2020; Khan et al, 2019; Michelle et al, 2018; MOHW, 2016; Gorman and Stoney, 2015; Hodge et al, 2007).

The Coate Inquiry focused on some proximal causes, decisions, and actions that led straight to identified failures in Victoria's Hotel Quarantine Program. The Inquiry did not try to examine the core underlying issues to any great extent, whilst the influence of ideology, belief systems, culture, and personal bias was left largely unexplored. However, despite the Inquiry's inability to deeply probe these issues, there is enough on what has been revealed in evidence and in the media to extrapolate a wide range of inferences and interpretations about possible relationships amongst the many causal, contributing and influencing factors (see later in Figure 15).

---

58 Although some documents, such as the National Health Emergency Response Arrangements appear to have not been updated since November 2011.

59 NSW Health resource page for emergency preparedness was current only as of June 2015, although the Public Health Emergency Response Preparedness Standards were updated in February 2019.

60 The Victorian State Health Emergency Response Plan was last updated in September 2017, but was due for revision in September 2020.

3
The approach to this review

Tracking the full extent of the various causal, contributing, and influencing factors that resulted in the Victorian Hotel Quarantine Program failure is a complex and daunting task. Whilst the Hotel Quarantine Inquiry (Coate, 2020a) through submissions and questioning of witnesses has revealed some of these issues, it has also been marred by obfuscation and misleading information by witnesses, and the omission of critical evidence by several key players. The Hon Jennifer Coate and Counsel Assisting have also been heavily criticised by a number of media commentators and widely on social media. The apparently superficial questioning of prominent witnesses (including Premier Daniel Andrews) and a lack of rigorous visible follow up to some revelations (such as earlier evidence being retracted, and the former Health Minister alluding to the Premier misinforming the Inquiry) has led to allegations that the Inquiry was not intended to be a "sword" to uncover the truth, but rather functioned as a "shield" to hide it.

This has to some extent been further compounded by indifferent reporting by some mainstream media outlets, which at times have appeared to be more 'Dan Andrews' Cheer Squad', than impartial journalists. It has only been the actions of a handful of journalists, in holding a torch to murky governmental processes and revealing error and misinformation, that pushed the Inquiry into being extended to undertake a more rigorous and probing exploration of some of the issues. It is equally eye opening that some of those journalists that dared to question Daniel Andrews' integrity and competence (such as Peta Credlin and Rachel Baxendale) have themselves come under attack, even receiving death threats, apparently from some of the Premier's supporters (Wahlquist, 2020). Despite these apparent problems, the Inquiry process has revealed a stunningly large range of systemic problems within the Victorian Government and its bureaucracy, in particular within and between the operations of a number of specific agencies. These appear to be problems that were not specific to just the Hotel Quarantine Program, or even to the broader management of the pandemic and its impacts, but have been manifest in a number of decisions and actions undertaken over the past several years. These are decisions that have resulted in both a fractured and highly vulnerable health system (Woodley, 2020a) and major leadership problems across different government departments. The pandemic has just proven to be a stressor that has revealed the already existing deep dysfunction, fragility, and vulnerability inherent within Victoria. These problems were not limited to just the internal operations of the State but were also apparent in the multiple examples of dysfunctional relationships between Victoria and the Commonwealth.

Although the Inquiry has allowed some shocking matters to be exposed, it has only focused on immediate causes, not attempting to unravel the deeper tangles of causal, contributing, and influencing relationships, and interdependencies. The submission of misleading, and in some instances possibly false evidence, and the unwillingness or avoidance of providing explanations about some decisions and actions, makes purely evidence-based analysis difficult, if not impossible. This means that to make any real sense of what happened and why it happened, reasoned suppositions and inferences have to be made. Where causal analysis in this case study relies upon such supposition and inference, reasonable attempts have been made to clearly identify those instances. Following this introduction, the book is organised into themes across five parts.

- **Part 1** provides an analysis of the general practices and current state of knowledge on capabilities, arrangements, decision-making, and activities that contribute to effective crisis management. This represents some of what we would reasonably expect to see in a well-executed response to a complex evolving situation, and provides some explanation of why this can fail. Part 1 provides us with the foundation for a subsequent analysis. of what may have and did actually occur within Victoria and the Andrews government, and how far from acceptable practice this was.
- **Part 2** provides an analysis of the wide range of decisions and actions that contributed to Victoria's hotel quarantine disaster, set against the generally accepted practices and concepts outlined in Part 1.
- **Part 3** details some of the failures that occurred after the quarantine breaches, such as the flawed test and trace system, that allowed widespread community transmission to occur. These failures ultimately contributed to 801 deaths and the single biggest denial of human rights in Australia's history.
- **Part 4** looks at some of the spiderweb of interconnecting causal, contributing, and influencing factors that together led to the range of disastrous decisions made within the Victorian Government and its bureaucracy.
- **Part 5** brings together the various themes explored in the previous Parts in order to facilitate reflection and questioning by the reader. The aim is to allow the reader to reconsider the presented material and draw their own conclusions about plausible causes of the hotel quarantine failure and subsequent catastrophic disaster.

Part 1

An analytical framework

4
The presence of systemic failures

The Coate Inquiry uncovered some compelling evidence of leadership failure and gross mismanagement within the Victorian Government and its public service. This evidence not only related directly to the hotel quarantine debacle and subsequent public health disaster, but also appears to be indicative of deep-seated systemic problems that have contributed to a number of other government failures during Andrews' premiership. This included continuing mismanagement of hotel quarantine well into 2021, the Belt and Road project with the Chinese Government, massive multi-billion dollar budget and time blowouts on multiple infrastructure projects (Simpson, 2021; Karpin, 2020, Sheridan, 2020), as well as alleged corruption within the Victorian Labor Party and Government and the conduct of multiple IBAC investigations, (including the potential association of Daniel Andrews), into alleged ethical failings and corrupt dealings associated with the United Firefighters Union (Johnston, 2022a; 2022b, Durkin, 2021; Johnston and Varga, 2021; McKenzie et al, 2021; Talbot, 2021), branch stacking (AAP, 2021a; Varga, 2021), misuse of public funds in the red shirts election scandal (Durkin, 2021; Johnston, 2021e; Woods, 2021) and for polling research (Tuffield, 2021e). With additional allegations of Labor's complicity in trying to obstruct, subvert, or compromise IBAC investigations (Johnston, 2022d; Clarke, 2021).

To understand the significance of the various decisions, behaviours, and outcomes associated with the failed Hotel Quarantine Program in Victoria, it is necessary to understand:

- Whether these failures were representative of single breakdowns, unique to just the management of the Program, or were they indicative of wider systemic failures within the broader Victorian Government.
- What constitutes expected and acceptable ways of leading, managing, and decision-making, especially during a critical incident or crisis.
- The influence of known poor governance and other practices within the Victorian Government, in contributing to the mismanagement of the pandemic response.

This Chapter provides an overview of these issues and establishes the foundations for subsequent exploration of what went wrong and why with the Hotel Quarantine Program.

Government mismanagement – apparently everywhere

There have been a lot of media reports in recent years, about the government's failures in decision-making, maladministration of government agencies, and the mismanagement of multiple areas of service delivery. It can always be argued that the media can sensationalise issues or only report with a certain political bias. However, when fully independent bodies, such as those tasked with overseeing the integrity and performance of these agencies, also start to report on significant government failures then we must sit up and take notice. When such investigations begin to reveal common patterns of failure across different agencies and in different aspects of their operations, then we need to look closely to determine possible deep causes of such widespread failures.

Gross mismanagement of major projects

The Victorian Auditor General (VAGO) has been extremely critical of the Andrews government's 'competencies' in managing major projects. A recent review looked at the delivery of individual major projects (where each project was valued individually at over $100m), finding that there were problems resulting in cost overruns of $6 billion on 42 infrastructure projects (Johnston 2021d; Offer, 2021; Skatssoon, 2021; Terrill, 2021; van Onselen, 2021). Whilst some of this massive loss was partially recovered by cost cutting and reduced scopes of other projects, there was still a $3.8 billion blowout on the overall budget. VAGO identified significant systemic problems in the government's management of major projects which included a "*tendency to underestimate costs and over-estimate benefits*" accompanied by a lack of understanding of the construction industry contributing to the project and financial mismanagement.

A number of contributing factors have been identified in these gross failures, including a lack of strategic thinking (particularly relating to material and human resource requirements), a lack of understanding about agency capabilities to undertake the work, an inadequate understanding of risk and mitigation requirements, and the inadequate provision of advice about critical knowledge gaps (VAGO, 2021b). In a separate review, the Auditor General also criticised the lack of transparency in major projects, with inadequate reporting to Parliament and to the public such that "*major projects performance is not timely, relevant or sufficient*" (VAGO, 2021a). That this could occur on major projects where one would assume the government's supposed best and brightest bureaucrats are employed is more than worrying. One must also wonder about the capabilities of those other public servants working on thousands of other less important projects, and how much waste and mismanagement is occurring on a daily basis.

These reports establish a theme, which appears to be common to many Victorian Government agencies:

- A lack of skilled expertise, advisory and operational.
- A lack of strategic capability.
- A lack of cognitive and decision-making capability.
- A lack of robust processes.
- A lack of transparency

Failings in the health system

What has become glaringly obvious, in the last few years, is that the range of factors identified in major project delivery failures, are some of those very same issues that played such key roles in the failure of the Hotel Quarantine Program. Many of these problems have been plainly evident within key agencies responsible for health within Victoria. In 2016, a government commissioned report found that health knowledge was not being *"shared and implemented widely"*; that the clinical care of many patients *"diverges from best practice"*; and that the Department of Health and Human Services (DHHS) exercised inadequate oversight and governance of the hospital system. The report also noted that DHHS had *"suffered a significant loss of capacity"*, with budget cuts and caps *"gutting many departmental functions"*, with a subsequent loss of *"talented staff"* (Duckett et al, 2016). Victoria's hospital system has been described as the "unhealthiest" in Australia as result, in part, of chronic underfunding (van Onselen, 2022).

A follow up review conducted by VAGO[61] in 2021 into clinical governance found that the Department of Health and Human Services[62] was *"not effectively leading and overseeing quality and safety across the health system"*. This included fundamental failings such as: inability to ensure that clinical practice

---

[61] Victorian Auditor-General's Office

[62] Which following the hotel quarantine debacle, was broken up into the separate Department of Health, and the Department of Families, Fairness and Housing (Jenkins, 2020a).

was operating safely, inabilities to detect trends and risks, no state-wide incident management system, and inadequate reporting (VAGO, 2021c). It is also plausible that leadership and management inadequacies also played a significant role in driving these degraded capabilities. No matter how talented and hardworking our frontline doctors, nurses, and paramedics are, there is little that they can change in the face of different priorities of senior bureaucrats and Ministers.

Another area of responsibility for DHHS was homelessness within the State. Homelessness had become such a serious social and health problem within Victoria, that the government provided over $1.4 billion for a number of programs to address the problem. Despite some benefits for some individual homeless people, the initiative has been criticised by VAGO for its "*poor planning, a lack of agreed goals and limited performance monitoring*" (VAGO 2021h). DHHS has been unable to determine whether this $1.4 billion worth of programs has actually had *any material effect* on reducing homelessness and its impacts.

Probity failings in procurement

Also in September 2021, VAGO released a report into 4 cases of alleged conflicts of interest in Victorian Government Procurement (VAGO, 2021d), involving:

- $86.4m for medical services for the Hotel Quarantine Program, awarded by DHHS.
- $35.2m paid to Unified Security for security services for the Hotel Quarantine Program, awarded by the Department of Jobs, Precincts, and Regions.
- $21 million for the Victorian Family Preservation and Reunification Response, awarded by DHHS.
- $199,260 for aboriginal archaeological surveying, awarded by Parks Victoria.

Whilst VAGO's assurance review could not find evidence of deliberate malfeasance or individual pecuniary self-interest, serious procurement breaches did occur. VAGO identified failures to follow policies and procedures, such that fairness and impartiality, transparency and value for money could not be demonstrated. Some of the contributing factors to these failures included staff non-compliances with policies and procedures, inadequate staff monitoring and reviewing of awarded contracts, lack of regard by staff into how conflict of interest might be perceived by the public, lack of understanding of procurement during critical incidents. All of which appeared to be driven by their inexperience in undertaking large procurements, general lack of awareness and understanding of procurement policies and procedures, and pressure (from above) that was applied to undertake the work in unreasonably short timeframes. Whilst an IBAC[63] report, in the same year, raised additional issues of inappropriate procurement practices within the Victorian Government, quoting one public servant "*Procurement decisions are open to favouritism [in] some circumstances*" (IBAC, 2021b).

General mismanagement and poor performance

Such continuing poor performance of Victorian Government agencies should come as no surprise. Other reviews by VAGO have shown that many areas of government do not comply with the resource management framework issued by the Department of Treasury and Finance. In particular, that these areas were unable to undertake analysis, measurement and reporting of the effectiveness and efficiencies of their services, whilst new improvement measures introduced in the budget papers had failed (VAGO, 2021e).

Even some of the of the Andrews government's 'star' initiatives, such as the digital delivery of government services which was meant to save money, reduce demand pressure, and improve customer satisfaction has failed to deliver. An independent review (VAGO, 2021f) showed that despite the quick role out of services such as the QR code reader for contact tracing, the program failed to deliver the wide range of services promised, did not achieve the promised costs saving, nor improved regulatory compliance. Some of the immediate causes of these problems were identified as the development of a poor business case, inadequate stakeholder management, and inadequate planning. Consistent with failures elsewhere in the pandemic response and across government generally, these were all failures to get even the basics right.

Some of the Victorian Government's mishandling of public policy issues has often been labelled as examples of the Left's hypocrisy, for example allowing the BLM protest to go ahead, whilst in the face of lower community cases stamping down on other protests expressing anti-government concerns. The pandemic response in Victoria has been littered with many other apparent

---

[63]Independent Broad-based Anti-corruption Commission.

hypocrisies in decision-making, such as declaring Crown Casino and other pokies venues as 'essential services', whilst forcing the closure of thousands of other (many of which were at much lower risk) businesses (Butler, 2020). Although this may be less hypocrisy and more a recognition of the continuing tax windfall that the gambling industry contributes to the Government's purse.

Following the government's refusal to publicly release the health advice that they received on these lockdowns, a number of civil court cases were launched in 2022 seeking compensation for loss of livelihood (Piovesan, 2022). For example, outdoor contract gardening (an isolated outdoor activity) was banned under the Victorian Government's mandatory restrictions, presumably because 'medical advice' judged the risk of lone worker outdoors to be much greater than crowds of people gambling indoors.

Probity and misuse of funds

The 2017-2018 Victorian budget provided $2m in funds for the Department of Premier and Cabinet (DPC) to establish a Migrant Workers Centre[64]. In setting up the Centre, DPC appointed a consultant to provide advice on arrangements for establishing and running the Centre. After this advice was provided, that same consultant was appointed as the Chair of the Centre and the operation of the Centre was subcontracted to the Victorian Trades Hall Council (VHTC).

VAGO investigated allegations that the VHTC had misused the funds provided for the operation of the Centre (VAGO, 2021g). The investigation found funds had been misused to provide staff for political campaigning in the 2018 and 2019 State and Federal elections. It was found that the Department of Premier and Cabinet did not undertake adequate monitoring and auditing of the contracts, and that even after being alerted to possible misappropriation of funds, the Department took no further action. The VAGO investigations also revealed that DPC failed to comply with its own procurement policies when it appointed the consultant, and that the DPC bureaucrat responsible for the consultant's appointment had undeclared conflicts of interest. This bureaucrat and the consultant had previously worked together at another government agency. It is uncertain what disciplinary action, if any, was taken in light of the VAGO report.

---

[64] To provide advocacy and education on rights for migrant workers that had been exploited, with the head contract to the Migrant Workers Centre Inc.

A systemic failure

This entire range of problems found by the Auditor General across different areas of Victorian Government operations indicate similar pervasive failings with similar apparent symptoms, causal, and contributing factors. These failures and factors appear to be very similar to the issues identified by the Coate Inquiry and are indicative of a deep systemic failure of leadership, governance, and capability. This raises serious questions about how could such a monumentally failed system of governance have arisen? How could the Andrews government have got things so consistently wrong for so long? Why was there so little interest in correcting these malpractices?

To answer these questions, we have to first establish a baseline understanding of what an effective system should look like, and then look at what can occur to cause such a deviance from 'acceptable normality'.

Head in the sand? Pandemic and planning preparedness

Was the Victorian Government really prepared for a pandemic of any sort prior to the start of 2020? Certainly, with the benefit of hindsight, it seems that whatever arrangements were in place or were 'waiting in the wings' were inadequate for the realities of COVID-19. However, was this just misfortune, or were these arrangements not-fit-for purpose in the first place?

A number of areas of the Victorian Government had in place pandemic/ widespread disease emergency plans from the early 1990's including the Department of Premier and Cabinet, Health Department, and Department of Agriculture[65]. During this time a number of multiagency exercises were conducted to validate the plans, with further testing in the 'fire' of several actual disease outbreaks. State and national multiagency response arrangements had been activated on several occasions for veterinary and potential zoonotic[66] diseases, including avian influenza, suspected foot and mouth disease, nationally significant fish kills, choroid blindness in kangaroos, etc. (Forsyth et al, 1992; Jones et al, 1997). Later experiences with the threat of equine influenza further consolidated this expertise. All of these experiences certainly built up a high level of large-scale disease outbreak experience within Victoria's bureaucracy, which consistently played a leading role nationally.

---

[65] The author was involved in the development and exercising of a number of these plans.
[66] Diseases transmitted from animals to humans.

Victoria was widely recognised as leading Australia in the planning, preparedness, and response to significant animal diseases and its overall approach to biosecurity, certainly up to 2008 (VAGO, 2008). This VAGO review also noted the effective relationship between the then Department of Primary Industries and the then Department of Health Services, which would have contributed to a high performing multi-agency disease outbreak response.
The commitment to disease disaster preparedness continued through the early to mid 2000's, and following the 2003 SARS pandemic, this saw a huge boost in activity. Almost all Victorian Government agencies refreshed their pandemic preparedness arrangements, including participation in the Commonwealth's pandemic planning workshops conducted by the Department of Industry, Tourism and Resources, and with participation in Exercise Cumpston - a national test of health system preparedness for pandemics (DOHA, 2007).

During this time the Commonwealth Auditor General released a report on the national preparedness for a pandemic (ANAO, 2008), alerting to the growing risk of a pandemic and emphasising the need for a continuing commitment to maintaining and improving preparedness. The ANAO Report concluded that Australia's health system was capable of responding well to a pandemic and that it could deal with the challenge of the *"unknown epidemiology of an emerging disease"*. ANAO also produced a number of lessons learned for future improvement of capability. This obviously recognised that preparedness needed to consider the prospect of other pandemic diseases in addition to influenza. A point that Victoria's subsequent pandemic *influenza* planning appears to have missed.

Some of the improvement recommendations in the ANAO Report make interesting reading, especially considering Victoria's continuing failures throughout most of the first two years of the COVID-19 pandemic. It now appears that Victoria followed an approach that was diametrically opposed to each of these proposed improvements, which included the need to:

- Change routine decision-making processes.
- Improve flexibility of pandemic plans and arrangements to better cope with changing severity of the pandemic and changing capability to manage it.
- Improve communication mechanisms.
- Preparation of public health policies and strategies ahead of any pandemic, as well as having public communications to *explain these measures prepared well in advance*.
- Open sharing of operational lessons learned.

- Establish nationally consistent arrangements.
- Better integration of general practitioners and pharmacies into preparedness arrangements.
- Building-in experience of command, control, and coordination into operations centres, and "ensuring seamless support for decision-making".
- "Ensure responses can be sustained over a prolonged period through planning for workforce training and surge capacity, scenario-based contingency planning and a continuing program of pandemic preparedness exercises".

It appears that either these lessons were not learned by Victoria or were quietly abandoned sometime in the years leading up to the pandemic.

In 2009 the national pandemic preparedness plan (COAG, 2009) was released, followed by the Victorian Health Management Plan for Pandemic Influenza in 2014 (DoH, 2014). The Victorian Plan was supposed to be updated based upon experiences of the 2009 H_1N_1 influenza pandemic as recommended in the Commonwealth's review of that pandemic (DHA, 2011). This review recommended specifically *"an examination of the policy on quarantine and isolation, including management, support systems and communication, be undertaken"*[67]. However, the Chief Health Officer admitted to the Coate Inquiry that this recommendation was never implemented. If this recommendation had not been ignored, Victoria would have had in place, at a minimum, a set of guiding principles upon which the Hotel Quarantine Program could have been based. Rather than what occurred, the largely uninformed planning and decisions that characterised the establishment of the Program.

Victoria's planning also only ever considered that quarantine (including for returning travellers) would involve *voluntary home-based isolation,* and in no way even toyed with the idea of mandatory detention as a quarantine approach. As late as 10 March 2020, just two weeks before the Hotel Quarantine Program commenced, Victoria's pandemic health planning still did not consider any quarantine possibilities beyond voluntary isolation in a person's own home (DHHS, 2020). This was despite the World Health Organisation issuing detailed guidance on the management of returning travellers and quarantine arrangements a *month before* Victoria updated its own pandemic plan (WHO, 2020).

---

[67] Coate, 2020a, p 219.

Although the Commonwealth's Pandemic Plan (DoH, 2019) noted that the use of hotels for quarantining of returning international travellers would be "problematic", the Victorian Government does not appear to have turned its collective mind towards what those problems could be, that is until it was much too late.

It is also interesting that Victoria persisted, for years, with exceptionally narrow preparedness and planning that was solely focussed on the prospect of pandemic influenza. Especially at a time when it was widely recognised that influenza was only one of a number of emerging and re-emerging diseases, with the potential to cause widespread outbreaks. Certainly, experts outside of Victoria were concerned about diseases such as SARS, MERS, dengue, Zika, Chikungunya, acute haemorrhagic conjunctivitis, West Nile virus, hantavirus etc., along with a huge number of other zoonotic diseases (USAID, 2021; Acharya et al, 2020; Gubler, 2017; Maurens and Faucii, 2020). Why would the Victorian Government persist with a primary pandemic plan that had an absolute focus on influenza, when over 30 new human pathogens had emerged over the preceding 30 years (Jones et al, 2008) substantially increasing the risk of a novel pandemic?

Was this already a sign that the Victorian Government's thinking was getting left behind the reality of a changed world?

In evidence to the Coate Inquiry, the then Secretary of DHHS stated that the Department had regularly undertaken emergency incident exercises that had specifically looked at the State Health Emergency Response Plan[68]. This included Alchemy in 2018 and Exercise Teapot in 2019, that both looked at infectious disease scenarios. However, the conduct of these exercises had been criticised, including by the then President of the Australian Medical Association, for failing to more broadly involve the wider medical profession outside of the Department.

The Inquiry concluded that lessons learned from exercising were *"not applied as they should have been"*, which was especially evident in the lack of practical pandemic planning within Victoria.

---

[68] Coate 2021a, p. 97.

5
An analytical approach

It is never good practice to just jump into looking at the causes of disasters without first having some form of analytical framework. Most Inquiries, however, do just do that, they start off with an idea of what went wrong, they then jump in and try to uncover evidence that supports that opinion. This invariably leads to a shallow understanding of the complex progression and interaction of events, to unreasonable reliance and blame on very proximal causes, or they become misdirected and deflected by the sensational and the easily recalled.

To provide a comprehensive and deep understanding of how the Victorian Hotel Quarantine Program disaster occurred, it is necessary to look at the available evidence through a different lens. An approach that allows a longer-term retrospective on decisions, actions, and behaviours, and one that allows the interrelationships of these factors to be explored. The analytical framework used in this and subsequent chapters is based upon many years of research into the pathology of catastrophic failures, and in looking at how organisational resilience and high reliability is pursued successfully (Gibson, 2020, 2023).

The over-arching analytical framework for this case study is based upon a thematic approach (Figure 1) based upon examining the effects of and connections amongst seven broad domains of factors:

i) Imperative drivers.
ii) Culture and leadership.
iii) Situational awareness and risk awareness.
iv) Governance and decision-making, including sensemaking.
v) Communication and information flows.
vi) People and team capabilities.
vii) Operationalisation.

All of these different domains interact with each other and influence the development, operation, and effect of each of the other domains. An effective system will experience feedback from its operationalisation, its outputs and outcomes, and undergo positive adaptation across the various domains (including imperative drivers) as a result. However, in reality, this is often problematic as both individuals and organisations can respond ineffectually to such feedback and be resistant to change. This will be especially the case where the imperative drivers have an unreasonably strong influence. Particularly where the drivers are ideologically based, establishing a significant psychological pressure to maintain those ideological beliefs even in the face of rational counter-argument or impending system failure.

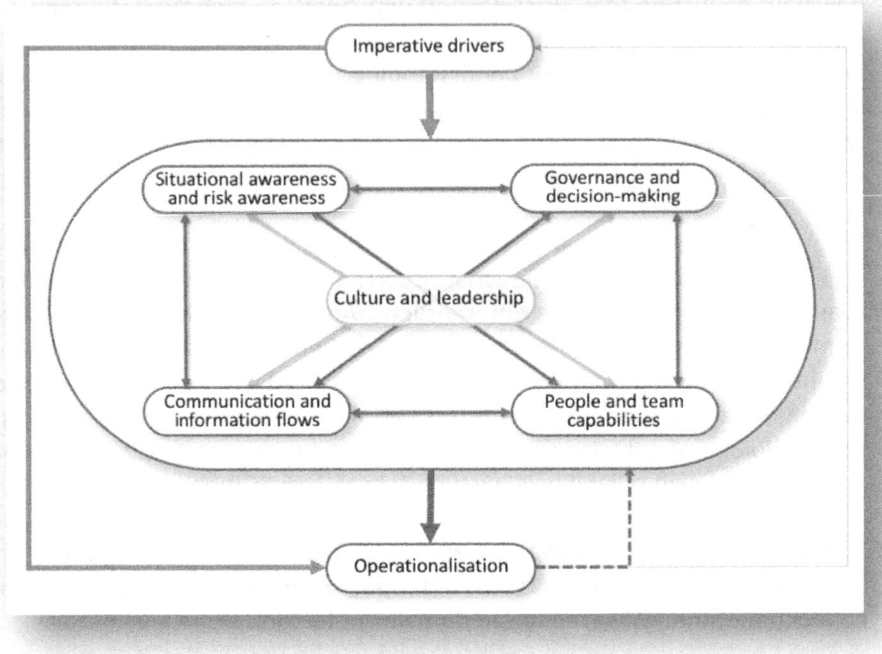

Figure 1 Factorial relationship model

In using any framework of this nature, it needs to be remembered that this is a simple representation of a highly complex system. As such the effects of manipulating one aspect of a system can have unpredictable and unexpected consequences elsewhere in the system. It is therefore often difficult to understand how a system works by just looking at individual elements in isolation. Much of how a current system works can only be gleaned from how it has worked in the past, using the benefit of hindsight, whilst at the same time understanding that past behaviour may not be a fully accurate picture of future behaviour. Although a poorly designed and poorly controlled system will tend to continue to perform poorly well into the future, unless some dramatic force of positive change is applied upon it.

We have to accept the need to look at the nature of these interactions over fairly long periods of time, be able to step back and recognise patterns of activity and behaviour, and extrapolate these patterns to circumstances where there is a lack of clarity. This requires that analysis is strongly founded upon evidence, and that any assumptions underpinning that evidence are surfaced and validated. The very nature of the Victorian Government's failure has resulted in much of the required evidence being hidden from public view or obscured by misinformation (potentially both deliberate and unintentional). This means that any analysis of what occurred must rely on plausible inferences. The reasonableness of the author's inferences is left to the reader to interpret and evaluate.

Imperative drivers

Imperative drivers are those factors that establish the underlying conditions that direct or influence the various assumptions, perceptions, thinking, decision-making, behaviours, activities, etc. These drivers are the key sources of the various conscious and unconscious biases that will continue to influence perception, sensemaking, and decision-making, both at an individual level, and within and across the various groups within the system.

Such factors may include:

- Basic underpinning *belief systems* that form the basis for overall purpose, intent, goals, etc., and are a critical driver and developer of values, individual biases, perceptions, and deep-seated assumptions (assumptions which are commonly about the world and how it functions).
- *Ideology*, which is established by the underpinning belief systems and the ideas, attitudes, and values that they generate (Erikson and Tedin, 2003). From the perspective of the Hotel Quarantine Program, the main ideologies were those that are highly likely to be political and social in nature.
- Historical *decisions and outcomes* that are the result of, or are significantly influenced by belief systems and ideology, and often act as a reinforcement for a continuation of the beliefs and ideology, even in the face of emerging counter-prevailing evidence. These are the decisions that ultimately strongly determine strategic direction and are critical to the establishment of the prevailing culture.

A problem with ideology?

Ideologies fulfil a number of important purposes in providing us with a cognitive and emotional framework that allows us to make sense of our world, give us a perspective on what ideally could or should be, and provide a guide and frame of reference on how to realise that perspective (White et al, 2019, Jost et al, 2009). Accordingly, ideologies and belief systems are an essential part of our psychological make-up. Although all ideologies have a degree of resistance to change, ideologies become problematic when that resistance is absolute, when the ideology cannot change even in the face of compelling and continuous contrary evidence.

An ideology is adopted when it aligns with and satisfies an individual's 'dominant motivations' (Jost et al, 2003). Ideological beliefs are usually rooted in strong emotion, along with affiliation and identity with a particular group. Once established, ideology is very difficult to change, irrespective of the facts that either dispute those beliefs or any progressive deviation of the ideology that may occur. Many individuals can hold onto erroneous beliefs over many years, and can often hold conflicting beliefs, effectively reconciling such cognitive dissonance, and continuing to support what they believe is the more popular stance[69] (Dusso, 2017; Nam et al, 2013). At the same time these individuals will seek reasons for dismissing other more reasonable alternatives (Aronson and Tavris, 2020), and any evidence that threatens those beliefs is frequently refused, disregarded, or irrationally disputed.

Even when there is some recognition of the unreasonableness of these beliefs, this very recognition can lead those individuals to further strengthen their conscious need for those beliefs, strengthen their disregard of the conflicting facts, and become even more outspoken advocates for their ideology (Gal and Rucker, 2010).

The pervasive effect of ideology

Ideology has a profound and pernicious effect on decision-making as well as affecting the way in which the other domains (in our analytical framework) develop and operate, serving to continuously undermine judgement (Manko, 2021; Wijtvliet and Dyevre, 2021; Hahnel et al, 2020; Weinshall et al, 2018; Newell and Matti, 2017; Weir, 2017; Yerka, 2013; Dietrich, 2010; Zorn and Barnes Bowie, 2010). Ideology imposes powerful cognitive and emotional

[69] Within their accepted group.

biases that can effectively coerce interpretation and reasoning, requiring far less factual information to support a congruent decision, than would otherwise be required to support a decision that conflicted with the prevailing ideology.

Whilst ideology has a major directional influence across the range of analytical domains (Figure 1), further adaptation and evolution of these intrinsic drivers (including ideology) are minimally affected by feedback evidence from the operationalisation of these factors.

Culture and leadership

There is a simple three element model of culture originally developed by Ed Schein (Schein, 2010), which has been subsequently modified into the 'buoy model' (Gibson and Gibson, 2023) to explain both sustainable and unsustainable cultural change (Figure 2). The model comprises 3 key elements:

- *The artefacts of culture*, which usually occur as a result of people's decisions, and which become visible through their actions and behaviours. This also includes representations such as pronouncements, policies, rules, published documents, the accepted norms, and explicit expectations. Like a 'buoy' these float at the surface and are visible to observers, but their 'position' is determined by the chain (values) and anchor (assumptions and beliefs).
- *Espoused values and goals*, which are usually not immediately visible, but can be expressed and hence are readily detectable. These values and goals drive the formation of cultural artefacts.
- *Underlying assumptions and deep-seated beliefs*, which are largely 'invisible' to others and are not often consciously recognised even by those who hold them. However, these assumptions and beliefs (conscious and unconscious) have a powerful influence on a person's and group's values and goals.

The buoy model posits that if the artefacts or espoused values and goals are subject to purposeful direction, change will occur, but its effect is likely to be only temporary. Eventually, the visible elements of culture will drift back to their original position, because they are 'anchored' by the deeper underlying and usually unconscious assumptions and beliefs. To achieve a longer term effective change in culture, it is necessary to pay attention to and shift this anchor, i.e., the deep underlying assumptions and beliefs.

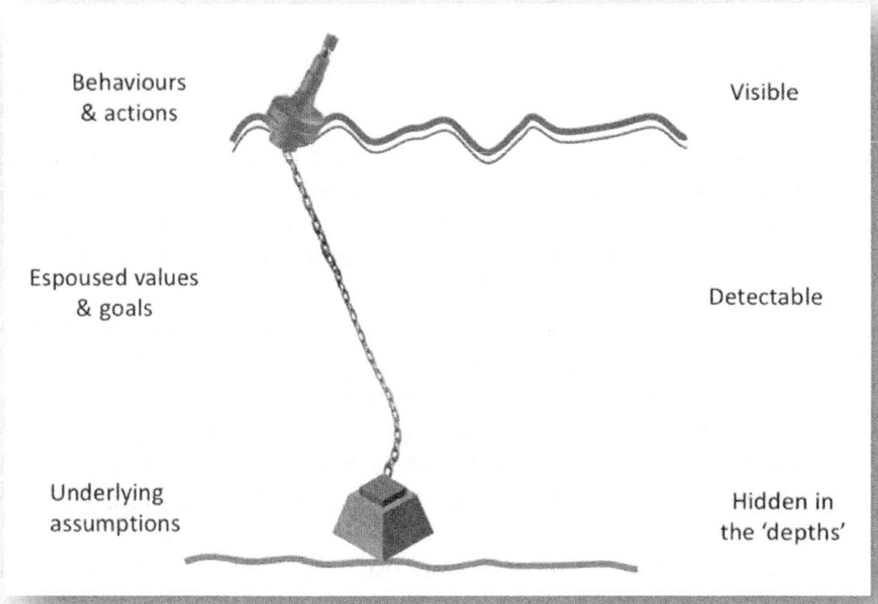

Figure 2: Buoy model of organisational culture[70]

Group ideology is a powerful determinant of an individual's beliefs and assumptions, and hence has a powerful influence on their behaviours, decisions, and actions. All three cultural elements will have an overall powerful effect on how decisions are made, how decisions are actioned, and how others are informed about those decisions. Societal and organisational culture will influence what information is attended to, how it is attended to, and how it is analysed. Culture will strongly influence individual biases and perceptions. Ultimately this means that decisions are rarely under full deliberate and rational

[70] Based on original discussions with Ivan Pupulidy, the then Director of the USDA Office of Learning.

control, and that cultural factors exert a strong, often unconscious, influence. That our thinking and decision-making is rarely fully rational may be surprising to some. However, the extent of potential unconscious influences is being revealed by a wide range of neuroscience and cognitive psychology research in recent years (Kitayama et al, 2019; Lin and Telzer, 2017; Saposnik et al, 2016; Gigerenzer and Gaissmaier, 2015; Grupe and Nitschke, 2013; Johnson et al, 2013; Lee and Harris, 2013; Starcke and Brand, 2012 Hilbert, 2011; Johnson and Busemeyer, 2010).

Organisational culture is a representative shared belief system and as such will be strongly influenced by the broader ideology within which it sits. Where ideological congruence becomes a key element of selection and advancement for senior leaders within an organisation, the dominant culture will be an even stronger reflection of the prevailing ideology. In recent years we have seen adherence to 'woke ideology' become a defining criterion in gaining and keeping employment in private industry, not for profit (Charters, 2021; Creighton, 2021; Klippenstein and Pardy, 2017; Young, 2017) and in government sectors (Stewart, 2020; Civil Service, 2017). Thus, those leaders expressing conformity with the prevailing ideology continue to climb the ranks of the bureaucracy, irrespective of their actual experience and competencies for the role. This in turn influences the predominant culture, creating an environment in which certain types of conforming decisions are preferred over those that are evidence-based but conflict with groupthink (Heneghan and Mahtani, 2020; Buoygues, 2019; Jhangiani and Tarry, 2014). Over time, it becomes easier for all decision-makers to conform with the groupthink culture and signal a concurrence with the ideology, rather than being identified as a 'heretic' and risk exclusion from the group.

When the prevailing ideology is misguided or perverse, leadership and cultural influence becomes similarly misguided and perverse further compounding poor decision-making (Moore, 2021; Ramaswarmy, 2021; Dowell and Jackson, 2020; Jamieson, 2020; Lewis, 2020a; Simpson, 2020; Smith, 2020; Stewart, 2020; Young, 2019). Thus, despite what official rules and obligations are in place, culture can have such a profound effect that results in these requirements and obligations being ignored.

Organisational culture and leadership will have a strong bearing on how others in the organisation interpret their surroundings, make sense of their environment, communicate and share this sense with others, and make decisions and act. Where the culture and leadership are congruent with the dominant ideology, this will strengthen that influence, conversely where ideology conflicts with culture and leadership, the influence of the latter can be significantly negated.

Cognition and emotion

The dual thinking system model posits that humans have evolved with a 'primitive' emotional thinking system that is automatic, fast, and efficient (includes intuition and pattern recognition), and a much slower, demanding, rational and consciously controlled analytical thinking system (Diedrich and Trueblood, 2018; Evans and Stanovich, 2013; Kahneman, 2011; Evans, 2008; Gilovich et al, 2002). In practical terms this means that a considerable amount of decision-making is made unconsciously (emotional system) but is subsequently 'rationalised' by the analytical system. In effect, the thinking and decision-making occurs outside of our conscious control, but once we start to become aware of the outcomes of this thinking, our conscious analytical system tries to rationalise the results by 'inventing' the reasoning after the fact.

Culture not only influences emotional thinking, it also exerts a powerful influence on how these unconscious decisions are subsequently rationalised (Yates and de Oliveira, 2016; Elwyn et al, 2010; Hopkins 2006; Kemp and Dwyer, 2001; Briley et al, 2000; Weber and Hsee, 2000). Thus, we often have far less rationale control of our decisions than we realise, being far more influenced by cultural and ideological cues, and the behaviours of others, than by pure factual considerations. Certainly, culture has been implicated in driving decisions and practices that contribute directly to organisational failure (Hald et al, 2020) including impaired ethical decision making, poor decisions about risk, poor prioritisation of issues and demands, poor and ineffective management, and insufficient capability development.

Organisational culture has also been shown to influence outsourcing decisions (Popoli, 2017) both consciously and unconsciously. Cultural influence is especially important where ethical decision-making is concerned (Hiekkataipale and Lämsä, 2017; Korać, 2016; Ford and Richardson, 2013; Huhtala et al, 2013; Nwachukwu and Vitell, 1997), and may overcome personal ethical and moral convictions in certain circumstances. It has been proposed that under major crises, microcultures may emerge in which ethical thinking is lost and "wise decision-making" is "corrupted" disregarding the longer-term implications (Mumley, 2019), even with leaders that are otherwise regarded as highly ethical.

Culture has a profound effect on how uncertainty is understood and how risk is dealt with, especially when highly asymmetric power balances[71] are a feature of that culture. Culture also affects how organisations learn from their experiences and how effectively they apply that learning. A 'poor' culture has been shown time after time to be one of the major determining factors in organisational failure and corruption (Hald et al, 2020).

Leadership and ethics

Leadership (at all levels of an organisation, but most profoundly at the top) strongly influences the underlying assumptions, the resulting values and inherent goals (including those not publicly espoused) of groups and individuals within an organisation. Major roles of leadership include making decisions and establishing a framework that guides the decision-making of others. A key aspect of this framework is its moral and ethical foundation. It has become increasingly apparent in recent years within government[72] that this moral and ethical foundation has been increasingly eroded (IBAC, 2021a, 2021b; Allen, 2020; Blanton et al, 2020; Buchan, 2020, IBAC, 2020; IBAC, 2019; Rainie and Perrin, 2019; Adams and Balfour, 2010).

Significant integrity issues within the Victorian Government's bureaucracy are regularly identified, by the media, by IBAC[73], in judicial reviews (Coate, 2020a) and in independent reports (Accountability Round Table, 2015). For example, the Accountability Round Table report states on its front page *"....especially the way government is conducted, its culture and quality, including the quality of its integrity systems. In Victoria they are a problem in their own right creating an environment that does not address or deter corruption but encourages it"*. With the continuing presence of significant indicators of integrity problems with the Victorian Government and its bureaucracy, it needs to be questioned what has actually changed since this report in 2015? Based on the public revelations of the last few years it appears that whatever has changed within government, it does not appear to have been for the better.

The growing phenomenon of 'ethical fading' is seen as one of the major contributors to a whole range of crises and scandals (Collins, 2019; Leigh, 2016; Bazerman and Tenbrunsel, 2011; Tenbrunsel et al, 2009; Tenbrunsel and

---

[71] In effect driving the 'perceived wisdom' (Kemp and Dwyer, 2001).

[72] Gradual degradation in ethical and moral foundation is increasingly evident in many 'western' democratic jurisdictions across the world.

[73] Independent Broad-based Anti-corruption Commission.

Messick, 2004). This concept embraces the ease with which ethical and moral considerations are overlooked once the brain is subjected to cognitive overload, as can so often occur in emergency and crisis situations. It is also based upon the very human predication to falsify (often without explicit awareness) in the need for self-preservation. In other words, in stressful conditions, ethical considerations are often the first to be abandoned and ***individuals are often blind to the extent to which they are comprising their own integrity,*** *especially when they feel threatened or are protecting their own self-interest.*

Ethical fading permeates many public sector (as well as private sector) entities, becoming increasingly insidious in the absence of strong ethical leadership. Countering ethical fading requires not just the right sort of leadership, it also requires strong governance frameworks that support ethical decision-making (Grimes, 2019). However, even the strongest governance framework is comprised when it is abandoned for the sake of expediency, allowing ethical fading to flourish.

The origins of ethical fading

Ethical compromise does not start with the impacts of a crisis. Like many of the failure pathways that contribute to a major crisis or disaster, ethical fading starts weeks, months or even years before the onset of any challenging incident. Indeed, ethical fading starts in the way that staff are recruited and is further reinforced by the way that staff are managed, rewarded, and promoted. Integrity may be given 'lip service' in key selection criteria but is rarely tested rigorously in the employment selection process. Merely asking the routine question *"tell me about when you had to deal with a difficult ethical problem"* does not really determine a candidate's integrity. One very respected executive headhunting firm had to pay significant compensation to their client, when after 6 months in the job it was revealed that the CFO they had placed had been terminated from their previous position for fraud.

Anecdotal evidence about the capabilities of HR professionals within the public sector, suggest that that there is not a sufficient understanding of good employment screening practices, and that eligibility and suitability testing is often superficial. In addition to the potential low quality of selection processes themselves, is the issue that even where 'good practices' are in place, they may be deliberately compromised by conflicts of interest and unfair preferential treatment. The media has regularly reported on appointments of public servants based upon their political connections or because they 'tick the box' on ideological grounds. Additionally, senior executives may themselves exert undue influence to subvert the selection process, as IBAC's 2021 integrity survey across the Victorian public service quotes one public servant: *'I've often seen upper management engineer recruitment processes to select their preferred candidate'* (IBAC, 2021b).

Effective leadership

Leadership during the pandemic

During times of crisis, individuals within organisations and (for societal crises) the citizenship at large look to their leaders for guidance, assurance, comfort, and perhaps above all else a truthful and accurate account of what is happening. In any crisis, but especially during the COVID-19 pandemic, political and organisational leadership should have had vital roles in establishing perspective and direction, and in making essential difficult decisions (Bundy et al, 2017).

Across multiple jurisdictions, effective leadership has either failed or been 'missing in action' during large parts of the COVID-19 pandemic (Bhalla, 2021; Bongiorno, 2020; Harris, 2021; Huanca 2020; Kauffmann, 2020; Li, 2020; McCauley, 2020; Murray and Meyer, 2020; Nye, 2020; OneSharedWorld.com, 2020; The Editors, 2020; Seerval and Shah, 2021) a not uncommon response when a 'mega crisis' occurs (Stern et al, 2020). However, Australia has fared better than many other democratic nations, with proactive leadership closing down international travel and substantially limiting the number of positive cases entering the community. When outbreaks from quarantine have occurred in other jurisdictions, in most cases quick and decisive action by State and Territory governments have limited the spread and impact of infections. Despite criticism being levelled at many of the Premiers and their governments, their leadership during the first year of the pandemic was fairly effective. They were able to contain early outbreaks to within days to a couple of weeks, and limit mortalities within Australia to a fraction of the population compared to the rates experienced in many other parts of the world.

However, leadership within the Victorian Government, in this same time period, came into particular criticism of its poor capabilities, lack of honesty and transparency, and its overall handling of the crisis (Bagaric, 2020; Carr, 2020; Coate, 2020a; Editorial, 2020; Hewitt, 2020; Karpin, 2020;). With the Premier, various Ministers, and senior bureaucrats coming in for criticism for ineffective leadership, poor decision-making, mismanagement, blame shifting, secrecy, and misinformation.

Crisis leadership

A range of traits and activities have been identified as important for crisis leadership during the pandemic, both from elected officials and from bureaucrats (Almohtaseb et al, 2021; Glenn et al, 2021; Haslam et al, 2021; Laur et al, 2021; Sadiq et al, 2021; Ahern and Low, 2020; Ball 2020; Forster et al, 2020; Graham and Goodhead, 2020; Kaul et al, 2020; Kerrisey and Edmondson, 2020; Nicola et al, 2020; Roberts, 2020; Rosa et al, 2020; Rutledge, 2020). These traits and activities include: alignment with core values, clear and honest communication, realistic situational awareness (including understanding uncertainty and risk), engaging in both short and long term planning, and establishing good governance and decision-making that can cope with high levels of uncertainty and ambiguity, creativity and innovation.

Effective crisis leadership also encourages distributed leadership, drives decision-making down to those with the best understanding of the situation and the best ability to make the decisions[74], and captures the perspectives of multiple stakeholders. Senior leaders, in a crisis situation therefore, need to position themselves as enablers of decision-making, rather than being the sole decider (Glenn et al, 2021).

Such devolved distribution and dissemination of leadership improves organisational agility and flexibility, allowing the organisation to quickly pivot and change direction as the rapidly changing environment necessitates. Studies indicate that the more a crisis represents a wicked problem, the more there is a need for such distributed leadership (O'Reilly et al, 2015).

Effective leadership during a crisis also requires humility from those in power, that they are able to recognise the value of others and are willing to listen to and take advice from them, removing the fear of blame, and establishing the equivalent of a 'just culture'[75]. By necessity this requires that senior decision-

[74] Also known as 'deference to expertise' in high reliability organising (Gibson and Gibson, 2023)

[75] The concept of 'just culture' was originally introduced into more advanced safety thinking over three decades ago. The concept recognises that failures (errors) occur not because of the fault of individuals (human error) but because of the variability of work systems in which those individuals make sense, make decisions, and operate.

makers make themselves available to their staff, and establish a high and continuing level of trust (Lewis, 2021).

However, successful leadership during the pandemic also rested substantially on the level of preparedness undertaken in the months and years prior to the pandemic (Windsor et al, 2020). No matter the public perception of the leadership, a lack of preparedness presents a substantial barrier to overcome during a crisis.

The pandemic has exposed fragility in many management structures, and has amplified leadership gaps in many organisations, with many leaders being ill-equipped for dealing with the realities of the new environment. Recent research indicates the need for three core leadership "pillars" for better dealing with a crisis (HBP, 2020):

- The need for effective sensemaking and the ability to make decisions under high uncertainty.
- Creating an authentic culture and establishing high levels of trust and empathy.
- Building their own capabilities and those of others with the new skill sets required for the late pandemic and post pandemic periods.

Situational awareness and risk awareness

Situational awareness under uncertainty

Situational awareness has been identified as a key determinant in establishing a common operating picture and in informing decision-making during crises and disasters (Okoli and Watt, 2018; Uitdewilligen and Waller, 2018; Van de Walle et al, 2016; Danielsson et al, 2014; Glick and Barbara, 2013; Schraagen and van de Ven, 2008; Sayegh, 2004).

A range of models have been developed to help explain situational awareness (Golightly et al, 2010; Endsley, 2000; 1995; Durso and Gronlund, 1999; Adams et al, 1995), which describe how an individual becomes aware of and pays attention to multiple factors that are present or emerging within their operating and decision-making environments.

These include as general elements:

- How attention is directed towards matters of interest or concern.
- How attention is aligned with individual and shared goals and priorities.
- How salient and novel information can divert attention, creating either heightened focus or distraction.
- How the information is processed in working memory[76], and how situational awareness can degrade as working memory's limited capacity is overwhelmed.
- How mental models, cognitive, and emotional frames affect the interpretation and sensemaking of the information, i.e., how an understanding of the current situation is gained.
- How current understanding can be used to project possible ways in which the situation could evolve in the future.
- How interpretive errors can compound, serving to further degrade situational awareness.

It is often forgotten that situational awareness is not a static one-time proposition. It is a continuing and dynamic process which considers the past, the present, and possible futures. Effective situational awareness involves constantly checking what is happening against our understanding and expectations, and then revising those expectations and understanding where differences become apparent.

It often goes unrecognised that an organisation that does not encourage and practice effective situational awareness in routine day-to-day activities is unlikely to suddenly acquire this capability[77] in the midst of a crisis. Effective situational awareness requires these individual and group capabilities to be developed, practised, and rehearsed as part of preparedness long before any actual incident arises (Kozasa et al, 2020; Koskinen-Kannisto, 2013).

---

[76] Working memory is short-term memory, lasting a matter of seconds to a minute or so. It is essential for processing incoming data, before it is stored into long term memory. Working memory has a very finite capacity, only capable of holding about 3 to 7 chunks of information at any one time (Wilhelm et al, 2013, Cowan, 2010, Gilchrist et al, 2008). Once this capacity is exceeded, further information is not processed into long term memory and is lost. Under stress (non-routine conditions, fatigue, etc) working memory capacity can be substantially reduced, and key information can be effectively 'ignored' or forgotten, and an incomplete operational picture is formed and relied on.

[77] Individual and team activities, training, experience, guidance, tools, and techniques that collectively build and maintain situational awareness.

There are a number of factors that can adversely affect situational awareness in the moment, including:

- The number of competing situational demands, for example, a 'high pressure' situation can increase workload and cognitive load. As situational awareness is highly dependent upon working memory, the introduction of new or increasing amounts of information in a stressful or rapidly evolving situation can quickly result in cognitive resources becoming overwhelmed.
- High complexity, high novelty, high volatility, and high uncertainty further add to cognitive load, and can also rapidly outpace situational awareness, requiring more cognitive resources to be allocated for continual refreshing.
- The speed with which conditions and information about those conditions change, compared to a person's ability and availability to make sense of that change.
- Personal issues such as exposure to other stressors (which also increase workload), fatigue, poor physical fitness and health, and even inappropriate diet, can all effect emotional and cognitive processing capabilities and impair situational awareness.
- Where a particular issue has high salience[78] and captures attention, to the detriment of other issues which are either unintentionally ignored or deliberately disregarded.
- Where there are multiple competing (often relatively low priority) demands which serve as distractions from important, and often more immediate issues. These demands become distractions, not necessarily because they have a high salience, but because they are perceived as less threatening or easier issues to tackle.
- Aberrant mental models (often because of unsurfaced and unchallenged assumptions) that influence and drive errors in situational assessment. It is also important to realise that although a particular mental model may be appropriate at a point in time, changing conditions can quickly invalidate that mental model.

---

[78] For example, something that is particularly prominent, noticeable, or that commands attention. When salience drives the focus of attention, then there are less cognitive resources available for other controlled cognitive and emotional functions including pattern recognition and use of memory to direct situational awareness. Therefore, in the presence of high salience stimuli (where that salience is misplaced, that is the salient stimuli do not reflect the key indicators for the developing conditions or situation), attention can be distracted and situational awareness becomes degraded (Gjøsæter et al, 2019; Nguyen et al, 2019; Endsley, 2015).

- Where holders of information do not effectively communicate, or miscommunicate to others, again this may be unintentional or done very deliberately.
- Social pressure, which either strengthens existing biases, or creates psychological stress to align with the social norms of the rest of the group.

One of the key issues during a crisis is the ability to recognise if the situation consists of simple routine problems (so called 'tame' problems), or if the situation is characterised by a number of wicked problems. A failure to recognise the distinction, and the assumption that only tame problems are present will invariably lead to shallow information collation and analysis and an inadequate situational awareness. Sensemaking and decision-making require a clear understanding about the situation being faced (Figure 3), i.e., what has happened, what is happening now, and what has not yet happened, but may or may not happen in the future. It is also critically important to understand what levels of certainty exist about the information being accessed:

- What is known and certain, such as verified facts?
- What is assumed or inferred, and has not or cannot be readily validated or reliably assessed?
- How stable is our current understanding, for example what changes could occur that would invalidate that understanding? Over what time periods could that change occur? How likely is such change?
- What areas of uncertainty remain?

In considering what situational awareness may have existed during past events, it is important to try to understand the conditions that were prevalent at the time, and how these conditions could have affected both individual and shared situational awareness. Individuals rarely '*lose*' situational awareness, their situational awareness is often appropriate to the conditions that *they can perceive, understand, and can do something about at a particular point in time.* In these circumstances, where it is claimed that "situational awareness was lost", it is more probable that attempts at situational assessment at the time did not have access to or did not use all of the available information. Situational awareness was not lost, it was always there, but just did not reflect the available reality of the prevailing circumstances at the time. The full extent of these conditions is then only apparent to us *with the benefit of hindsight* (Dekker, 2015a; van Winsen et al, 2015).

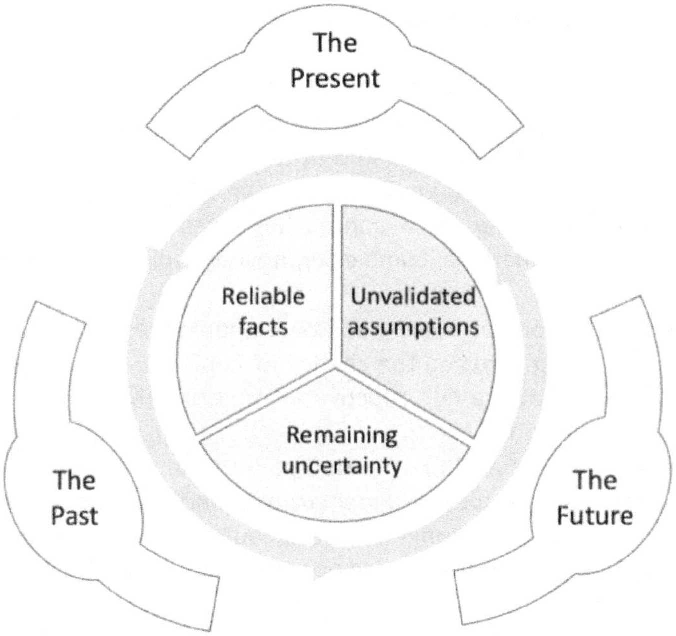

Figure 3: the basis of situational analysis and awareness

Understanding risk

It is all well and good developing effective situational awareness, however, using it to make sense and make meaningful decisions is a different issue. In any environment, uncertainty can be constraining. Not knowing how a situation could evolve, or which decision option represents the best chance of success are constant real-world problems. This is where an understanding of uncertainty and effective assessment of risk can significantly improve sensemaking and decision-making. In many crises and disasters, it is apparent that the issue of uncertainty is largely misunderstood and ignored, and that risk assessment is undertaken poorly if at all.

There are a whole range of issues with the current (Standards-based) methodologies used for risk management (Aven and Ylönen, 2019; Hodge, 2019; Monat and Doremus, 2018; Aven, 2017; Minksy, 2016; Ball and Watt, 2014; Kaplan and Mikes, 2012; Hubbard and Evans, 2010; Hubbard, 2009), which are amplified when dealing with situations characterised by high uncertainty and complexity. There are a variety of reasons why risk assessment (and by extension risk management) is often ineffective in these situations (Gibson and Gibson, 2023), including:

i. *Problems with the risk management process:*
   - Traditional (Standards -based) methodologies are based on linear thinking[79], involving linear (step-by-step) processes, that can work well in the simple linear environments for which they were originally designed. However, such approaches often struggle increasingly as system and situational complexity, novelty, volatility, and uncertainty increase.
   - The applications of these traditional approaches commonly have an overwhelming focus on the chance of familiar types of future events occurring. They are not effective at exploring the speculative, or the highly novel and uncertain.
   - There is a great deal of attention paid to the effectiveness of known controls, as they operate *under current conditions* (i.e., the conditions for which they were originally designed). There is little consideration about how such controls could operate under very different high stress conditions, such as could occur during a major prolonged incident. There is little consideration of vulnerability, both inherent (in the design and current operation[80] of a system), or that could emerge once a system is placed under increasing stress.
   - In those situations where risk management is undertaken, there is often a huge focus on generating lists of risks, which tend to be analysed and treated in isolation of each other, without considering potential interactions and interdependencies with other risks, associated factors, and outcomes.

---

[79] Involving so called 'Cartesian-Newtonian thinking, named after the 17th Century French philosopher Rene Descartes, and English polymath scientist Sir Isaac Newton.

[80] This includes the concept of the 'normalisation of deviance'. Over time most processes are modified away from the original design, with the introduction of 'band-aid' fixes and other workarounds. These deviances become accepted as part of the normal way of doing things, and are usually expedient, they help to get the job done. Whilst everything may be fine under normal (relatively low stress and stable) conditions, such processes have increased fragility once conditions change to the unexpected. This is further amplified by the lack of recognition of the gap between the expected work practices ('work as imagined') and the actual 'deviant' work practices - 'work as done' (Vaughan, 2016). The converse of this is where people continue to operate processes long after the environment has changed, processes that do not work as intended under the new conditions and do not achieve any meaningful value (Alvesson and Spicer, 2016), the so called 'stupidity paradox' a very common phenomenon within a multitude of government agencies.

ii. *Problems with the analytical tools for risk:*

- There is a belief among many risk practitioners that making a subjective estimate (read 'guesswork') about the consequence of some potential future situation and combining that with a subjective estimate of likelihood (again, read guesswork) constitutes effective risk assessment. Such types of assessment are undertaken even in situations that are not probabilistic and for which there is no precedent upon which to base likelihood.
- This almost total reliance on the 'consequence x likelihood' relationship ignores a whole range of other risk assessment approaches and tools that could be better applied to high uncertainty situations.
- Expert judgement about risk is often substituted by reading a risk rating off an untested, misunderstood, and often plagiarised[81] risk matrix. Although the use of the risk matrix in most cases is completely unsupported by any scientific validation, its use continues in many risk assessment applications where it is often worse than useless, and in some situations can be outright dangerous (Gibson and Gibson, 2023; Monat and Doremus, 2018; Goerlandt and Reniers, 2016; Duijm, 2015; Way et al, 2014; Kontovas and Psaraftis, 2009; Smith et al, 2009; Emblemsvåg and Kjølstad, 2006).

iii. *Problems with the application of risk assessment /risk management:*

- Risk assessment is often reduced to an overly simplified tick-box exercise, lists of risks are arbitrarily rated, and this rating is then used to *justify* decisions *post hoc* (if used at all for anything beyond 'ticking a box'), rather than more meaningfully used to *inform* or provide a frame of reference for decision-making.
- Alternate and more relevant methodologies and tools are available, but the average 'risk manager' has neither the experience nor the expertise to apply these tools in any meaningful way.
- The decision-maker often does not have the skills and expertise to understand anything beyond a simplistic 'risk assessment product', or to use it within effective decision-making.
- The decision-maker may be functioning completely adequately under routine conditions, but when faced with turbulence and complexity, they have insufficient cognitive resources to handle such changing conditions and deal with the growing ambiguities. Useful risk

---

[81] It is fairly common to see risk matrices copied from one organisation and then applied in multiple other organisations (across different sectors) with little or no attempt to customise their use to different contexts, or to validate the thinking underlying the construction of the matrix.

information, which may be seen as too complex or an additional burden, is consequently ignored.

- Analysts and decision-makers often have an inflated sense of their own competence, and at the same time are oblivious of their own shortcomings, a commonly experienced phenomenon known as the Dunning-Kruger effect (Ehrlinger et al, 2008; Pronin, 2007; Dunning et al, 2003; 1990).

Governance and decision-making

Good governance and leadership are well recognised enablers of an effective crisis and disaster response (Khan et al, 2018), and as drivers for integrity, collaboration, and decision-making before, during, and after a crisis. During the pandemic, one of the key differentiators of effective decision-making has been the judgement on when to act quickly (which may result in unanticipated severe consequences), or to wait until more information becomes available in the hope that there will be more certainty on outcomes (which can be equally problematic, as the situation can spiral out of control before decision-making even starts). For example, throughout the pandemic, some political leaders have been criticised for acting too precipitately on invoking lockdowns, whilst others in similar situations have been subject to criticism for delaying the decision (McHugh, 2021; Shanahan, 202; Lathouris, 2020). There seems to have been little appreciation, by mainstream media or the general public, that the search for the 'good option' may not be feasible in a complex crisis such as the pandemic. Good decision-making in these circumstances is often about choosing the 'least bad' option.

The leadership and management of large-scale critical incidents does not just happen because of normal capabilities, routine processes, and day-to-day management arrangements. In Australia, as with most developed nations, there are many decades of experience gained from failure as well from success in dealing with emergencies, crises, and disasters. Certainly, within government, the ability to manage major disruption has been recognised as a key requirement for at least the last two decades, and this has seen a significant growth in formal activities such as disaster recovery, business continuity, issues and crisis management, and incident and emergency management (Gibson and Gibson, 2023).

Systems and frameworks, such as AIIMS[82], have been established nationally to provide governance, guide decision-making, and manage resources in complex evolving emergency and crisis situations. Whilst at state level, such governance mechanisms have been enshrined in legislation, plans, and procedures.

However, it appears that this experience was not capitalised upon effectively during the Hotel Quarantine Program, proven command and control mechanisms such as AIIMS and the State's emergency management structures and expertise seem to have been sidelined or forgotten at key times during the crisis.

Lessons learned and not learned

The drivers and pathology of major crises and disruptions have been the subject of decades of research and are now reasonably well understood[83] and, along with the experience of managing real incidents, have helped to inform continually improved preparedness over this time. However, there is also a considerable wealth of research that shows that lessons may be 'identified' but are consistently not 'learned', and that the same mistakes in managing major incidents and crises are encountered repeatedly (Dyson, 2020; Kurtz, 2020; Cionek et al, 2019; Goyal and Howlett, 2018; Allington et al, 2012; Phillips, 2008; Rostis, 2007; Tarakji G., 2992; Sisemore, 1991). The failure to learn lessons has occurred with all types of incidents and incident responses, including health disasters and especially during the recent pandemic (Wankmüller, 2020).

There are a range of reasons why lessons are not learned effectively, and why the mistakes of the past continue to be repeated. However, rather than just a case of 'lessons not learned', it is more often that the *'right* lessons are not learned' because a shallow causal analysis often 'blames' proximal reasons

[82] Australasian Inter-service Incident Management System, a common systematic approach for control, command, coordination of resources during an emergency or disaster, originally based upon the US Incident Management System approach.

[83] Gibson and Gibson, 2023; Sharma, 2017; Alcalde Cuesta et al, 2016; Gans, 2016; Dekker, 2015b; Doloi and Crawford, 2015; Gibson and Pupulidy, 2015a, 2015b; Lee, 2015; LGiU, 2015; Noujoumi et al, 2015; Gibb et al, 2014; Hiles, 2014; Leslie, 2014; Moloney, 2014; Quinlan, 2014; Tichy, 2014; Bircham and Connolly, 2013; Carillo-Castrillo, et al, 2013; Smith et al, 2013; DMTR, 2011; Bharosa, 2010; Cramm, 2009; Mooren et al, 2009; Smits et al, 2009; Goldhammer, 2008; Light, 2008; Bernstein, 2006; James and Wooten; 2005; Wright and van der Schaaf, 2004; CAIB, 2003; Kadam, 2003; Carlson and Doyle, 2002; Rosenthal et al, 2001; Rosenthal, 1989; Petersen, 1978; Heinrich, 1931.

rather than the complexity of the underlying causes[84]. There are a range of factors involved in the failure to effectively learn the lessons (Jacobsson et al, 2019; Drupsteen and Hasle, 2014; Rasmussen et al, 2013; Lundberg, 2012; Hovden et al, 2012; Fahlbruch and Schöbel, 2011; Dekker, 2009; Sanne 2008; Cheverau et al, 2006).

These factors include:

- Problematic lessons learned processes:
    - absence of effective processes for investigating, analysing, and capturing lessons;
    - lack of appropriate skills for undertaking analysis of experiences, resulting in poorly formulated and misleading insights and lessons;
    - a poor understanding of the range of analytical tools that can be applied to lessons identification and sensemaking;
    - lessons provided in a manner and format that restricts and prevents actual learning;
    - a lack of understanding about incident pathology, resulting in attention focused on misleading 'causes' whilst failing to appreciate the role played by other causal, contributing, and influencing factors;
    - Impracticality and irrelevance of some of the improvement recommendations that arise from the lessons learned process.

- Issues with leadership and decision-makers:
    - leaders that perceive little value in lessons learned;
    - competing and more immediate priorities for attention[85];
    - the imperative for quick (shallow) wins rather than longer term meaningful change;

---

[84] This is a not uncommon outcome of Inquiries and Royal Commissions, which often do not go beyond immediate 'causes' in their findings. The very approach taken by Royal Commissions and other public inquiries creates an internal conflict in their aims ('uncover wrongdoing' vs 'lessons learned') which inhibits or deflects deep open learning (Wilkins and Phillimore, 2019; Eburn and Dovers, 2015). Those called before such inquiries are placed into a position where they have to defend their decisions and actions, and protect their self-interest, rather than provide a comprehensive account of what occurred and why. That is before the influence of political motives behind their establishment and their actual independence is considered (Hogan-Doran, 2019).

[85] A short term focus on performance can be a potent driver for diverting and misplacing attention (Bircham and Connolly, 2013). There can be little personal gain from implementing lessons learned when an organisation's recognition and reward systems are focussed on other short term performance indicators.

  - insufficient experience, knowledge, and competencies to understand and apply lessons;
  - decision-makers inappropriately prioritise lessons;
  - wilful decisions to not participate or ignore lessons.

- Situational barriers and constraints:
  - organisational time and resource constraints that hinder implementation of lessons learned;
  - situational complexity hinders effective analysis;
  - resistance of individuals to identify errors (particularly their own);
  - communication barriers that restrict the flow of information;
  - the existing mental models of those involved that constrain analytical and intuitive thinking about the incident and response;
  - organisational culture that influences individuals' trust and willingness to participate in the lessons learned process;
  - general comfort with the status quo and a resistance to change;
  - fundamental lack of understanding of normalisation of deviance and the perpetuation of beliefs that 'work as imagined' represents reality.

Governance

There has been considerable research, as well as practical experience in recent years, into the governance and management of disasters and other major incidents (Kovács, 2019), including its codification into the major activities of planning, preparedness, response, and recovery (Cozzolino, 2012). With these activities being strongly focused on developing an 'all hazards' capability (Penta et al, 2017; Adini et al, 2012; Ayub et al, 2007), that is theoretically capable of dealing with a wide variety of different emergencies, crisis, and disasters. However, such a broad sweeping approach has been criticised for its potentially less effective capability than a specifically targeted approach (Gregory, 2015; Donahue et la, 2012; Hausken et al, 2009).

Following a disastrous wildfire season in California in 1970 in which 16 people died, there was significant criticism regarding the effectiveness of the emergency response (reviewed in Rowley, 2008). These criticisms included (reviewed in Gibson and Gibson 2023):

- *"The absence of a standard overarching incident management structure"*.
- *"Difficulties in obtaining current, centralised, and accurate information"*.

- *"Reduced ability to conduct centralised planning and prioritising for the deployment of scarce resources".*
- *"Communications problems between different agencies".*
- *"Agencies using different structures, technical languages and unique terminologies that created further confusion".*

It was out of this disaster that the first codified national incident management system (IMS) evolved in the USA, and was subsequently adopted and customised by Canada, Australia, New Zealand, and several other jurisdictions (with the notable exception of the UK). This system is codified in its current form as the Australasian Inter-service Incident Management System - AIIMS (AFAC, 2017), and has been adopted by agencies in the Commonwealth, States, and Territories. Although the system is not perfect, it has been used successfully by government agencies in a wide range of different emergencies and crises, and is being increasingly adopted into and further adapted by the private sector (Gibson and Gibson, 2023).

One of the key aspects of an effective response under an IMS is the concept of unity of control, that there is one person in overall charge of the management of an incident, and that everyone involved in the incident understands and acknowledges that controlling role (Figure 4). AIIMS embodies most of the generic IMS concepts and structure, but is often displayed as a more traditional hierarchical structure with all subsidiary functions reporting to a single incident controller. The key benefits of such an approach (rather than having just a collection of agency representatives meeting as the incident management team) is that everyone present has a defined role, some span across the incident and across multiple agencies (such as 'planning' and 'logistics' functions, whereas others are focused on specific front-line activities (operational and tactical response). Such an approach has proven to be highly effective in a wide variety of different types of incidents because:

- Everyone understands their own role and how they fit into the bigger response picture.
- Everyone understands the roles of others (including limits of responsibility and authority) and how these other roles fit into the bigger response picture.
- Priorities are clearly established and assigned to specific roles, which reduces unnecessary repetition and avoids turf wars.
- Key decisions and actions are not forgotten because of misassumptions that someone else is responsible.

- The incident controller is not overwhelmed by 'people management' distractions in the incident management team, because the structure deliberately limits the span of control to about 5 to 7 subordinates.
- Specialist subject matter experts are involved as 'advisors' as required, rather than becoming part of an overly large and unwieldy decision-making machine.

AIIMS, when combined with each jurisdiction's legislative arrangements, should provide a comprehensive set of arrangements for major incidents and prolonged crises and disasters.

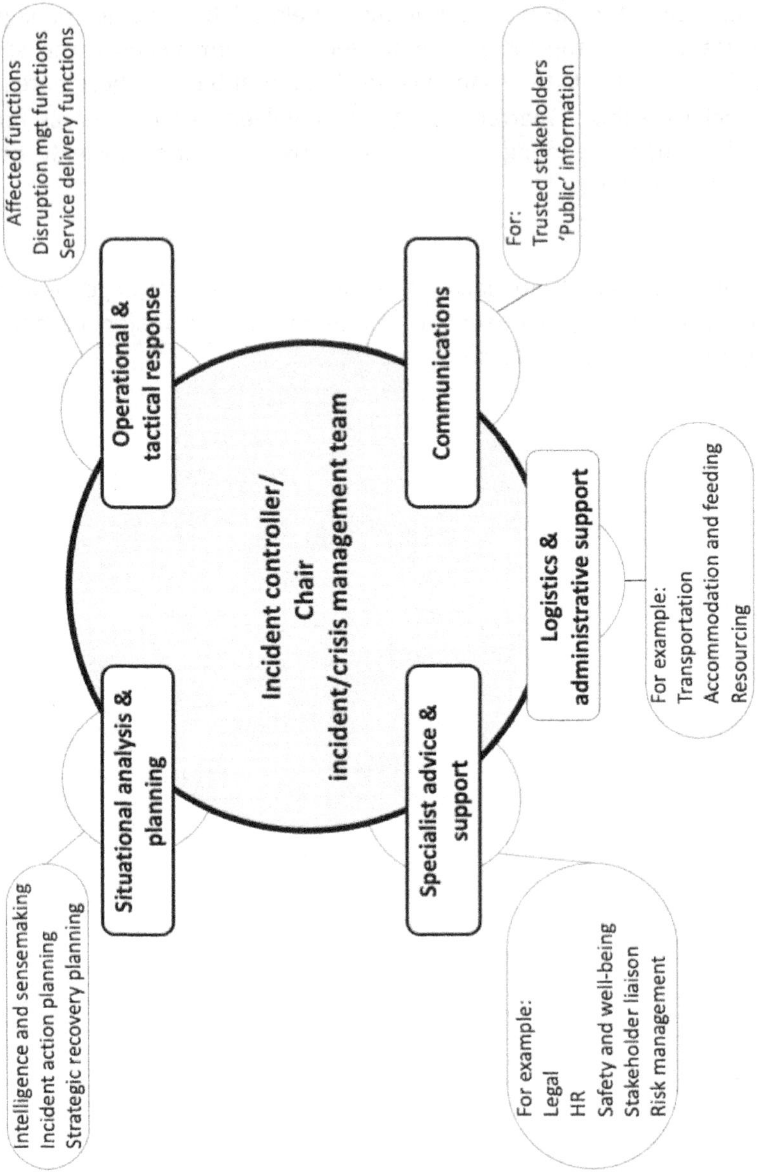

Figure 4: a generic incident management system[86]

[86] Adapted from Gibson and Gibson, 2023.

Victoria's Emergency Management Act, 2013, established certain agencies to be nominated as either 'control agencies' or 'support agencies'. The State's Emergency Management Manual (EMMV-which was in effect until September 2020, and hence covered the first period of operation of the Hotel Quarantine Program and its subsequent catastrophic failure) provided a guidance table allocating control[87] or support agency status for different types of incidents. For example, in the case of a "plague or an epidemic" the control agency was either DHHS[88],[89] for human disease, or DEDJTER[90] for animal or plant disease. It should also be noted that DHHS was also identified as the State's lead agency for advising on and securing accommodation for *displaced "individuals, families, and households*" (EMV, 2020).

These arrangements, AIIMS and EMMV were specifically developed to facilitate control, command, and coordination, and to help ensure interoperability, effective decision-making, and effective communications during a multi-agency response. One of the key outcomes from such an approach is to establish a common operating picture for all agencies involved in managing a situation, and in particular to establish shared situational awareness and sensemaking. These are capabilities that are especially important during a prolonged public health emergency (Brooks et al, 2016). The importance of developing an effective common operating picture, and the consequences of failing to do so were significantly illustrated during the 2010 H1N1 influenza pandemic (Fraser and Blumenstock, 2020). This lack of a common operating picture, in the case of H1N1 in the USA, resulted in substantial issues with the distribution of vaccines, whilst in the case of COVID-19 in the USA, this lack of a common operating picture was implicated in the significant problems encountered in the testing program.

Central to these arrangements is establishing clear accountabilities, a vital element in an effective emergency, crisis, or disaster response (UNDRR, 2019;

---

[87] The primary agency for responding to and in overall charge of the management of the incident)

[88] Department of Health and Human Services, which retained responsibility for human disease incidents under the State Emergency Management Plan that came into effect on 20 September 2020, with responsibilities in particular for 'health emergency response', 'health protection', 'operational management', 'intelligence and information sharing', etc.

[89] Following the revelations of serious dysfunction within the DHHS following the Coate Inquiry, the Department was broken up into two separate entities: the Health Department and the Department of Families, Fairness and Housing (Burton 2020; Jenkins, 2020a).

[90] DEDJTER: Department of Economic Development, Jobs, Transport and Resources. Under machinery of government changes, control agency responsibilities were transferred to the newly formed Department of Jobs, Precincts, and Regions established in 2019.

Amaratunga et al, 2016), and in doing so seek to avoid authority being contested (Moynihan, 2008), and avoid any confusion about which agency and individual is in overall control. All of which seems to have forgotten or ignored in the debacle of setting up the hotel quarantine program and other aspects of the pandemic response.

Public inquiries

Victoria, along with other jurisdictions has had plenty of opportunities to get the emergency management governance arrangements 'right'[91]. Over several decades there have been a number of major crises and disasters, with Royal Commissions, Inquiries and investigations time after time identifying the same problems in governance and accountability, situational awareness, decision-making, risk assessment, inter-agency coordination, and communication (Binskin et al, 2020; Government of South Australia, 2020; Walker 2020; Snow, 2018; Sapat and Esnard, 2016; Thawley and Comley, 2015; Teague et al, 2014; Funabashi and Kitazawa, 2012; Holmes, 2012; 2011; Jerrard, 2012; National Commission, 2011a; 2011b).

Whilst public inquiries often establish the 'facts', reveal some institutional failings, and provide some insight into 'causes' and 'fixes' (Mintrom, et al, 2021; McCallum, 2019), they can just as frequently obscure the underlying issues and provide unsuitable shallow simplistic solutions for deep complex problems (Burton 2021a; Henriques-Gomes, 2020; Prasser, 2020; Suraweera and Ofner, 2020; Shepheard, 2019; Ireton, 2018; Lane, 2018; Hill, 2017; Peplow, 2017; Craven, 2015; Black and Mays, 2013; Lauder, 2013; Chia, 2009; Boin et al, 2008; Walshe, 2005; t'Hart and Boin, 2001; Rodger, 1985). It has also been argued that some inquiries (such as the Coate Inquiry) provided little more insight than could have been achieved instead by an independent review by an infectious diseases expert, and achieved within a few weeks and at a fraction of the cost (Burton, 2021b). It may even be that public inquiries reveal as much 'untruth' as they do the actual truth (Berg, 2014), and can be easily manipulated for political gain.

---

[91] Historically, many different jurisdictions appear to be neither learning the 'right' lessons from their own experiences, or from the experiences of other jurisdictions, with the same sort of failures occurring in different types of disaster. The Victorian Government has had a wealth of historical experience and lessons learned on which to draw. However, the findings from the Coate Inquiry show that that the Andrews government made the same types of mistakes repeatedly.

Recommendations have been made in multiple jurisdictions regarding improving governmental capabilities for managing crises and disasters, and in each instance have been responded to by a public declaration of acceptance and an intent to rectify the problems. However, that the same repeated issues keep arising in crisis after crisis does question whether lessons have indeed been learned. Are the problems with implementation, or that the 'right lessons' have not been identified in the first place? That is, have the root causal, contributing, and influencing factors not been effectively determined? In both cases it also raises the questions about whether the appropriate competencies are in place at all levels of analysis and decision-making with those involved in the end-to-end lessons learned processes.

Decision-making

Within governments and government agencies, decision-making largely occurs as a result of processes that are variously rational, intuitive, emotional, or political in nature (Elbanna, 2017). In high uncertainty situations such as in public health emergencies, decisions often have to be made under conditions of high uncertainty, significant time constraints, and resource limitations (Khalid et al, 2020). Pandemics, such as COVID-19, are certainly characterised by uncertainty and confusion (Juliano et al, 2021), which can confound already existing sub-optimal decision-making processes.

Further amplifying these limitations are the common tensions that exist between political interests and operational requirements in a disaster or crisis response (Bosomworth et al, 2017; McConnell and Stark, 2002). Added to which are a range of self-protection, self-promotion, and unmanaged conflicts of interest of some of those involved in making decisions during a crisis or disaster.

Decision-making under high uncertainty

Most day-to-day decision-making, undertaken in relatively certain and stable environments, is strongly rational and script based. However, under high uncertainty, such routine decision-making capability often proves inadequate, with a marked persistence in following increasingly irrelevant scripts. Effective decision-making under high uncertainty requires an ability to leave these scripts behind as and when required, and engage in more intuitive[92] and improvisational thinking and decision-making (Tabesh and Vera, 2020; Hadida et al, 2014; Certo et al, 2006). Intuition and improvisation do not just occur in a vacuum, and to be effective need to build upon relevant deep experience and an appropriate analytical frame (Okoli and Watt, 2018; Miller 2018; Leigh 2016, BINBS, 2013). An example of such a frame is using an 'inquiry mode' approach (see below). However, some caution does need to be applied to relying upon intuition. In the absence of an adequate experiential grounding and a deep knowledge base (particularly under crisis situations when the emotional system can predominate), such intuitive thinking can be misleading and result in ill-considered decisions. In other words, without the involvement of sufficient expertise, a significant reliance on intuition can be dangerous.

The dual thinking system has been proposed as a useful model for how thinking and decision-making occurs. Decision-making involves neural networks that are located in many different parts of the brain, with the prefrontal cortex and the amygdala playing important controlling roles in rational (analytical) thinking and emotional thinking respectively (Rutishauser, 2016; Rudorf and Hare, 2014; Virlicks, 2013). Under routine conditions, both thinking systems are operating (Diedrich and Trueblood, 2018; Evans and Stanovich, 2013; Kahneman, 2011; Evans, 2008; Gilovich et al, 2002), but under high stress (such as high uncertainty, complexity, and volatility), the emotional system can predominate, meaning that rational, logical thinking and memory formation degrades (Goodman et al, 2017; Scwabe and Wolf, 2013). Conversely, some individuals react to such a crisis by trying to revert to the highly familiar and comfortable routine and overly rational thinking mode, depressing or ignoring any expert intuition, pattern recognition and insight that may arise.

Effective decision-making in a crisis requires both analytical and emotional thinking (Holmes, 2018), for example employing a recognition-primed decision-making (RPD) approach (Schakel and Wolbers, 2021; Treurniet and Wolbers, 2021; Cumin et al, 2020; Neiva and Borges, 2019; Bouafia and Zahari, 2017; Leland, 2009; Klein, 1998). This form of decision-making relies on the rapid matching of patterns (held in the memory and derived from experience) with patterns detectable in an evolving situation. From this recognition of

---

[92] Intuitive thinking and decision-making are based upon applying a high level of knowledge and experience to rapid and often unconscious pattern recognition from the available information, where past conditions, decisions and successful solutions are extrapolated and applied to similar current situations. This 'intuition' is often the key difference between the novice and the expert, giving the expert the ability to sort out the important signals from the background noise, rapidly recognise their importance, and apply those solutions that have worked previously in comparable situations.

meaningful patterns, the expert decision-maker can then draw upon a repertoire of associated options (based upon their experience and knowledge).

This allows a decision to be made quickly, under high uncertainty and for ill-structured problems, without the need for a lengthy comparison of different options. A preferred option can then be subjected to a deep analysis by using cognitive simulation to determine how the option could play-out in real life and assess its suitability for addressing the problem. An RPD approach is often used as a natural way of making decisions in incident management teams (Crichton et al, 2008) and when applied by an expert can be highly effective. However, under high uncertainty and in the hands of the inexperienced, RPD will often result in poor decisions and outcomes. The RPD concept illustrates that even with a comprehensive suite of shared information being available, under crisis situations in particular, prior specific expert knowledge and experience is essential in making rapid and effective decisions (Li et al, 2020).

All decision-making is based upon assumptions, which are often hidden, not just from others but from the individual decision-makers themselves. Decisions have an absolute dependency upon assumptions, but when these are unsurfaced, unchallenged, and unvalidated they often lead to the collapse of effective decision-making (Sim, 2016; Halal, 2015, National Commission, 2011a; 2011b; Daly and Walsh, 2010; Barabba, 2011; Lucas and Goh, 2009).

Group decision-making under high uncertainty

A model first developed more than twenty years ago can also help explain how different approaches to decision-making can significantly affect outcomes in conditions of high uncertainty and crisis. This model promotes the concept of two key modes of decision-making (Garvin and Roberto, 2001; Leppänen et al, 2018):

- ***The advocacy mode***: which invokes a shallow and narrow mode of analysis, and is usually based upon the assertion of an opinion with little evaluation or justification. Such an approach can be a combination of both asserting and persuading others about a favoured position and defending that position from challenge (often by discouraging or dismissing contrary views). The advocacy mode can be particularly common within public sector decision-making and can become a default position when faced with rapidly moving and high uncertainty situations, especially in the presence of significant power imbalances within a group.

- ***Inquiry mode***: which invokes a more collaborative, explorative, analytical, and problem-solving approach. Decisions are informed by evidence, and based upon reasoned argument and constructive criticism, and by its very nature encourages contrary and conflicting views. The inquiry mode takes time and effort and requires a suppression of hierarchical power along with a requirement for effective critical thinking and complex problem-solving skills. Such skills appear to be uncommon capabilities within many public sector institutions.

It is highly unusual for group decision-making to only involve a single mode (advocacy or inquiry), most such decision-making features a combination of both modes, although one mode will often be overrepresented. The benefits of adopting an inquiry mode for decision-making have been well illustrated in several governmental crises, including US President John F. Kennedy's approach during the Cuban missile crisis (Mintz and Barr, 2021), generally acknowledged as one of the greatest policy decisions in world history. Conversely, JFK is also seen as making one the worst decisions in modern history, to direct and support the invasion of Cuba by Cuban exiles resident in the USA, that resulted in the Bay of Pigs disaster (Hansen, 2013). This disaster owed its genesis to advocacy and 'groupthink' amongst JFK and his advisors (Dixit, 2019; Feuerherd, 2019; Dueñas , 2017). In the lead up to the April 1961, military invasion of Cuba (by Cuban exiles directed by the US Government). Where any attempt to take a deep considered analysis of the situation, or to allow any dissenting opinions against supporting an invasion of Cuba, were both equally suppressed. The decision to invade was effectively made before the 'decision-making process' was undertaken, which drove "an assumed consensus" amongst all of those involved, with no one dissenting or questioning the decision[93].

JFK and his team appeared to have learned from their earlier decision-making failures and were able to successfully switch to inquiry mode decision-making in time, to resolve the Cuban missile crisis some 18 months later. Their decision-making approach ensured there was no preconceived 'solution' that drove discussion, that the best ideas surfaced and were considered (using "constructive conflict" and "open inquiry"), and that competing options were fully considered (Mullane, 2017; Allison and Zelikow, 1999; Allison, 1969). The result was a combined naval blockade and political solution, instead of the alternative for direct military action against Cuba and the Soviet Union, which would have seen a likely escalation to nuclear war.

---

[93] The development of such a situation will become an important consideration when we explore the decision to use private security at quarantine hotels, later in this book.

Other major policy failures, including many of those associated with the invasions of Iraq and Afghanistan (and the subsequent 2022 disastrous withdrawal) appear to have route causes in similar "assumed consensus" amongst key decision-makers (Dorani, 2018; Henderson, 2018; Mintz and Wayne, 2014; Badie, 2010). As will be discussed in later Chapters, these historical decision-making catastrophes appear to be remarkedly close to the situation in which the major decisions about the Victorian Hotel Quarantine Program were made. Here, groupthink, consensus assumptions, and advocacy mode decision-making appeared to have been the predominant *modus operandi*. It seems that ministerial and senior bureaucratic decision-makers in Victoria were not great readers of history, and that the government was unwilling or unable to learn from its own many previous failures in decision-making.

Whilst adopting an inquiry mode is important in supporting intuition during a crisis, intuitive thinking can in turn be a vital contributor to an effective inquiry mode approach, especially in adopting a strategic mindset (Lindberg and Krasnici, 2020).

Democratic countries, which would be expected to better promote an inquiry mode of decision-making generally fare better in crises than non-democratic nations where advocacy mode decision-making predominates (Ben-Ami, 2020), although there will of course be a wide range of other influencing factors at play. It is also interesting that those western democracies that have been criticised for a more authoritarian and less transparent approach (those that would be expected to adopt a more advocacy-oriented approach), are also those same jurisdictions with more apparent failures in their decision-making.

Advocacy mode decision-making tends to produce 'simplistic' solutions to highly complex problems, and often occurs because of undue ideological influence (Peters, 2021; Rauch, 2021). Advocacy mode decision-making can be shown to have been at the heart of a number of 'crises by mismanagement' such as the two space shuttle disasters (Vaughn, 2016; Maclean, 2004; CAIB, 2003; Rogers, 1986). Situations where a heavily biased and ill-informed decision was allowed to overrule the need for a more considered analysis

Studies have shown that issues such as over self-confidence, restricted information flows, and low transparency are major factors in failed decisions (Ardebili and Padoano, 2020), factors that often predominate in advocacy mode decision-making.

One of the key aspects of leadership in dealing with crises and wicked problems is that leaders are able to encourage effective participative decision-making, and in particular that they both promote and personally demonstrate inquiry mode decision-making (Karelaia and Van der Heyden, 2020).

Decisions in the public health context

The problems with making and implementing decisions in the high uncertainty of a public health emergency should be well known from published accounts (Setiawan, 2019; Parker et al, 2009), and should serve as cautionary tales for all senior decision-makers. Although it can be difficult to ensure the success of *decision outcomes*, it is eminently feasible to ensure the quality of the decision-making *process.* However, it is also well known that the decision-making and responses to public health emergencies are often poor-quality processes, do not always follow the scientific evidence, and can be strongly influenced by political and other societal factors (ECDC, 2019). The key parameters for success in public health decision-making should be no surprise:

- Robust situational awareness and risk assessment to develop an up-to-date and informed common operating picture.
- Decision-making and action planning that is evidence based, to develop mitigations to risks that could have an effect (both direct and indirect) on human health. Ideally, this should occur through arrangements such as an Incident Control/ Incident Management System (e.g., AIIMS). As decision-making is occurring under high uncertainty, it needs to be highly adaptive to respond to changing situations and new emerging information (ECDC, 2017; Lurie et al, 2006), without simply rushing into making decisions in conditions that are highly volatile and turbulent. Starting slowly, not only helps to plan the process, but also helps to 'quiet' the amygdala and lessen the effect of a potentially dominating emotional thinking system.
- Effective communication and consultation, which conveys information about the situation, the risks, the decisions, and the implementation of the required actions, thereby elevating situational awareness and promoting shared sensemaking.
- Process control, including monitoring to ensure that information is flowing to those that require it, that decisions and action plans are being mobilised and implemented as required, that risks are acceptable, that no unacceptable new risks have been introduced, that resources are being utilised effectively and efficiently, and that the outcomes from the action plan are being achieved.

Non-decisions

The concept of non-decisions has been explored for several decades (Milsom et al, 2020; Bratteteig and Wagner, 2012; McCalla-Chen, 2000; Zelditch and Walker, 2000; Rose and Davies, 1994; Moriss, 1987; Debnam, 1975; Bachrach and Baratz, 1970; 1963). Broadly, 'non-decision-making' involves those in positions of power influencing, manipulating, and suppressing decision-making, whilst providing a façade that decision-making is unbiased and evidence-based. Thus, non-decisions are frequently encountered when a large and unaccountable power imbalance exists (Brisbois et al, 2019). Several types of non-decisions have been recognised:

- Where actors deliberately manipulate disclosure and discussion in decision-making to what they regard as acceptable "safe" issues, and thereby reducing the chance of the powerful decision-maker being challenged.
- Where decision-making is restricted to only a preferred or limited range of options, whilst other feasible options are deliberately excluded because of incompatibility with the prevalent ideology and values.
- Where discussion of issues and options (particularly in a public forum) is diverted to other matters so that a decision is not made.
- Where individuals who do not have the requisite experience, knowledge, or competences are placed in the role of decision-maker, deliberately excluding those with the relevant knowledge and expertise.

The concept of non-decisions is often applied to political self-interest that keeps issues off the agenda (Sharkansky and Friedberg, 2002), and can be seen where problems are too complex to fix easily, where those making policy lack a sufficient understanding of the issue, and where there is a failure to deal with coordination issues across multiple agencies. The forcing of non-decisions can occur through enforcing compliance on a minority view onto a group of decision-makers, resulting in a failure to pursue certain ideas or lines of enquiry. This usually occurs because those in powerful positions:

- Use or threaten force, intimidation, or harassment.
- Use or threaten punitive actions or other sanctions.
- Provide or offer inducements and rewards.
- Delegitimise or invalidate the importance of certain ideas or issues before consideration by decision-makers.

- Introduce barriers that prevent certain ideas, information, or issues being available to decision-making.
- Deliberately conceal essential information.
- Divert focus by overwhelming decision-making with unnecessary information and discussion.

Non-decision making may also occur because of serious clashes of personality, either between powerbrokers and decision-makers, or within groups of decision-makers.

Reversibility of decision-making

There is a core concept about decision-making in high-risk situations and where wicked problems are manifest, and that is the concept of 'reversibility of decisions'. This is not a new concept, and over the last 30 years or more a considerable volume of literature on the subject has been published (Schmitt; 2018; Bullens, 2013; Bullens et al, 2013; Hafner et al, 2012; Bullens et al, 2011; Frey, 1981).

Decisions can be regarded as being either reversible (the decision and implementation path can be easily changed after the original decision), or irreversible – a decision that is very difficult (almost irreversible) if not impossible to change after it has been made. Most of the decisions that we make in routine situations are reversible, and for the small number of day-to-day decisions that may be irreversible the consequences are small enough to be ignored or absorbed. The difference between the two types of decisions is therefore generally unimportant for routine decision-making, and accordingly we become quickly habituated to treating all decisions as if they were reversible.

However, under conditions of high uncertainty, high volatility, novelty, and complexity, (ideal wicked problem conditions, and the situation with establishing and running Victoria's Hotel Quarantine Program), decisions are *much more likely to be irreversible*. Making irreversible decisions requires a very different skill set and different cognitive framing than is used in business-as-usual situations. Decision-making, under non-routine conditions, must be approached in a very different way (Ansell and Bartenberger, 2016). Treating irreversible decisions as reversible decisions, and rushing in with an incomplete understanding of the context and problem space can literally have fatal outcomes.

In situations where decisions are likely to be irreversible, greater caution and heightened analysis is required (Belizaire. 2021; LaRiviere et al, 2018; Bezos, 2015; Kalra et al, 2014). Many non-routine situations will require both reversible and irreversible decisions to be made, and will need different decision-making processes to be used at different times. Recognising which decisions can be made quickly using routine decision-making and which decisions require more deliberation and a different approach is key to dealing with high uncertainty. Those involved in decision-making need to recognise when they are faced with an irreversible decision, and need to be able to switch their decision-making approach, from one mode to the other. When faced with an irreversible decision, adopting an effective approach involves:

- Ensuring that the problem that the decision-making is trying to solve is the actual problem that needs to be tackled. This requires that a deeper understanding of the problem space is achieved before the decision itself is fully articulated.
- Taking time to follow a robust decision-making process and allowing opportunity for reflection before agreeing on a final decision.
- Accepting that decisions need to be led by data and information, and that irreversible decisions require a much broader and deeper consideration of what is relevant and important data and information.
- Being aware of the potential influence of biases, conflicts of interest, power imbalances, advocacy mode effects, and other coercive forces on the decision-making process.
- Ensuring that assumptions are comprehensively surfaced, challenged, and validated, or modified or abandoned when necessary.
- Considering the nature and effects of uncertainty on decision making (for example through an assessment of risk).
- Stress testing preferred options under plausible future potential conditions (given the high levels of prevailing uncertainty, the likelihood of such conditions developing can become increasingly irrelevant, more focus being placed on consequences and the ability to control the potential situation).
- Determining the vulnerabilities of options, and the conditions under which such vulnerabilities could manifest.
- Evaluating the extent to which these vulnerabilities could be addressed, or their impacts managed, and the degree to which chosen options could be modified over time as the context changes.

Decision-making and behavioural insights

Over the last decade or so, many jurisdictions, internationally and within Australia, have recognised the potential benefits of using behavioural insights to inform and help deliver government policy, particularly where complex problems and solutions are involved (BETA, 2023; Drummond, 2021; Hallsworth et al, 2018; Halpern, 2015; Oullier, 2013).

Behavioural insights make use of a range of scientific disciplines including anthropology, cognitive psychology, behavioural economics, etc. to help understand how people (such as the general public) make decisions and how they behave. This insight can then be used to craft public policy and improve understanding of how the public will engage with and respond to official information. The use of behavioural insights has been successfully applied in many areas of health, and the World Health Organisation (WHO) has successfully promoted its use in a wide range of projects, including in the management of the COVID-19 pandemic (WHO 2021b). Within the UK, behavioural insights have been widely applied to improve outcomes in health care and public health (Chadborne, 2018), for example through its EAST Framework[94] (Snijders et al, 2016).

This seems to be exactly the sort of assistance that one would reasonably think should be available to help design and operate a hotel quarantine program and for the management of any subsequent community outbreaks. The Australian Government has had an established specialised health behavioural insights capability that long predates the pandemic (Health Department, 2021). The Victorian Government established a Behavioural Insights Team in 2015 within the Department of Premier and Cabinet (ANZSOG, 2021; DPC, 2019), with several projects being undertaken in the health portfolio (VicHealth, 2021; Halpern, 2016). However, from publicly available information, it appears that little, if any use was made of behavioural insights capability in setting up Operation Soteria, the breach response, or in any of the subsequent reform activities for hotel quarantine. Although the government did spend millions of dollars of public money on private consultants researching the popularity and political impacts of the lockdowns (Johnston, 2021b; Parsons, 2021), with suggestions that this information may have been more influential on decision-making than actual health advice. As of June 2022, the Andrews government

[94] EAST: **E**asy (making the best option the default option – i.e., reducing behavioural friction by removing barriers), **A**ttractive (attracting attention), **S**ocial (making preferred behaviours more visible) and **T**imely (introducing changes at the most appropriate times).

was still fighting in the courts to keep this information secret (Johnston, 2022c; Sunraysia, 2022).

A new government agency, Insights Victoria, was established in August 2020, but its existence was kept secret from the public until it was revealed in a Freedom of Information request from a major newspaper (which the government attempted to deny). The agency, which apparently reported directly to Daniel Andrews, appeared to provide less of a behavioural insight development capability and more of an intelligence function. Gathering and analysing data on the Victorian people, including social media use, credit card spending and health information. Whilst government bureaucrats can apply to access the data on a need to know basis, Daniel Andrews' Private Office has apparent free access, opening up the real opportunity for its misuse for political purposes (Aldred, 2022).

There is nothing wrong with a government uplifting its data insights capability (and many governments do so), good policy decision-making absolutely needs to rely on access to good data. However, the apparent ease with which this agency and its data could be used for political purposes is disturbing. Whilst the government's attempts to keep the operation of the agency secret, especially since it reports directly to the Premier, is sinister to say the least.

The lack of public disclosure about any use of behavioural insights during the pandemic response does raise issues that require answers. Were behavioural insights ignored by key decision makers in the Victorian Government (which could indicate negligence), or were such insights being secretly used for covert political reasons, which would seem to be highly unethical to say the least.

Normalisation of deviance

The concept of normalisation of deviance was popularised as an explanation for one of the key causes leading up to the Challenger shuttle disaster (Vaughan, 2016), when contract engineers' warnings about the potential for rubber seal failures were disregarded by NASA leadership. The concept of normalisation of deviance entails the accumulation of unofficial shortcuts (deviances) in decision-making and processes, that overtime progressively become the accepted norm (Lapinski and Rimal, 2005).

Although such 'deviances' appear to be an easier way of operating under routine conditions, they introduce heightened fragility, and can result in catastrophic outcomes when conditions change to the non-routine. Such normalisation often remains unrecognised, and the belief persists in senior management that decisions and processes are undertaken as originally intended ('work as designed') or according to the understood authorised processes ('work as imagined'). Such false assumptions are sometimes strengthened by uninformed, incorrect, or misleading information about what is happening ('work as reported'). There is often a significant gap between management's beliefs or perceptions (Figure 5) and what is actually happening in reality ('work as performed').

Normalisation of deviance, as well as degrading capability can also result in unfounded assumptions perpetuating and warning signals, (both about changing conditions and about the effectiveness or ineffectiveness of decisions) being missed or ignored.

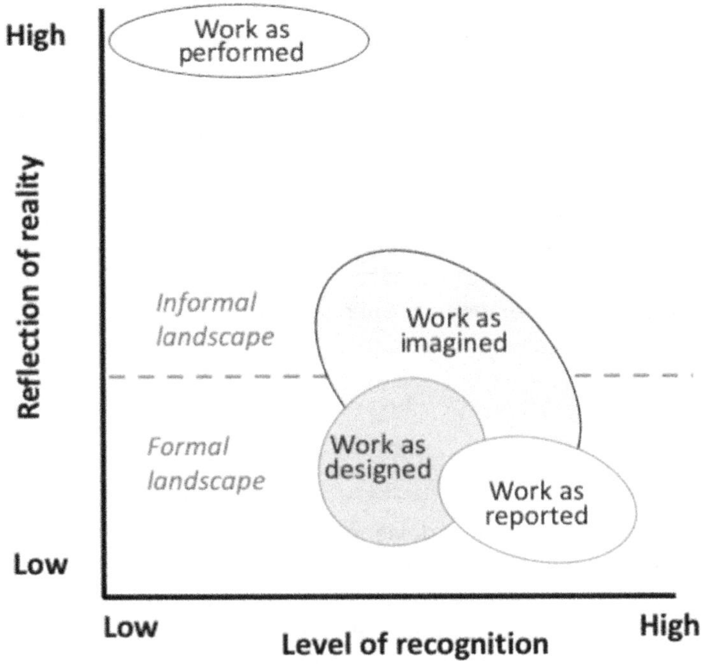

Figure 5 Normalisation of deviance

Normalisation of deviance is likely present throughout the Victorian Government and its agencies As more demands and stress are placed upon the bureaucracy, the more deviance that is likely to occur, and the more such deviance will be normalised into readily accepted, bur fragile, practices. Whilst normalisation of deviance has probably contributed to many of the government's overall long term performance problems, it is highly likely to have been a major factor in the Hotel Quarantine Program disaster.

Communication and information flows

During public health emergencies, effective communications rely heavily upon local context knowledge, upon credible and trustworthy relationships (Sanford et al, 2020), and upon the informal knowledge and networks that arise from these relationships. The success of a crisis management team is almost always critically dependent upon these information and communication flows (WHO, 2017). During a public health crisis, understanding risk is paramount, not just for those that must deal with health hazards, but for all of those making key decisions (Wang et al, 2020; Seeger et al, 2018).

The need for transparency and disclosure during a crisis or disaster, particularly a public health crisis, has been highlighted as an important element of sensemaking and response (Spalluto et al, 2020; UN/DESA, 2020; Albu and Wehmeier, 2013; O'Malley et al, 2009). This is especially the case in multiagency responses where, for a variety of reasons, holders of certain information can seek to withhold a full disclosure from other agencies and individuals. This is more often a desire to promote or protect parochial interests (e.g., 'knowledge is power') than it is for legitimate confidentiality or security concerns. In some situations, the lack of transparency can itself cause its own additional crisis involving public backlash and outrage beyond the original crisis (Mattera, 2020; FAU, 2019; Knaus, 2019; Parker, 2019; DeFazio, 2019; Torossian, 2019; Kiley, 2017; Zhou, 2016; Ohlheiser, 2013; Padgett et al, 2013).

Within government entities, transparency (or its lack) has been associated with three determinants (Fairbank et al, 2007):

- *Personal factors*: including an individual's[95] conviction or beliefs about the need for transparency, balanced with the fear about how transparency could be used against that individual or the organisation.
- *Organisational factors*: including how governance arrangements, culture, and internal messaging support the principles and practices of transparency, or conversely encourage secrecy and an absence of disclosure.
- *Resource factors*: including organisational structures, communication channel availability and access, capabilities, competing priorities, and time availability, and the importance given to transparency and openness.\

Transparency and trust (which itself is often amplified by transparency) have been shown to be important factors in helping to manage uncertainty and fear during a pandemic (Menon and Goh, 2005). Transparency means that information is truthful, representational, and meets the expectations of stakeholders (Balkin, 1999).

People and team capabilities

Most effective emergency, crisis, and disaster responses are not facilitated by individuals working in isolation, but by teams working collaboratively (Gibson and Gibson 2023), with these teams demonstrating:

- "Rapidly developing individual and shared sensemaking (within the team and with other teams) and to make agreed decisions within the contextual timeframe".
- "Formal and intuitive synchronisation of interdependent tasks by the different team members".
- "High levels of trust, collaboration, and improvisation".
- "Understanding and acceptance of error as a learning opportunity".
- "Ability to immediately receive feedback on individual and team decisions and actions, and to rapidly act on that feedback".
- "The migration of leadership within the team as situational change demands different expertise[96]".

---

[95] Usually a senior public servant or ministerial position.

[96] Also known as 'deference to expertise'.

However, many leaders and decision-makers assume that teams will just perform as and when required, with little thought to their development on the way (Gibson and Gibson, 2023). Teams that may be performing in an acceptable manner during business-as-usual, are unlikely to perform well under the demands of a crisis unless their capabilities, resourcing, and direction are accounted for as part of preparation. High performing teams do not just arise naturally, they require developing and nurturing. There is a considerable amount of literature on the development of high performing teams, with examples in:

- High reliability organisations (Oeij et al, 2017; Riley et al, 2010; Burke et al, 2007; Baker et al, 2006).
- Elite sports (Morgan et al, 2015; Finn and McKenna, 2010; Green, 2005; Baker et al, 2003).
- Healthcare (Stout et al, 2017; Salas and Rosen, 2013; Riley et al, 2011; Riley et al, 2010; Jain et al, 2008; Benn et al, 2007).
- Military (Goodwin et al, 2018; McGinn, 2015; US Army, 2015).
- Law enforcement (Bradley and Jancewicz, 2016; Wesnser, 2015; Hess and Hess, 2012; More and More, 2012),

High levels of trust and autonomy are both characteristics of high performing teams and essential factors that facilitate high performance in individuals. Trust and autonomy are both rapidly degraded in cultures that are perceived as toxic or overly micromanaged (Williams, 2019; Aubrey, 2012; Mohr et al, 2011; Härtel, 2008; Appelbaum, 2007). Which highlights the critical role that culture plays in sustaining all of the key traits associated with high performing teams, and in particular for a culture that is founded upon values shared across the team (Satell and Windschitl, 2021). Research (Pentland, 2012) has also highlighted the essential contribution of (high energy, high engagement, high exploration) communication to establishing and maintaining high performance teams.

Leadership

Leadership is not necessarily restricted to senior political figures and senior executive management (in fact it could be argued that such leadership has often been notable by its absence in these two groups) but is by its nature present at multiple levels of an organisation. However, crises frequently invalidate existing leadership systems (Rego and Garu, 2007), and a very different set of competencies and experience is often required in the high novelty, complexity, turbulence, and uncertainty of a crisis. The best available information has to be actively sought out (situational awareness), the most appropriate cognitive and emotional capabilities need to be used (shared sensemaking), risk needs to be recognised and decisions need to be made as close to the 'sharp end' of the crisis as possible, by those with the best capabilities to do so. An effective leader recognises when they are not the best suited to a particular situation and will allow and encourage others to take the lead, even on a very temporary basis, a concept known as deference to expertise.

Deference to expertise

Leadership which accepts and promotes 'deference to expertise' not only more effectively delegates responsibilities, it also helps to establish a culture where more junior staff are not afraid to speak up and identify problems and errors in the way that things are being directed and done (Godlock et al, 2017). However, in some situations a lack of care and an over-reliance on certain 'deferred experts' (i.e., deferring to an individual based upon their status, rather than to their actual expertise) can create a "prima donna syndrome" (Dekker, 2014). When such prima donnas arise, they are often characterised by an unwillingness to follow the established rules, an avoidance of accountability, and a rejection of any negative feedback. Further, their self-portrayal of specialist 'expertise' often goes unchallenged and overrides other legitimate organisational concerns. The presence of 'prima donnas' can result in competing information or opinions being disregarded, and lowered team effectiveness through their "corrosive" effects on team cohesion.

'Prima donnas' usually demonstrate high levels of 'psychological entitlement' for greater power and greater rewards, with this sense of entitlement contributing to lowered situational awareness and cognitive processing (Harvey and Martinko, 2008). Thus, the very fact that they are so relied upon as the 'expert', serves to reduce their complex problem solving and decision-making capabilities.

Emergent leadership

One of the features of a well-managed crisis is that effective leadership often emerges in unexpected places, where it was previously not officially assigned or recognised (Feddersen, 2020; Rowland et al, 2020; Anderson, 2018). Such emergent leadership has been shown to be especially important in public health crises and disasters (Nyenswah et al, 2016), and a key factor in influencing the performance of a current response (Sanford et al, 2020).

There is a deeply embedded cyclical relationship that often occurs during a crisis, where emergent leadership is inhibited, resulting in impaired situational awareness, sensemaking, and collaborative decision-making. Impairment of these factors then serves to further inhibit the formation of emergent leadership, creating and establishing a 'vicious cycle' that leads to further amplification of the crisis.

In recent years, in multiple western democracies, there has been an increasing politicisation of public health leadership (Halverson, 2021; Abbas, 2020; Cowper, 2020; Frieden et al 2020, Hart et al, 2020; Huang 2020; McCracken and Ahmed, 2020; North 2020; Roper, 2020; Wan and Blake, 2020; Zaza, 2020; Sundin, 2019; Bekker et al, 2018; Gostin 2018; Phillips and Green, 2015; Chokshi and Stine, 2013; Goldberg, 2012; Brown, 2010; Meadowcraft, 2008), suppressing emergent leadership, adversely affecting the quality of leadership decisions, and ultimately producing undesirable outcomes.

Crisis leadership performance

During and in the wake of a crisis, the performance of leaders is judged not only by peers and masters (political and otherwise) but also, especially in government, by the general public. Such 'assessments' are generally shallow in nature (Boin et al, 2013; 2008) based upon 'symbolic performance', and judging leaders to be either 'good' or 'bad', in what can become either a blame game or unquestioning faith. Reality is far more nuanced, again a bad outcome does not necessarily mean, in every instance, a bad process, and many good and bad outcomes are achieved despite any particular leadership capability and performance.

For example, during the height of the pandemic there was much media praise for the then New Zealand Prime Minister's (Jacinta Arden) leadership in responding to and limiting the impacts of the pandemic. Whilst undoubtedly fulfilling one of political leadership's requirements - building public confidence, the reality may be very different from the broadsheet and broadcast hyperbole and bias. A recent factual analysis shows the reality to be less impressive than the media commentary would have us believe (Windsor et al, 2020). Indicating that New Zealand's cultural values rather than its political leadership have had far more influence on New Zealand's success in its response to COVID-19 response. A phenomenon also seen in other jurisdictions.

There are multiple factors that will determine the effectiveness of crisis leadership, beyond the cognitive, emotional, and experiential capabilities of the leaders and senior decision-makers themselves (Benlahcene et al, 2020; Boin et al, 2013; 2008), and that affect different parts of a crisis' progression (Keen et al, 2020; Liu et al, 2020; Kupucu and Ustun, 2018; Persson et al, 2017; DuBrin, 2013; Stern, 2013; Kapucu and Garayev, 2011; Boin and t'Hart, 2003), including:

- Those that affect leader/decision-maker situational awareness:
    - the availability of information about the situation – is the available information useful? Are best endeavours made to actively make *enquiries* about, *access*, and *use* the information?
    - The extent to which situational awareness is developed collectively and shared (Nofi, 2000);
    - the rate of change in the situation (dynamic vs stable), and the speed of onset and approach of changing conditions;
    - the complexity of the developing situation;
    - the novelty of the developing situation and the degree to which it can be pattern matched to previous experience;
    - the degree to which future change can be predicted or anticipated, including to what extent can historical experience inform the present and help to envision the future?
    - the timeliness of leaders/decision-makers in recognising changing conditions;
    - the ability and willingness to seek out and recognise deviations from the expected context (Roe and Schulman, 2008), including error seeking behaviour;
    - the existence of a culture that not only facilitates but encourages collective situational awareness (Weick and Sutcliffe, 2002).

- Those that affect the performance of leader/decision-maker sensemaking and decision-making, including:
  - the level of uncertainty and ambiguity associated with the available information;
  - the level of trust in the sources of information and confidence in the quality and integrity of that information;
  - the presence of and reliance on assumptions, especially where these assumptions are unsurfaced or unchallenged;
  - the courage to make decisions in the face of remaining significant uncertainty;
  - the timeliness of decision-making in relation to the speed of onset and rate of change of the pertaining conditions.

- Those that affect enaction and delivery of outcomes:
  - the presence of systems that allow the timely and sufficient surveillance and monitoring of changing situations, emerging conditions, and the effectiveness of enacted decisions;
  - the willingness to actively deal with the outputs of this surveillance and monitoring, to adjust objectives, modify or abandon previous decisions, and change direction as required;
  - the willingness and ability to develop and maintain collaborative relationships, including with those that may have been previously viewed as competitors[97] or antagonists;
  - the ability to recognise, accept the necessity of, and invoke workarounds, that in turn elicit other undesirable issues that will need to be managed.

- The nature and extent of the outcomes achieved, including unintended outcomes:
  - the extent to which the hazards, threats, and risks associated with pursuing a decision and achieving the intended outcomes were recognised and understood;
  - the achievement of clarity and transparency, such as the extent to which the following were acknowledged and shared with others:
    - an understanding of the recognised hazards, threats, and risks,
    - knowledge about institutional capability and vulnerabilities,
    - the recognition of priority objectives,
    - the symbolic versus practical nature of pronounced outcomes.

---

[97] Such competition is also manifest within the government/public sector, not only in competition for resources, but also for status, recognition, preferences, privileges, promotion, and other rewards.

Effective crisis leadership

Effective crisis leadership (Dirani et al, 2020; Bogusky-Halper, 2020; Brower, 2020; Koehn, 2020; Luscombe, 2020; McGuinness, 2020; Obrenovic, 2020; Veil, 2020; Wooten and James, 2008) requires:

- *Clarity of values, purpose, and direction*: if leadership achieves nothing else, it absolutely has to establish what needs to be done, why this has to be done, and how this is to be done.

- *Maintaining a moral and ethical capacity*: one of the first casualties of a crisis can be the abandonment of the ethical and moral compass for the sake of expediency (Gentlin, 2020; Goyette, 2020; Johnson, 2019; Jurkiewicz, 2017; Parnell et al, 2013). Often, when the "end justifies the means" we embark upon a journey that results in an abrogation of certain human rights and loss of long held freedoms, for uncertain long term gains.

- *Empathy*: the ability to develop a real understanding of how the crisis is perceived by others and how both the crisis and the leadership decisions will affect these others, physically, emotionally, and psychologically. It is not enough to just understand, nor is it simply a case of expressing sympathy. Rather empathy needs to be incorporated into decisions, communications, and actions.

- *Trust*: needs to be built, nurtured, and maintained. Trust in the leader helps build the courage and confidence of those without power, allowing them to participate, speak up, and make decisions without fear of the consequences of doing so. However, trust goes both ways, and the effective crisis leader has to be able to establish trust with others. In non-routine situations an effective leader is willing to listen to others and take their advice, to give up some of their 'power', and encourage others to take on more responsibility. The issue of trust goes beyond hierarchical relationships within teams, and needs to be a key feature of the relationships between different leaders and different teams. An absence of trust can only lead to dysfunctional relationships and the loss of 'crisis leadership'.

- *Clarity of authorities, accountabilities, and responsibilities*. One of the key expectations of an incident management/command system is that there is an absolute clarity about who makes what decisions and who takes what actions. This helps to ensure that everyone undertakes their required duties, everyone else knows who is doing what, and there are clear chains of decision-making and authority. This also allows for when any disruption in the chain of command occurs, providing clear alternatives should a particular senior decision-maker not be available. In particular, such clarity can be a major factor in helping to mitigate the risk of 'turf wars' breaking out when confidence and decisiveness are premium requirements.

- *Thinking and decision-making in a vacuum*. Most crises are characterised by an acute shortage of certain types and amounts of data and information that would normally be available for routine decision-making. As well as coping with this uncertainty, decision-making also has to deal with high levels of ambiguity and paradoxes[98] (Carmine et al, 2021), a natural reaction to which is to try to reduce or remove them before making a decision. Counterintuitively, it seems that more effective decision-making can be achieved through an ability to 'embrace' these paradoxes and ambiguities, and to seek out errors and failures (and learn from them), rather than to avoid them (Fraher and Grint, 2018).

- *Learning and adaptation*: as a crisis progresses, it is important that leaders do not just learn, but learn the right things, being able to separate out the meaningful information from the random 'noise' that accompanies every crisis. Decisions, their implementation, and outcomes need to be monitored in as close to real time as is feasible, with errors and misalignments sought out, recognised, accepted, and adjusted for (Fraher and Grint, 2016).

Rapid feedback capability is absolutely essential within any non-routine situation. In dealing with the wicked problems that many public health crises present, the existence of some level of error and failure will always be part of developing and implementing a solution. Wicked problems are rarely solved by putting in place a single obvious solution, and initial decisions often subsequently prove to be inadequate. Decisions may need to be reversed, changed, or built upon multiple times before effective solutions begin to be mobilised. Inadequate leadership always tries to hide errors and deny failure, and when mistakes become apparent to others and can no longer be denied, the default position is almost always to blame somebody else. By doing so, such leaders rarely escape the consequences of their actions. The problems they have sought to hide continue to fester, almost certainly guaranteeing the

[98] For example, the need to maintain good governance, control, and discipline during a crisis, versus the need to be flexible, agile, and adaptable.

emergence of even bigger problems in the future. Many superficially effective leaders continue this behaviour of denial hoping to have moved on to other ventures before the problem 'explodes' uncontrollably.

Many 'failures' that result in crises and disasters are strongly associated with decision-making undertaken by 'novices' rather than by 'experts'. This is not meant to imply that junior staff are novices, whilst senior executives are by default experts. The distinction between the two is as dependent upon the context in which individuals are placed, as it is dependent upon the *specific relevance* of the experience and competencies of those involved. Government bureaucracies are replete with senior executives (novices) that clearly do not have the knowledge, skills, and experiences for their substantive roles, let alone the required capabilities for managing the high complexity and uncertainty of a crisis. Novices rely on rigid rules and scripts that allow little freedom for exercising professional informed judgment. They follow prescribed processes, even when these processes make little sense or are outpaced by changing conditions. Novices possess certain traits that force their reliance on inflexible scripts that in turn reinforce their traits (Figure 6). This can be exceptionally problematic for novices, allowing them to become strongly committed to an inappropriate course of action. Without the cognitive or emotional resources to either meaningfully recognise their predicament or to question and challenge their direction and choices.

At the opposite end of the spectrum to these novice traits are those that characterise high expertise, traits that allow individuals to exploit other ways of problem-solving and decision-making rather than just following inflexible scripts. Effective leadership and decision making in a fast-moving crisis requires expertise that is not commonly found in the ranks of those that prosper in a highly script and rigid rules-based environment. Whilst some individuals may possess such skills innately or through real life experience, they are more usually developed through education and practice. Capabilities that require foresight, commitment, and resourcing in order to develop over time.

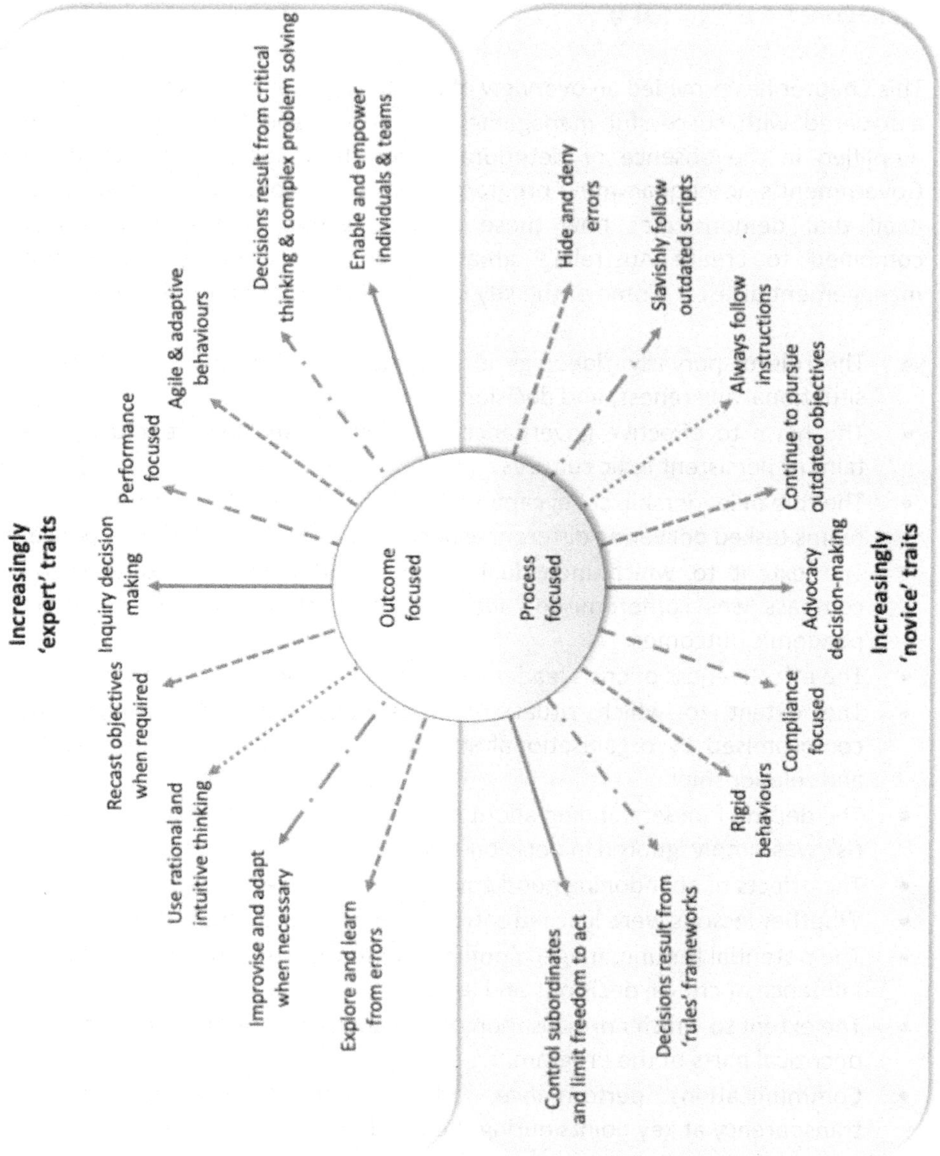

Figure 6: Expert vs novice traits

Chapter summary

This Chapter has provided an overview of attributes, capabilities, and practices associated with successful management of crises, and how crises can be amplified in the absence or deterioration of these factors. The Victorian Government's hotel quarantine program debacle is a contained case study in itself that demonstrates how these various factors (and their absence) combined to create Australia's greatest ever public policy and health management disaster. Some of the key themes form this Chapter include:

- The role of pervasive ideology in influencing agency and team culture, situational awareness, and decision-making.
- The harm to effective governance and decision-making created by the taint of persistent toxic cultures.
- The role of leadership style, capabilities, and ethics on the performance of teams tasked delivering different aspects of Victoria's pandemic response.
- The extent to which individual leaders' and decision-makers' moral compass was compromised, and the effect of this ethical fading on pandemic outcomes.
- The effectiveness of crisis leadership during the core of the pandemic.
- The extent to which situational awareness and sensemaking was compromised by organisational structures, bureaucratic arrangements, and relationships.
- The depth of understanding about important risks, or the extent to which risk was simply ignored in decision-making.
- The effects of abandoning good governance practices.
- Whether lessons were learned satisfactorily, or were simply disregarded.
- The potential for unmanaged conflicts of interest to be present, and their influence of critical decisions and actions.
- The extent to which normalisation of deviance was present in the delivery of critical parts of the Program.
- Communications performance, and reasons behind the lack of transparency at key points during the pandemic response.
- The level of trust apparent through the various interactions and relations that would have been critical for the delivery of a successful program.

The various themes explored in this Chapter will be revisited in the remaining Chapters to help explain how The Victorian Government could so completely fail in its top priority: to protect the people of Victoria.

Part 2

Analysis of the hotel quarantine failure

6
The analysis

Why are decisions made that result in tragic outcomes

We will probably never know the fundamental reasons why certain decisions associated with the Hotel Quarantine Program were made in the way that they were. The Andrews government appears to have made a determined effort to keep various aspects of the pandemic response closely guarded secrets. Certainly, the Coate Inquiry did not probe deeply into the underlying causal factors that drove and influenced these decisions.

This was not unique to just the Coate Inquiry. In fact, many similar Inquiries, Royal Commissions, and investigations can be criticised for only seeking out proximal causes (often blaming someone for a decision made or action taken) without seeking to really understand the development and flows of underlying conditions that led to those decisions and actions. In doing so, formal inquiries infrequently address and provide sustainable solutions to deep underlying problems. Many inquiries uncover similar factors time after time, irrespective of whether they are looking into bushfires, floods, child abuse, health disasters, or other catastrophic incidents (Binskin et al, 2020; Government of South Australia, 2020; Walker, 2020; McClellan et al, 2017; Jerrard, 2012; Holmes, 2011, 2010; Teague et al, 2010). The actual value provided from many such formal investigations and inquiries for developing sustainable lessons learned should be carefully considered. Yet whatever the effectiveness or failure of these approaches, we as individuals or as part of organisations fail consistently to learn from the past, even when meaningful lessons are identified and made available.

Where a decision can be identified that directly contributed to a catastrophic failure, the natural reaction is to blame someone. However, in many circumstances this is unfair and unjust, as decisions are usually made with the best of intentions and using the best information that was available at the time. Although there will be some circumstances where such blame may be warranted. Especially where an individual wilfully ignores or disregards information, covers up their errors and in doing so creates even bigger problems, or makes decisions not with 'good intent' but to instead further their own interests. Such instances are blatant conflicts of interest and often represent egregious failures in moral, ethical, and legal duty of care.

The purpose of this case study is not to assign blame to any individual or group, involved in front line decisions and actions. In the lead up to the hotel quarantine debacle, decisions were made that were inadequate and inappropriate, and such flawed decision-making continued throughout the unfolding crisis and into its aftermath. Criticisms and accusations have also been laid by several commentators about capabilities of and decisions made by some of those involved in conducting the Coate Inquiry. Whether the hotel quarantine failure was a result of long-term systemic failure in the government and bureaucracy, or was a result of incompetence and conflicting interests in the immediate lead up to and during the pandemic, is a matter of exploration and discussion for succeeding chapters.

Thinking beyond the evidence

As a result of the Coate Inquiry's inability to probe deeply enough, and the apparent avoidance of a full and honest disclosure by some of those involved in the Hotel Quarantine Program's critical decisions, it is not possible to conclusively determine all of the underlying factors. It is therefore difficult to establish the extent to which different individuals undertook 'best endeavours', displayed incompetence, or were wilfully negligent in their approach and decision-making.

It is left to the reader to make their own judgements, which by necessity must look to and beyond the Coate Inquiry's evidence, balancing the known facts with the possible events and actions that may reasonably be believed to have occurred. Each reader must decide what did and could plausibly have happened (or did not happen), and evaluate the network of relationships within the range of potential underlying conditions. It is not possible to say definitively what did happen, and because of either the unintentional or deliberate obfuscation of many of those involved, it is only possible to explore what could plausibly have occurred.

Each reader therefore needs to evaluate the potential relationships to determine which were causal (including contributing and influencing factors), and which were correlations, coincidences, or were merely spurious. Questions especially need to be asked about what did drive and influence *each* key decision associated with the Hotel Quarantine Program disaster and the subsequent government pandemic response.

For example, to what extent did the following occur:

- An inadequate or inappropriate situational awareness and sensemaking because the decision-maker:
    - did not have the access to the required information;
    - was overwhelmed by the demands of the situation and the volume of available information;
    - was faced with a situation that was changing so rapidly they were unable to maintain sufficient and current situational awareness;
    - rejected the information provided;
    - lacked the cognitive expertise and professional experience to understand and interpret the available information;
    - relied on other (inadequate, inaccurate, inappropriate, or misleading) sources of information;
    - was deliberately prevented by others from establishing effective situational awareness.

- A decision-maker that did not have sufficient expertise and experience to:
    - develop appropriate situational awareness or sensemaking about a developing situation;
    - make a meaningful analysis of a highly complex situation;
    - understand that some issues represented 'wicked problems' and required a very different approach to their resolution;
    - have the cognitive and emotional means to bring together the resources to resolve these wicked problems;
    - recognise that not all decisions were reversible and therefore required different approaches to making those 'irreversible' decisions;
    - to make sense of the technical information they did have access to, and to make reasonable decisions informed by their technical knowledge and specialist experience.

- A decision-maker believing that they had little flexibility, because:
    - the speed with which conditions were changing severely limited their choices;
    - cultural and other institutional imperatives strongly directed their decision-making;
    - to follow their own judgment seemed substantially out of lockstep with the attitudes and judgements of their peers or superiors;

  - they either received directions from others, or understood or believed such directions to have been issued;
  - there was opposition, either real or perceived, against other potentially more effective options.

- A decision-maker had already accepted the need for a certain outcome, and self-directed their decision-making to achieve that predetermined outcome, because this outcome:
  - fulfilled a higher priority ideological objective;
  - provided a self-interest advantage;
  - established a 'safe position', for which the decision-maker believed they would not be criticised;
  - was believed to be the most acceptable outcome to those in more senior positions of authority and power.

As subsequent Chapters delve more deeply into the decisions and actions taken by elected officials and the bureaucracy, these issues highlighted above should be continually referred to by the reader.

An approach

The following analysis of the Victorian Hotel Quarantine Program failure does not follow a traditional incident investigation methodology. Such methodologies are based upon linear thinking and linear problem solving. These types of approaches can work well in situations where mechanistic (linear) systems are present and where simple linear cause-and-effect relationships prevail. However, when human factors such as situational awareness, cognition, emotion, and decision-making (and their complex interactions) are increasingly involved, the system becomes increasingly non-linear (complex) and traditional analytical methods increasingly struggle to provide any sensible analysis (Pupilidy and Vesel, 2017). The failure of the Hotel Quarantine Program is typical of many other such catastrophic failures[99].

[99] Such as the Deepwater Horizon oil rig blow out (National Commission, 2010a), the Mercedes Benz A Class crisis (Puchan, 2001), the North American mass blackout (US-Canada PSOTF, 2004), Enron collapse (Anon., 2007; Millon, 2003), Columbia space shuttle disaster (CAIB, 2003), and many more incidents.

The proximal causes of the Andrews government failure (as with many other catastrophic disasters) resulted from people trying to balance a range of competing information, priorities, obligations (such as legal requirements. operational directions, and potential political influence), and conflicting options, in an environment of high novelty, complexity and uncertainty. All of which were underpinned by systematically and systemically flawed contributing decisions, behaviours and actions over the months and years preceding the pandemic. As the analysis will explore further, these proximal causes were underpinned by a complex web of questionable relationships, decisions, behaviours, and actions that stretched back to the early days of Victoria's incumbent Labor government.

One of the key factors in this tragedy appears to have been an overriding assumption that the Hotel Quarantine Program was just another routine problem that could be solved using routine thinking and routine processes. For example, DJPR approached their responsibilities as though this was just another simple logistical exercise, with little or no understanding of the unique requirements needed for managing a complex public health situation. Once Operation Soteria was underway, their apparent hubris[100] blinded them to the need to continue to adapt as the situation started to evolve in unexpected (but nevertheless highly predictable[101]) ways. Similar thinking seems to have been common throughout the Victorian Government's mismanagement of the Hotel Quarantine Program.

It must also be remembered that the failure of the Hotel Quarantine Program was not just the 801 tragic deaths resulting from quarantine breaches, but the abuses and impacts on those forcibly detained, and on those frontline staff that had to endure unacceptable conditions that put their safety, health, and wellbeing at risk. The prosecution of Victoria's Health Department by WorkSafe indicates the extent to which workers' health and safety were apparently disregarded. Whilst a report by the Victorian Ombudsman showed that not only did alleged human rights abuses occur within the Program, but also occurred in record numbers as a result of the Andrews government's decisions made during the pandemic (ABC News, 2021b; Ombudsman; 2021; Piovesan, 2021c; Tuffield 2021a; IMCL, 2020)

---

[100] The leaked self-congratulatory video produced by Global Victoria about their role in the Hotel Quarantine program illustrates the level of hubris in existence at the time, and the complete lack of awareness about their unsuitability for a project of this nature (Sky News, 2020c; The Australian, 2020). An example of the Dunning-Kruger effect in action.

[101] At least it should have been predictable to anyone with a basic understanding of infectious disease control.

Governance and decision-making

There were a number of pivotal decisions that were central to the Victorian Hotel Quarantine Program failure, turning what could under other circumstances have been a limited quarantine breach, into what has been called Australia's greatest public administration failure (Kemp, 2020; McCulloch, 2020). These decisions are tightly interlinked:

- The decision to place high risk quarantine facilities into hotels in highly vulnerable Melbourne CBD[102] locations (the issues associated with this decision are considered in Part 3).
- The decision to use private security for first tier control of on-the-ground quarantine arrangements, a decision that was inconsistent with the approach undertaken by other States and Territories which used police and military personnel.
- The decision to reject the Australian Government's offer of substantial Australian Defence Force (ADF) personnel, again a decision out of step with other jurisdictions.
- The decision to appoint a seemingly inappropriate and incapable security provider (Unified Security Group) to undertake major responsibilities for providing quarantine hotel security.
- The decisions to assign critical responsibilities to agencies that were outside of their normal scope of operations, and with requirements that sat outside of their knowledge base and capabilities.
- The decisions to appoint a number of individual officials to roles for which they were clearly not competent, experienced, or otherwise suited.
- The decisions to ignore expert advice and to sideline or exclude technical experts from key roles.
- The decisions associated with establishing and resourcing a manifestly ineffective and incapable contact tracing and testing system that was rapidly overwhelmed, by even the early stages of community transmission.
- The decisions to chronically under fund and under resource Victoria's public health system and hospital system over many years, which would severely compromise the State's ability to cope with increasing pandemic cases.

These decisions did not stand in isolation. They were influenced and driven by earlier decisions made by the Andrews' Labor Government in the years and months before the pandemic. In doing so they established the basis for the

---

[102] CBD: central business district.

decisions made during the pandemic, and from which initial quarantine breaches would evolve into a tragic public health disaster.

The Coate Inquiry has found the Hotel Quarantine Program disaster to represent a monumental failure of both good governance and of acceptable government (Coate, 2020a). However, the Coate Inquiry has itself failed to convincingly determine the root causes of these manifest failures[103]. The unwillingness of responsible individuals to come forward and be transparent, the apparent obfuscation and factually incorrect responses by some witnesses, and widescale 'memory failures' of various Ministers and bureaucrats, means that many of the contributing factors to the Program's failure will not be made public. By necessity, this analysis must make some inferences and suppositions about the circumstances leading up to these key decisions. The reader is left to undertake their own analysis and exercise judgement about what may or may not have occurred.

[103] Such as the now widely criticised and discredited conclusion about the 'creeping assumption' of the decision to use private security.

7
The decision to use private security

How pivotal was the decision to use private security in the Victorian Hotel Quarantine Program? Whilst using police and ADF would not have guaranteed against a quarantine breach[104], it is highly likely that the myriad of problems that arose from the use of private security would not have occurred. The Inquiry found that the use of police, instead of private security, would have minimised the risk of an outbreak occurring[105].

The origin of the decision

The Coate Inquiry states that whilst no individual can be identified as making the decision about private security, and that this decision was made at a meeting of officials at the State Control Centre (SCC) at 4.30pm on 27 March. The Inquiry also makes the case that the (now former) Police Commissioner, Graham Ashton, was highly influential in that decision (although he was not present at this 'decision-making meeting' held at the SCC). Apparently, the insinuation was that private security was used because Victoria Police did not want to take on the primary on-the-ground role at the quarantine hotels. Whilst there may have been some such preference for police not taking on this role, there is compelling evidence that suggests other players were far more influential in the decision to use private security.

The Inquiry also suggested that, under this 'police influence', the appropriateness of using private security became an accepted position with no single person having sole responsibility for that decision. This constituted the so called 'creeping assumption' and collective decision-making[106] previously alluded during the Inquiry. All that is really apparent is that multiple Ministers and senior public servants suffered a collective inability to recall who made this key decision.

---

104 And experiences later in the pandemic in other jurisdictions show that such breaches could occur.

105 Coate, 2020a p. 201.

106 Collective decision making, where apparently the decision to use private security crept up on a group of senior bureaucrats, without them being aware of an actual decision being made, and without any identifiable person being responsible. Whilst in some circumstance this could occur, it is highly implausible given the evidence of other events leading up to this 'decision'.

This raises several questions that still require resolution:

- If such a 'creeping assumption' occurred, how did such an assumption arise?
- How did a consensus viewpoint on this multi-million dollar spend of public money on outsourcing arise?
- An 'assumption' is something that is accepted without proof, how plausible is it that $40+ million and the safety of people's lives would be committed to, based on a mere assumption?
- An assumption is based on beliefs, in which case which individual held the belief that private security should be used, and on what grounds was that belief based?
- If Chief Commissioner Graham Ashton had that belief (as was alleged, but with little real evidence), what situations gave rise to him developing those beliefs. Was this based on a resistance to Victoria Police being used in such a role? Or did he believe that others in more powerful positions desired such an outcome?
- How could such an assumption prevail in Victoria, when that assumption ran counter to the Prime Minister's early announcement about the availability of ADF personnel to assist in the Program, and was likely discussed in National Cabinet?
- How could such an assumption be held by only the Victorian Government, when no other jurisdiction appears to have held a similar assumption?

The Health Minister at the time (Jenny Mikakos) told the Inquiry that the suggestion of a creeping assumption was "implausible" (Kolovos, 2020a). Whilst an examination of the evidence presented to the Inquiry and matters subsequently revealed by the media seems to be inconsistent with the Inquiry's conclusion on this matter (see below).

What influenced the decision?

Several pieces of 'evidence' point to the *possibility* of either Victoria Police command or alternatively someone close to Premier Daniel Andrews influencing key decisions being made about hotel quarantine arrangements. How realistic is it that such influence could have occurred and that relevant experts did not resist such influence? Could sufficient pressure have been placed upon some decision-makers by those in more senior positions?

The use of private security certainly had the potential to create a number of temporary jobs, an economic objective that would have been perceived as an easy win for the Government. This could have been a strong influence on whoever made the decision to use private security, either by direct pressure or bring perceived as an attractive government objective. Such a political outcome could easily have become a more potent driving force than public health priorities and the need to manage community risk effectively.

There is certainly a precedent for those in power to ignore expert advice in pursuit of ideological or political ends. This was demonstrated in the long running saga and break-up of the CFA[107] within Victoria. Senior officials that stood up to Premier or resisted the proposed changes were either dismissed or 'resigned' their positions, including the Emergency Services Minister, the CEO of the Country Fire Authority (CFA), the recently appointed Chief Fire Officer, 20 plus other senior officers, and the entire CFA Board (SBS, 2017; Wakeling, 2020). Whilst the replacement Chief Fire Officer, Steve Warrington, resigned after refusing to sign-off on certain requirements[108] associated with the breakup of the CFA (Marozzi and Willingham, 2020; Reiss, 2020), along with the resignation of the MFB's[109] Chief Officer (AAP, 2019). This was followed by the resignation of the CFA's Deputy Chief Fire Officer (Stephanie Rotarangi), only part way through her contract. That the decision to break up the CFA was politically motivated (rather than to create a more efficient service) appears even more convincing.

To add to the potential for collusion, IBAC subsequently launched an investigation (Operation Richmond) into possible secret deals between the Victorian Government and the United Firefighters Union, including assertions about the Premier Daniel Andrews possible involvement (McKenzie and Sakkal, 2022; Sakkal, 2022; Carey and Towell, 2018). The investigation which commenced in 2019, has been subject to legal action blocking the release of the report (Johnston, 2023a, 2023b). With indications that the legal actions have been resolved, it is now expected that the Operation Richmond report will be released sometime in 2024.

It is highly plausible that if such a coercive culture persisted within government during the pandemic response, and within the Hotel Quarantine Program in

---

[107] Country Fire Authority

[108] Claims have been made by the ABC and SBS that the United Firefighters Union was allowed significant power (by the Andrews government) in the development of these requirements.

[109] Metropolitan Fire Brigade/ Metropolitan Fire and Emergency Services Board.

particular, then anyone who believed that the Premier had made a decision about private security would plausibly be fearful of expressing any dissension.

The power and influence of Victoria Police?

If the Inquiry's findings are accurate, then Victorian Police Chief Commissioner Graham Ashton played a major influential role in the decision to use private security instead of using police and ADF personnel. Indeed, Graham Ashton's text referring to a DPC deal about the use of private security indicates his proximity to the time of the decision and suggests a close nexus in decision-making with Ashton and those close to the Premier. This raises two important questions how influential was Victoria Police's position on the decision to use private security? And to what extent was Victoria Police's position subject to political influence and interference?

Could Victoria Police (VicPol) really have been that influential that they were able to drive government decision-making in breach of long standing democratic principles? The existence of the strong relationship between police and the Labor Government has been spoken about by commentators and journalists for many years. Indeed, *"whatever VicPol wants, VicPol gets"* has been a frequent catchphrase used by some senior Victorian Government bureaucrats. To what extent did such an apparently widespread perception have a basis in fact?

Victoria Police has had substantial influence within Government, both through its Command and through the Police Association's political power (Halse, 2011; Finnane, 2000). The Police Association even demonstrated its political influence during the previous Liberal government's tenure, with secret deals being made over changes to legislation (Le Grand and Ferguson, 2012). More recently, during the pandemic, allegations have been made that it was pressure from the "police unions" that caused Daniel Andrews to refuse military assistance from the Commonwealth (Smith, 2020). Whilst the Victorian Government granted extraordinary powers to police during the pandemic, unparalleled by any other state and unprecedented in Australia's history (Roskam, 2020b; Hickey and Nedim, 2020; HRW, 2020; Lewis, 2020b; VEOHRC, 2021). At the same time the Victorian Government has allowed police to use apparently excessive and unreasonable force, including the use of pepper spray and ballistic weapons on unarmed protestors (MALS, 2021).

Aversion to using police?

To what extent was the prospect of using sworn police personnel to enforce quarantine an unpopular option within Victoria Police? Certainly, it appears that Victoria Police were more comfortable with some group, other than themselves, being responsible for first tier protective duties at quarantine hotels. An understandable preference, given that Victoria Police had been subject to increasing workload demands in enforcing the government's imposed COVID restrictions on businesses and on the public. Imposing additional resourcing demands for policing quarantine hotels would have certainly stretched limited capability even further, perhaps critically given the very real prospect of some form of civil unrest arising.

Any option that would have prevented a significant additional work overload would have been acceptable, if not welcomed by Victoria Police. In fact, Victoria Police gave evidence to the Inquiry that using police 24/7 at quarantine hotels was regarded as an inefficient deployment of resources. However, there was also no evidence that the potential benefits of using Victoria Police in a wider role beyond enforcement was even considered[110].

Could police command's concerns about 'inefficiency' have overridden the need to manage substantial public health risks? Alternatively, could there have been concerns that Victoria Police members would be unnecessarily exposed to COVID-19 infection, with the resulting substantial loss of policing capability for the State? Certainly, such concerns appear to have existed, since it was claimed that "a full risk assessment" was conducted for police to work at quarantine hotels with the subsequent development of detailed safety procedures[111]. Although, this did not lead to the implementation of an onsite police workforce. If such a risk assessment was conducted, why then did police not raise similar concerns about security guards becoming infected? Was there some assumption that working in the private sector conferred some extra immunity or risk mitigation against COVID-19?

Despite Victoria Police undertaking a risk assessment for their members' involvement at quarantine hotels, there is no evidence of anywhere else within the Victorian Government conducting a robust risk assessment on the obviously much greater risks of using private security instead of police. Someone, somewhere, made that fateful decision either in ignorance of the risk, or in the disregard of such risk. If the decision to use private security emanated from

---

[110] Coate, 2020a p. 201.
[111] Coate, 2020a p. 201.

within the police service, then it was a decision that put police self-interest above the interests of the Victorian public.

Whilst Victoria Police influencing political decision-making remains possible, there is no evidence about how this could have occurred. Conversely could Victoria Police command, along with other senior bureaucrats have been subject to undue influence from elsewhere?

Victoria Police, influenced or independent?

Concerns over police independence has a long history across multiple jurisdictions within Australia, as well as in Canada and the UK (Tomazin, 2019; Roach, 2018; 2017; Killey, 2017; Stenning, 2016; 2011), involving both sides of the political divide. Apparent political interference with policing has become increasingly evident in many western democracies, including in Victoria. This came to the forefront during the pandemic, in what many have seen as an over extension of police authority in acting against political protests and in enforcing their respective government's emergency restrictions (Campbell, 2021; Joint Committee on Human Rights, 2021; Martin, 2021; West, 2021; Bell et al 2020; Bowcott, 2021; Human Rights Watch, 2020a; Sumpton, 2020). Some 83 countries have been implicated in using the pandemic to justify widespread human rights abuses, including the suppression of free speech and the disproportionate use of police powers (Human Rights Watch, 2021).

Frequent allegations have been made about the Labor government's political interference in Victoria Police, especially during Daniel Andrews time as Premier. A former Deputy Commissioner of Victoria Police (Sir Ken Lay) has made multiple allegations relating to toxicity and corrupt behaviours (Le Grand and Cooper, 2019; Varga, 2019). This included an allegation that political staff working for former Labor Premier John Brumby and Police Minister Bob Cameron had asked the Deputy Commissioner to manipulate crime data to make it appear more favourable on the eve of a State election (Le Grand and Cooper, 2019).

Victoria's former Chief Commissioner (Ashton) has been subject to particular claims of a lack of independence from the Andrews government (Hutchinson, 2017), including:

- The appointment of previous close confidents of the Premier into senior positions within Victoria Police. For example, Graham Ashton's Chief of Staff was previously Daniel Andrews' Chief of Staff[112], an appointment that caused outrage at the time (Ferguson, 2016). Even more controversy arose when this Chief of Staff was subsequently appointed to an Assistant Commissioner role as head of the new "Gender Equality and Inclusion Command" (Lewis, 2019).

- Allegations into the political policing of demonstrations during COVID-19 restrictions. For example, the 'Black Lives Matters' (BLM) protests were not only allowed to proceed despite breaching restrictions, the tepid official response apparently amounted to de facto approval and support by both Victoria Police and the Andrews government (Baxendale, 2020c; Begg, 2020; Ferguson 2020; Kolovos, 2020d). A significantly different response was shown in New South Wales were the police initially sought to prevent the BLM protests from occurring, then making several arrests when the protests went ahead. Interestingly, Victoria's tacit acceptance of the societal need to protest, (but only when the purpose aligned with the Andrews government's ideology), did not extend to protests that where critical of the Premier and his policies (Ferri, 2020). Those involved in anti-lockdown and anti-mandated vaccine protests faced the use of excessive force, fines, arrest, and forced entry of their homes by police. Even some independent journalists, that were critical of the Victorian Government and of the standard of policing at these events, were arrested or pepper sprayed by police.

It also appears that some other Victoria Police enforcement operations during the pandemic were forced by political decisions, rather than by police or expert health advice or requests. Premier Daniel Andrews at various times alluded to some of the more onerous lockdown restrictions, such as the 8pm curfew, were out in place at the request of police or public health experts. However, during the Coate Inquiry, the Deputy Health Commander (Professor Michelle Giles) openly contradicted Daniel Andrews' stance (Vinall. 2020). It quickly became apparent that the curfew decision was not based on expert medical or scientific

---

112 Whilst Daniel Andrews was in opposition. The Chief of Staff is the closest adviser, and runs the political private office for their leader.

advice, or at the request of Victoria Police (Baxendale, 2020a; 2020b). When the Premier was challenged on the truthfulness of his statements and confronted by the denials of police and the Chief Health Officer, Andrews refused to reveal who made these decisions on harsher restrictions. Instead trying to deflect media attention with responses such as it made *"the job of the Victoria Police easier"*, still implying that the curfew was a police operational requirement.

The Premier was later forced to admit, despite his earlier denials, that the curfew *was his* decision (Chung, 2020). Perversely, it later emerged that this further removal of human rights had made no difference to the spread of COVID-19 (Tuffield, 2021d).

During the Inquiry, Graham Ashton (then Chief Commissioner) stated that whilst private security was a *preference* for Victoria Police, they did not make *the decision* on private security. It is therefore highly plausible that Victoria Police was subject to significant political influence and interference during the pandemic response (Cater, 2021a; Phillips,2021; Drummond, 2020; Roskam, 2020b), and that such influence or interference became a key factor in the private security decision. The question then becomes how could such political interference have occurred, and to what extent could Daniel Andrews (or those close to him) have been involved?

The decision-making sequence

The Coate Inquiry proposed that the private security decision was made at the 4.30pm SCC[113] meeting held on the 27 March 2020, and that no single person was responsible. Rather the decision to appoint private security arose from a collective process with multiple parties involved. Astonishingly, the identity of these parties has not been resolved, nor can any Minister or bureaucrat remember being part of a decision-making process.

However, when some of the actual evidence presented to the Inquiry and various irregularities uncovered subsequently by journalists (Credlin 2020a; 2020b; 2020c) are considered, the plausibility of this conclusion needs to be questioned. There are several pieces of evidence that appear incompatible with the Inquiry's conclusion, including:

---

[113] SCC: State Control Centre.

- A decision on private security was a matter of discussion earlier in the day, several hours before the SCC meeting, as revealed in various text messages and meeting notes.
- That the Premier himself stated at a press briefing, *well before the SCC meeting* that private security would be used. However, part of the Inquiry Report[114] appears to deflect attention from the Premier's statement by listing *"The remarks made by the Premier, and the corresponding media release"*, but then curiously omits the Premier's comment about private security made in his statement to the media. Although his actual words on the matter are buried elsewhere in the Inquiry Report.
- The transcript and audio record of the SCC meeting shows that there was no decision-making about private security as an option that occurred at this meeting. There was nothing that occurred during the meeting that remotely resembled a decision-making process about private security. When the use of private security was mentioned briefly during the meeting, it already appeared to be an established fact, accepted by those present. The transcripts indicate that the key players at the SCC meeting already knew that this decision had been made prior to the meeting being held, and it appeared that the option of using private security *was final and not up for debate or discussion about alternate options.*
- The chronology of key events (Figure 7) leading up to the 4.30pm SCC meeting clearly demonstrates opportunities for when the decision on private security could have been made.

[114] Page 119.

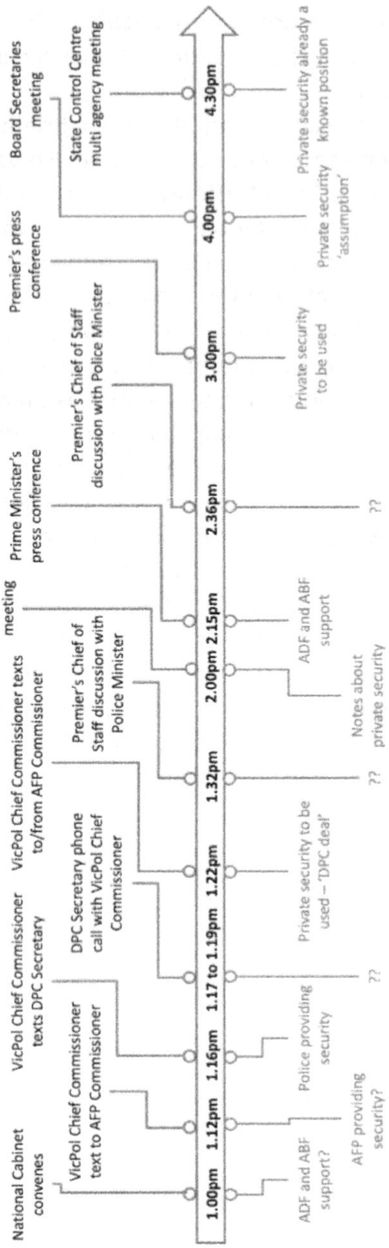

Figure 7: chronology of key events in the decision-making about the use of private security[115].

[115] ADF: Australian Defence Force; ABF: Australian Border Force; DPC: Victorian Department of Premier and Cabinet

A decision surfaces

How plausible is it that the Premier or those close to him played a key role in making this critical decision about using private security. The broad sequence of events early on 27 March 2020 included:

Late morning/early afternoon: Evidence indicates that initially Victoria Police command believed that police would be providing first tier protection at the quarantine hotels. However, this understanding changed following a conversation between the Police Chief Commissioner and one of the Premier's closest advisors.

12.06 pm: An email is sent from a senior executive in DPC[116] to DJPR staff seeking detailed information about hotel and other accommodation[117]. This email states that this is an urgent request *from the Premier* and that the information was going to be provided to the Premier's Private Office. This indicates that despite the Premier's protestations to the contrary, he appears to have been very closely involved in the micromanagement of the setup of the Program.

1.12 pm: the Police Chief Commissioner (Graham Ashton) texts the AFP[118] Commissioner about the possibility of using AFP officers at hotels, the use of private security did not appear to be a primary option that was being considered by VicPol at this time.

1.17pm: Chris Eccles (Secretary of the Department of Premier and Cabinet[119]) left the Premier and walked out of the National Cabinet[120] meeting to speak with the Premier's Chief of Staff, the content of which conversation remains unknown. The Chief of Staff was never asked, during the Coate Inquiry, to provide evidence or answer questions about any role that she may have played in decisions on the day.

---

[116] DPC: Department of Premier and Cabinet; DJPR: Department of Jobs, Precincts and Regions.

[117] Although the use of private security was not mentioned in the email.

[118] AFP: Australian Federal Police

[119] And close advisor to Premier Daniel Andrews.

[120] The National Cabinet convened at 1pm to discuss the hotel quarantine arrangements. During this meeting, all jurisdictions (without Victoria's future adherence) had agreed on a model of relevant state police and ADF to provide security and enforcement.

1.17pm: at about the same time as the conversation with the Chief of Staff, Eccles holds a phone conversation with the Victoria Police Chief Commissioner for just over two minutes. Originally under cross examination during the Inquiry, Eccles denied any such communication had occurred, but a later examination of phone records showed that the call did occur. Following the revelation of the phone call, Eccles resigned his position. After these revelations by the media, The Chief Commissioner of Victoria Police provided a fresh statement in evidence to the Inquiry in which he recalled that Eccles had told him that private security would be used at the quarantine hotels (Coë, 2020). This recollection was supported by the content of the text message sent from Ashton to the AFP Commissioner immediately after this phone conversation with the DPC Secretary. However, Eccles continued to deny any knowledge of the private security issue in cross examination during the Coate Inquiry.

1.19pm: a member of Premier Daniel Andrews' Private Office talks to DPC officials about 'security' (Sakkal, 2021b).

1.20pm: Chris Eccles speaks with Simon Phemister, Secretary of DJPR about the details of the Quarantine Hotel Program, including hotel rooms, cleaning, logistics), but surprisingly neither of them (when questioned at the Inquiry) could recall private security being discussed.

1.22pm*:* The Chief Commissioner of Victoria Police engages in a sequence of texts with the Australian Federal Police Commissioner (Reece Kershaw):

- Ashton: *"ADF will do passenger transfer and private security will be used"*.
- Kershaw: *"OK, that's new"*
- Ashton: *"I think that's the deal set up by our DPC"*[121].

1.35pm: Simon Phemister meets with Claire Feebey and other officials to begin detailed planning for the Program. Ms Feeby's notes from the meeting record that she will be in charge of everything including "security", and also mentions "Police and security".

It appears that the 1.17pm phone conversation between Eccles and Ashton results in a change in the Chief Commissioner's understanding of the security arrangements for the hotels, which suddenly moves from using police to using private security. The language used is also curious. Ashton does not text that it was a DPC '*decision*' but a DPC "*deal*", an odd word to use in this context. Unless of course Ashton believed that an agreement (i.e., a commercial deal) had

[121] Department of Premier and Cabinet.

already been made with a private security company to provide such a service. The truth of which is unlikely to emerge until an inquiry with real coercive powers (such as a Royal Commission) is eventually held.

2pm: An online MS Teams meeting was held with the Victoria Police Chief Commissioner (Graham Ashton), Emergency Management Commissioner (Andrew Crisp), and the Minister for Police (Lisa Neville). Notes written during the meeting by both Ashton and Crisp reveal that a decision had apparently been made about using private security in a primary role (Maiden, 2020). Other verbal evidence provided during cross examination[122] stated that on Ashton seeking confirmation about the arrangements, that Andrew Crisp confirmed the (already made) decision that private security would be used. It was also confirmed that there had been no consultation with Ashton or Neville on this decision. Although Crisp had earlier denied under cross examination that he knew about these arrangements at the time of the meeting. As Queen Elizabeth II famously said about a different controversy "*recollections may differ*".

Did the phone conversation with Chris Eccles lead the Chief Commissioner to believe that the Premier wanted private security to be used? Once journalists had uncovered this phone call (made part way through the National Cabinet meeting where hotel quarantine arrangements were being discussed). the new evidence clearly shows that:

- It does appear that Graham Ashton did believe that some 'deal' had been done by those close to the Premier to use private security.
- Over a period of six minutes Ashton went from not knowing about private security to informing a Federal Police colleague that private security would be used[123].
- The phone call from the DPC Secretary to the Chief Commissioner occurred during this six-minute time period (Durkin et al, 2020), when Ashton's understanding of the hotel security arrangements was changed.

The Inquiry drew a different conclusion from this evidence, and discounted the Chief Commissioner's position on when he believed the private security decision was made. Certainly, Graham Ashton's belief seems to align more closely with the evidence, than the does the Inquiry conclusion.

---

[122] Transcript of proceedings involving Graham Ashton, P-1669.

[123] Revealed in a message written by Ashton at 1.22pm on 27 March to AFP Commissioner Reece Kershaw.

The Premier's understanding of the arrangements

Although Premier Daniel Andrews made strenuous denials about being aware of the decision to use private security, or that he would even be involved in any operational decisions about the Hotel Quarantine Program, the available facts suggest otherwise. The Premier was forced on other occasions to admit he had previously provided misleading information (for example about the 8pm curfew decision). Publicly available evidence from the Coate Inquiry indicates that the Premier and some of his staff could have been *directly* involved in arrangements for the Hotel Quarantine Program during the 27th of March, when the key decisions were made:

- Although the Premier's Chief of Staff (Lissie Ratcliff) denied her involvement in the private security decision, later evidence (including the "secret text messages"[124]) *"reveals Ms Ratcliffe was central in plans to implement the program"* (Durkin et al, 2020), and shows her and the Premier in communication on 27th March about detailed operational aspects of the quarantine arrangements and her contacting the Minister for Police at 1.32pm and 2.36pm on that day (within the time periods when private security arrangements were likely being communicated). Ms Ratcliffe was never called to give evidence before the Inquiry and the nature of those conversations remains undisclosed.
- During Friday 27th March the Premier was also in contact with the CEO of Logistics at LinFox[125] regarding helping with the hotel arrangements. After the telephone conversation, the Premier texted his Chief of Staff: that the CEO of Linfox was happy to assist with these arrangements and LaManna[126] was happy to feed people. So, despite the Premier's protestations that he did not take an active role in operational matters to do with the set-up of the quarantine hotels, some text messages released by the Coate Inquiry indicated otherwise.
- There is no satisfactory explanation for why the Premier would talk about the use of private security 90 minutes before the decision was supposed to have been made at the SCC meeting and hours before he was supposed to have been told about private security. At 3pm on 27th March at a televised media briefing the Premier stated *"Police, **private security**, all of*

---

[124] Coë, 2020.

[125] Linfox is a large logistics solutions company, founded by billionaire Lindsay Fox. Premier Daniel Andrews has an allegedly very close relationship with the Fox family, including with Lindsay Fox's son Andrew (Flower 2021d; Le Grand et al 2021)

[126] LaManna is an independent supermarket and café in Essendon, some 20 minute plus drive from the quarantine hotels.

our health team will be able to monitor compliance in a much easier way, in a static location, one hotel or a series of hotels" (Andrews, 2020c). Yet no one knows or 'can recall' how the Premier came to know about private security, or who might have briefed him on the matter. As the Premier himself admitted under cross examination, he would not have spoken about private security unless he knew about its possible use in the Program.

The State Control Centre's role

Despite the Inquiry's deliberations, there is no actual evidence that the decision to use private security occurred during the 4.30pm SCC meeting, or occurred as a result of a loose collective effort. The audio recording and transcript of the SCC meeting does *not* show any development of an assumption (creeping or otherwise) to use private security. On the contrary, there was *no actual 'discussion'* about private security and there was *no actual decision* made to use private security during the SCC meeting. It appears that it was *already accepted* that private security would be used, before the virtual meeting commenced, and remained un-questioned throughout the meeting.

Prior to any 'discussion' on security or hotel arrangements in the meeting, Andrew Crisp[127] who was chairing the meeting had to leave to take an urgent call from the Premier[128]. Private security was only mentioned three times during the entirety of the meeting, twice without Andrew Crisp being present.

The very first time that private security is mentioned during the meeting (at 24 minutes 50 seconds into the meeting) was in response to being asked about security arrangements, Mick Grainger[129] stated "*But then in terms of security, there would be private security, and then the police would have a role perhaps around that as well, but we'd have to work through what that looks like"*[130]. This is not a decision, it is a statement of fact about a decision already made, prior to the SCC meeting, to use private security.

---

[127] Emergency Management Commissioner. Transcript of SCC meeting held on 27 March 2020, submitted in evidence to the Hotel Quarantine Program Inquiry. Accessed at: https://www.quarantineinquiry.vic.gov.au/exhibits.

[128] Line 15-34 page P-9. Transcript of SCC meeting held on 27 March 2020.

[129] Assistant Commissioner, Victoria Police.

[130] Line 20-22 page P-12. Transcript of SCC meeting held on 27 March 2020, submitted in evidence to the Hotel Quarantine Program Inquiry.
Accessed at: https://www.quarantineinquiry.vic.gov.au/exhibits.

The second mention of private security is from Claire Febey[131] (at 25 minutes into the meeting) *"as you say there are different steps in security, and some of it should be for example increasing the provisions of private security"*.

Overall, this brief exchange about the use of private security lasted for less than 30 seconds.

The third mention of private security occurred following Andrew Crisp's second exit and return to the SCC meeting[132], when he raised the matter (at about 53 minutes 10 seconds into the meeting): *"Sorry, can we get — again, apology, I missed, I had to step out again — but in terms of security at accommodation, have we covered that? Is it private security, Victoria Police? I understand that the preference of Victoria Police or the Chief Commissioner is that private security be the first line of security"*. Mick Grainger affirmed that was police's preference. The following exchange then took place[133] at about 53 minutes 40 seconds into the meeting: *"MR CRISP: So I'm just curious as to who's going to take responsibility around contracting private security? Is that DJPR? Claire? "MS FEEBEY*[134]*: Yes, I understand that's for us to take up"*.

Again, it appears that Andrew Crisp knew about the use of private security from outside of that meeting. He was not present during the first two mentions of private security but was sufficiently aware enough that private security was to be used that he sought confirmation on the matter when he later returned to the meeting.

These brief exchanges represent the entirety of the 'discussions' about private security at the SCC meeting. Where in any of this is an actual decision being made? The entire discussion covering private security, which lasted for under a minute, is about confirmation of prior decisions and the very superficial sharing of information, hardly a decision-making process.

The overall conduct of the SCC meeting was overwhelmingly about reporting on, confirming, and coordinating *decisions that had already been made prior to the SCC meeting*, including for airport arrangements, transport, accommodation, private security, etc. This was not a meeting about weighing the costs and benefits of different options and making critical decisions. Nor

---

131 Claire Febey at the time of the Program was the Executive Director, Priority Projects in the Department of Jobs, Precincts and Regions.

132 He had again been called out of the meeting.

133 Line 40-42 page P-22 Transcript of SCC meeting held on 27 March 2020.

134 Claire Febey, the newly appointed Executive Director Priority Project Unit, Department of Jobs Precincts and Regions.

was it about challenging various decision options. This meeting was predominantly about confirming and sharing information across agencies, about *what was already decided.*

The Inquiry's conclusion about the decision to use private security guards was that *"there were those with influence who contributed to an understanding being reached that private security would be used"*[135], which was then formalised as a decision at the SCC meeting. The Inquiry's conclusion requires us to believe that four brief mentions (taking about 40 seconds in total) represents a decision-making process about using private security, that:

- Was out of line with the approach being used by the other jurisdictions, and hence was a decision without precedence at that time.
- Went contrary to earlier statements out of National Cabinet.
- Represented a huge commitment of over $40 million public money.

Just how plausible is the Inquiry's conclusion that a decision to spend $40 million on private security took just 40 seconds with no actual discussion occurring, or even alternate options being raised? A decision is a conclusion made after considering options (at its most basic, "do we do this, or do we do something else?"). The conversation about private security was not a decision, it instead appeared to be just some restatements about a much earlier decision that was already known by those attending the SCC meeting, and that they were totally unwilling or unable to question.

It is also very interesting, that despite his later denials, it appears that the Dan Andrews was very closely involved in operational aspects of the Program. Why else would he have so urgently need to talk with Andrew Crisp, that he had the Commissioner pulled out of the critically important SCC meeting?

---

[135] Clause 133, page 132. Coate 2020b.

Was the Premier involved in the decision?

The Premier and those closest to him have denied any involvement in this decision about private security. However, there have been multiple occasions on which individual integrity and credibility have been questioned, during this crisis. The Premier has made repeated denials about various aspects of hotel quarantine matters, including that no offer of ADF support was made for the Program. For example, the Premier told a Victorian Parliamentary Inquiry that it was *"fundamentally incorrect to assert that there was hundreds of ADF staff on offer and somehow someone said no"*, and has repeatedly denied that offers of ADF support were made.

However, at a joint media conference, in which the Premier participated, after the National Cabinet on 27 March, it was stated: *"It has also been agreed that the Australian Defence Force will be engaged to support the implementation for these arrangements"* (Sky News, 2020c).

More convincingly, documentary evidence presented to the Coate Inquiry appears to contradict the Premier's assertions and have raised further questions about his credibility in the matter (Chung, 2020; Harris, 2020; Moore 2020; Taylor 2020a; Willingham and Handley, 2020; Wooten, 2020), and show that there were multiple communications, including:

- Emails between the two most senior officials reporting to the Prime Minister and the Premier respectively clearly showing that this offer was discussed.
- Later letters between the Prime Minister and the Premier, which apparently contradict the Premier's account.
- The Emergency Management Commissioner (Andrew Crisp) had requested ADF support to replace private security, but this was rescinded by Victoria the next day, apparently after communications between the Prime Minister's Private Office and that of Daniel Andrew's Private Office (Moore, 2020). The Premier later admitted that some 16 hours after Andrew Crisp had made the request, the decision to rescind this request was made by Victoria's Crisis Council of Cabinet chaired by Daniel Andrews himself (Baxendale and Varga, 2020).
- The former Health Minister Jenny Mikakos made a statement to the Inquiry that the Premier's evidence about private security should be "treated with caution" (Kolovos, 2020a). Following the release of the Inquiry Final Report on 21 December 2020, the former Minister then made a statement about the lack of transparency in the Inquiry, stating that the

> Inquiry has *"failed to ask key questions"* and highlighting that some of the Premier's phone records had been redacted in their entirety and made subject to a non-publication order (Barron and Flower, 2020; Piovesan, 2020). The Premier then refused point blank to release his phone records, which would have either helped to support his assertions, or have helped to confirm his complicity.

How probable is it that the Premier would have had some knowledge of, or involvement in the private security decision, given his apparent hands-on involvement in other aspects of the Program on 27th March and his announcement about private security some *90 minutes before* the decision was apparently made at the SCC? It even appears that the Premier may have given a de facto admission that the decision to use private security was made earlier in the day of the 27th March, *if not before* (Baxendale and Varga, 2020).

How much weight should be given to the Premier's denials about his involvement in or prior knowledge about the private security decision. Notwithstanding the media commentary about the lack of transparency about government decisions, the Premier's integrity has been called into question on multiple other matters. There were multiple occasions when the Premier's truthfulness about decisions (such as the 8pm curfew) being based upon medical and police advice have been challenged, with Premier eventually being forced to admit the truth about some of his earlier misinformation. In the case of the curfew, Daniel Andrews was later forced to admit that the curfew was his decision and was not requested by either Health or Police. Since then, the government has made strenuous efforts to block the release of other documents relating to medical advice on the mandatory lockdowns, even in the face of directions to do so by the Victorian Information Commissioner and the Courts. (Clarke, 2021a; Goldin, 2021; Piovesan; 2021d).

A similar pattern of behaviour seems to have persisted over the following years, leading right up to the time when he finally resigned. In the wake of his resignation, Daniel Andrews' credibility (along with some other senior Ministers) was again questioned following revelations about the decision to cancel the Commonwealth Games which were to be held in regional Victoria (AAP, 2023; Durkin, 2023; Ferguson and Freri, 2023; Hansard, 2023; Johnston; 2023; Sakkal and Rooney, 2023; Willingham, 2023)

There is increasing evidence that the use of prolonged lockdowns may have been a serious misstep (Pak et al, 2021), that in many jurisdictions their effectiveness at reducing COVID-19 related death rates have been exaggerated, and their overall benefits have been minimal. Countries that did not impose prolonged mandatory lockdowns have fared no worse than, and at times better than those countries with such lockdowns, but with very different longer term economic, employment, social, community health, and mental health outcomes (Creighton, 2022; Herby et al, 2022).

Similarly, in January 2022 it was revealed that government decisions on vaccine booster shot mandates, crowd capacity increases at the Australian Tennis Open, and the suspension of IVF procedures were made without medical advice, with no consultation with the Chief Health Officer or his team on these matters (Meehan, 2022). There have been suggestions that Andrews and his Ministers listen to health advice only when it is aligned with their interests, and ignore the advice when it is not (Benardi, 2020).

Concerns have also been raised about the legitimacy of some of the health advice that has been provided. Allegations have been made that the government and its bureaucrats have misstated statistics in support of several decisions that have been made. In the case of justifying wearing masks outdoors, that they have exaggerated the risk of outdoor transmission some 50 times higher than reality, with their claims of 5% transmission versus the much lower 0.1% transmission shown in international studies (Goldin, 2021). The decision to enforce the wearing of masks by children in school has been especially contentious, with conflicting studies and claims about their effectiveness (Busby, 2022; Kavanagh, 2022a; Heneghan and Jefferson, 2022; McKeever, 2022; PHO, 2022; Tang, 2022; Bell and Traxler, 2021; DOE, 2022; Broadfoot, 2021). Again, statistics have been apparently misstated by the Chief Health Officer in support of the mandate, with it being claimed that 8% of UK children had absences due to COVID when they returned to school, when the actual absentee rate was below 1% (Cameron, 2021).

Was the decision-making process about private security robust?

The decision to use private security in quarantine hotels is most remarkable for an almost complete absence of any evidence that anything resembling an actual robust decision-making process was in place. Even the most rudimentary look at risk exposures associated with using private security should have set off sufficient alarm bells that some serious consideration of alternate approaches or the imposition of additional controls should have occurred. It appears that multiple decisions were made that were based on unrecognised and unvalidated assumptions, where risk was either not considered or was purposefully ignored. All parties involved, from the Premier and responsible Ministers, to senior and middle ranking bureaucrats all deny any participation in or knowledge of the decision to use private security. That the decision-making was wholly either incompetent, or alternatively was driven by another agenda, where public health was a secondary consideration, are both plausible conclusions.

Whilst the Coate Inquiry concluded that no person could be blamed for the decision to use private security, decisions such as this do not suddenly materialise out of thin air. Someone had to identify private security either as an option or as a mandated requirement. The first person that we know to have mentioned private security is the Chief Commissioner of Victoria Police, shortly after speaking to the DPC Secretary (who left the Premier in the National Cabinet meeting to do so). The next person to publicly mention private security was the Premier himself. On the balance of probabilities, a decision to use private security was made or discussed sometime in the hours before the 4.30pm SCC meeting.

From the pure perspective of the known chronology, individuals that appear to be the closet in time to this crucial decision time period were:

- The Premier, Daniel Andrews.
- The Premier's Chief of Staff, Lissie Ratcliff.
- The Department of Premier and Cabinet Secretary, Chris Eccles[136].
- The Chief Commissioner of Victoria Police, Graham Ashton.
- Minister for Police, Lisa Neville.

All of whom have denied any direct involvement in the decisions, and who all appear to have suffered similar memory lapses over the same time period[137]

[136] Who resigned in the aftermath of misinformation provided to the Inquiry.
[137] Apart from Lissie Ratcliff who was not called before the Inquiry and therefore could not be asked questions about her memory of the events.

Problematic risk assessment

Even in the absence of the most basic documentation of the key decision-making process, and the inability of the Inquiry to identify what, when, and by whom key decisions were made, it appears that there was little if any consideration of risk about the use of private security.

This raises three key questions which have yet to be answered:

- Was the need for risk assessment, in the presence of substantial uncertainty, likely harm, and known serious vulnerabilities, simply ignored?
- Were the outcomes of risk assessments (either formal or informal) simply rejected or disregarded because they conflicted with a predetermined and desired outcome to use private security?
- Was the process for risk assessment used within Victorian Government agencies simply unfit for purpose, and no robust analysis was available?

Ignoring the risk

Since the real decision-making process about the use of private security for first tier protection remains unknown, we may never know how risk was considered, if at all. It is not unknown for government programs to be implemented hurriedly (for example over a weekend) and for the presence of risk to be ignored.

Such a scenario occurred in the Labor Rudd Government's 'pink batts' Homeowners' Insulation Program, which resulted in the tragic deaths of four workers, multiple serious injuries, and hundreds of house fires, along with allegations of widescale fraud. The program was instituted during 2009-2010, in an attempt to counter some of the effects of the earlier global financial crisis of 2007-2008.

In this particular case, the desired outcome (the need for an economic stimulus) overrode any real consideration of safety-related risk. Whilst the opportunity to learn from the problems and experience of other overseas jurisdictions on similar programs was dismissed on the grounds of expediency. The Royal Commission into the 'pink batts' program (Hanger, 2014) identified a number of failings and learnings which have direct relevance to other types of government programs[138], including:

- The existence of conflicting aims in a program that "inevitably" give rise to tension and conflict. For example, the need for an urgent response versus the need for "careful planning over time".
- The allocation of responsibilities to a government agency that was "ill-equipped to deal with a program of its size and complexity".
- The political appointment of key leadership positions within the program (in the case of the 'pink batts' program, by Prime Minister Rudd), rather than a robust selection based upon the most experienced and qualified for the job.
- A failure to "identify and manage the risk".
- Allowing resources to be used that were "unsuitable and dangerous".
- Relaxing training and competency requirements, and instead substituting poorly specified supervision requirements.
- Allowing on-the-ground activities to commence without a "robust audit and compliance regime" in place.
- Divesting responsibility for monitoring health and safety arrangements to other entities.

Each of the above points could be applied equally to the Victorian Hotel Quarantine Program debacle in a case of lessons *definitely not learned*.

The risks of using private security

The risks of using private security in the context of the Hotel Quarantine Program should have been obvious. Although Victoria Police and others seem to have been comfortable initially with the use of private security (in general), this 'comfort' seems to have been entirely based upon their past experience of working with private operators on *sporting and other events*. However, no one in police or government seems to have considered the difference between security guards working in a high risk health environment (quarantine hotels) and undertaking crowd control at a football match. Sporting events and massed gathering are contexts for which many private security officers are specifically trained and are contexts that private security companies are usually familiar and experienced in working within.

---

[138] And would have provided incredibly useful learning for planning the hotel quarantine program.

Conversely, it has long been recognised that inexperienced security guards cannot be simply dropped into a health setting and be expected to function effectively and safely. Security guards in hospitals require highly specialised training, with nationally recognised competencies and training programs in place (Australian Government, 2019; 2014). Many of the reputable security companies offer ready (specially) trained 'healthcare security guards'. On top of which, before starting work, these security guards receive additional intensive induction training from health professionals which includes detailed instruction on infection control within a health care setting.

None of this should have been a surprise to decision-makers within the Victorian Government. A 30 second internet search would have provided a wealth of information on security in health care, including training, standard operating procedures, and even advice and reviews undertaken by the Victorian Government itself (Victorian Government, 2017). Before the pandemic, to place security guards into a high risk environment in a hospital, without even the most basic training would have been regarded as wilful negligence. How different then was the placement of untrained security guards into the high infection risk environment of a quarantine hotel?

Anyone with even a basic understanding of private security contracting understands that, when a highly experienced and highly competent security company takes over a guarding contract, the transition process requires weeks if not months of careful management if it is to be successful. Even before such transition takes place, good security operators spend weeks planning and resourcing the transition. Almost anyone that has managed a new outsourced security contract will have experienced multiple non-compliances with the terms of the contract and other serious operating problems during the transition and subsequent settle-in period. Effective transitions are not achieved in a matter of a few days, even for highly familiar types of work.

Furthermore, one of the most basic requirements is that the security provider has a safe work management system, detailed standard operating procedures (SOPS), and an appropriately trained workforce in place before starting on-the-ground work. Capabilities that seem to have been absent in Unified Security's case. Any competent contract manager would be expected to review and approve these SOPS and the quality of security personnel assigned to an outsourced contract. Such assurance is not a luxury or 'nice to have', it is an absolutely fundamental activity in managing a security contract. Expecting that a private security contract can operate well from day one, without effective monitoring and oversight begins to look like gross negligence. To expect that such private security providers and their employees could instantly and seamlessly transition into a public health quarantine operation was at best naïve, smacks of incompetence and at worst is grossly (even wilfully) negligent.

A problematic industry

Although there was an apparent 'comfort' with using private security contractors, warning bells should have been ringing from the very first mention of using such outsourcing in the Program. Significant problems within the private security industry were know publicly for some considerable time before the pandemic, including the existence of some rogue operators, poorly trained employees, a highly casualised and low paid work force (forcing many security guards to have multiple other jobs elsewhere), extreme cost minimisation measures (short cuts), along with poor health and safety compliance. Even the most basic competent risk assessment should have identified the huge level of risk associated with the use of private security as the Victorian Government intended. Was such a risk assessment simply not conducted, or was the risk reporting simply ignored by those involved in the key decisions and management of the Program?

One of the reasons for establishing the government's preferred supplier panel for security outsourcing was to pre-evaluate the suitability and reliability of selected reputable security firms in order to avoid some of the known problems and risks within the industry. In the year before the pandemic, the Victorian Government itself had raised its concerns about these serious problems within the security industry, and in 2019 had announced a future review into the industry (McGinn, 2019a).

Despite the fact that there are many private security companies that are responsible, trustworthy, and perform well, the industry as a whole does not carry such a reputation. In the years preceding the pandemic there were substantial concerns about serious vulnerabilities within the security industry, such as:

- The overall ineffective regulation of the industry, and questionable compliance with requirements.
- Poor quality training and inadequate skills maintenance of guards and supervisors, including issues with the quality of the training content leading to security-related qualifications.

- Questions about integrity and probity within the industry, including occurrences of serious misconduct, with a number of cases involving fatalities.
- The generally low education levels, poor competencies, and inadequate language skills of many of those employed as private security guards.
- The relatively low levels of remuneration and poor job security of many security guards operating in a hugely casualised workforce. This included the necessity for many security company employees to work multiple other jobs[139] (such as taxi/Uber drivers, food delivery drivers, in supermarkets, etc.).
- Inadequate on the job supervision.
- Security guards operating under unsafe working conditions, including the lack of provision of adequate equipment.
- Uncontrolled subcontracting and sham contracting of guards.

Unfortunately, there is no evidence that the Victorian Government undertook any serious competent consideration of risk, control effectiveness, or vulnerabilities before decisions about private security were made. This is surprising given that the problems with the security industry were known to and discussed amongst officials at the time[140]. To believe that Ministers and senior bureaucrats were not generally aware of problems within the industry stretches credulity too far. For a senior public servant or Minister not to realise that using private security could be problematic, they would have to have been living under a stone for the last decade. Premier ***Daniel Andrews himself announced an election commitment in 2018 to review the private security industry,*** and many of the known vulnerabilities had been picked up in the scope of the Victorian Government's intended reform of the industry (Victorian Government, 2020). Prior to the commencement of the Hotel Quarantine Program the Victorian Government[141] "*was on notice of those vulnerabilities, including the risk of inadequately trained staff, underpayment of wages and poor working conditions...*"[142].

---

[139] Which would substantially increase exposure to any guards that became infected during a pandemic, and massively increase the likelihood of significant community transmission occurring.

[140] Coate, 2020a p.170.

[141] This includes even the Premier admitting that he had prior awareness of problems within the security industry – Coate, 2020a p. 196.

[142] Coate, 2020a p. 195

Each of these known vulnerabilities subsequently played out during the early stages of the Hotel Quarantine Program, and became important contributing factors in the subsequent disaster.

It appears that decision-makers ignored these problems whilst in pursuit of objectives that had little to do with protecting public health. The choice of the agency that took charge of putting in place these quarantine arrangements (Department of Jobs, Precincts and Regions) rather than the Department of Health and Human Services perhaps gives a clue to what the true priority for the Victorian Government was at the time.

Misunderstanding the risk

It is now apparent that the risks of using private security in a public health quarantine setting were not adequately explored or subsequently managed. However, for the sake of argument let's make an assumption that risk was considered in decision-making (although there is little evidence to support such a bold assumption!). This then raises the question: *'If risk was considered, was the risk assessment process appropriate and adequate?'*.

Most Victorian Government agencies have in place risk management arrangements that are directly based upon the commonly used international Standard (adopted by Australia) for risk management: AS ISO 31000: 2018[143]. Many of these individual agency risk management arrangements are a direct adoption of the Standard, with little real customisation[144] by agencies to align with their own unique strategic and operational contexts. Although these risk management arrangements may function acceptably in relatively simple routine environments, standardised approaches (such as those based upon ISO 31000 and COSO[145]) are known to have a number of serious flaws (Gibson and Gibson, 2023), which can be further amplified by the way in which the Standards are interpreted and implemented.

---

143 Standards Australia, 2018

144 An informal review (by this author) of publicly available Victorian Government agency risk management methodologies revealed a number of serious conceptual problems and inconsistencies with the Australian Standard and better practices, questioning the appropriateness and accuracy of risk assessment conducted within those agencies. Numerous implementations of ISO31000 have been found to be almost unworkable, and produce misleading results that are commonly accepted by senior bureaucrats without questioning.

145 COSO: 2019

These types of methodologies can struggle in environments of high complexity and high uncertainty. To address some of these recognised problems, Standards Australia released a completely new Standard for disruption-related risk[146] in late 2020. Similarly, the International Standards Organisation recently published a technical specification on emerging risk Standard to further address some of the substantial shortcomings of the current ISO 31000 Standard, and has commenced a process for a revision and updating of the Standard. The Coate Inquiry did not investigate these matters, but they are valid lines of inquiry that should be explored and learned from, before similar failures in decision-making occur in the future, for example:

- To what extent are the risk management approaches used in government agencies fit-for-purpose under routine and under non-routine conditions?
- Are the significant limitations of current approaches sufficiently understood by analysts, advisors, and decision-makers?
- Are the agency's risk professionals sufficiently experienced and skilled to be able to use a range of different risk assessment tools beyond the very basic consequence/likelihood estimation promoted by ISO31000 (which often devolves into little more than just guesswork)?
- Is information about uncertainty and risk being developed and presented in ways that provide a sufficient basis for informed decision-making about complex and wicked problems?
- Do decision-makers have the right mix of experience and skills to interpret and make sense of risk-related information, and make effective decisions under deep uncertainty and high complexity?

Whilst there may have been some discomfort in the uncertainty surrounding the consequence and likelihood of potential future events that could arise from the use of private security, it appears that little was done to address this discomfort. It would have been a highly feasible approach to consider the well-known vulnerabilities within the security industry (that were apparently ignored), and ensure that controls were established from the very start of the Program to address those vulnerabilities. Either these issues were never looked into (which seems highly likely) or were just simply ignored for the sake of expediency in the face of ideological and political pressures.

In which case, the decision to use security in the front line role was not just a failure of risk management, it was an egregious failing of the decision-making process itself. This demonstrates that the Victorian Government and its various agencies need to consider adopting better decision-making approaches that

[146] Also relevant to a wide variety of different types of high consequence-low likelihood risk.

incorporate fundamental methodologies for better understanding vulnerability and uncertainty. Blind acceptance of a flawed methodology should no longer be tolerated.

The disregarded risk of using private security

The Inquiry concluded that the original intent of using private security to provide static guarding was not unreasonable[147]. However, this is a reasonable assumption only if effective systemic and sustainable controls could have been implemented, and the level of risk reduced to an acceptable level, by ensuring:

- The appointment of experienced, reliable, capable, and well-resourced security companies, with a strong commitment to the health and safety of their employees.
- Organisational cultures were in place that were positive, open, and supportive, allowing security guards to raise concerns and report on errors without fear of reprisal.
- Security workforces could deploy experienced and highly competent security guards that displayed high levels of personal integrity and commitment.
- High quality and consistent specialist technical training could be provided that aligned with the requirements of the work to be undertaken.
- Work practice controls could be established, including infection control, hand hygiene, social distancing, provision and correct use of PPE (personal protective equipment), etc.
- Clear objectives and directions for the work to be undertaken could be established.
- Robust workforce supervision would be in place that ensured procedures were followed, that non-conformances were detected, reported, and corrected in a timely manner
- Highly dependable assurance arrangements were working in a way that ensured that all key controls were operating as required, systematically and consistently.
- Continuing reappraisal of risk and adjustment of controls would be undertaken, especially when changes in work requirements could introduce new hazards, threats, and vulnerabilities.
- Governance mechanisms would be implemented that allowed concerns and uncertainties to be freely raised with the controlling agency.

---

[147] Coate, 2020a p.195.

That there were multiple and continuing failures to establish these controls effectively in several of the high risk quarantine hotels is obvious in hindsight. For some of the security providers this proved to be an unsurmountable issue. Yet a passing familiarity with the security industry should have raised serious concerns about the feasibility of achieving even these basic control requirements.

A number of senior bureaucrats, in giving evidence to the Coate Inquiry stated that they thought the use of private security at quarantine hotels was appropriate given their experience of private security guards being used at *major events and at Parliament House.* For these officials to not recognise a difference in context between using private security at a cricket match or checking office doors had been locked, and using them in a high infection risk quarantine facility was unbelievably naïve.

If this situation was only a failure to manage risk in the appointment and operation of private security for the original intended limited duties, then this would be bad enough. However, private security was quickly used for duties well beyond their initial scope, work for which they were manifestly unprepared and untrained to undertake. This scope creep introduced exponentially higher levels of risk, for which there was no consideration of improving control effectiveness. That this could occur to workers potentially exposed to a highly infectious disease such as COVID is not just almost beyond belief, it is downright horrendous.

It is now known that the decision to appoint private security in such a role was one of the key contributing factors to the disaster that was to unfold. Yet, even as these private security guards were performing their duties at the hotels, there was still time, a window of opportunity to change the course of history. However, in typical form, decision-makers within government ignored the warnings about emerging problems within the quarantine hotels and carried on regardless.

Within 24 hours of the commencement of quarantine operation on site, leaked emails showed that there were serious concerns about the performance of private security guards. One public servant (from within DJPR[148]) emailing DHHS and Emergency Management Victoria requesting urgent assistance, stating that

"We request that Victoria Police is present 24/7 at each hotel starting from this evening. We ask that DHHS urgently make that request as the control agency".

148 Department of Jobs, Precincts and Regions.

This was followed by a second email, on the second day of the Program raising concerns that the private security guards were "not adequate' for the work they had to undertake (Jenkins, 2020b).

If someone is in informed about and becomes aware that there are serious control failings and unacceptable risk, but then fails to undertake reasonable measures, surely that constitutes gross negligence?

The decision to appoint Unified Security

Once the decision was made to use private security contactors in the quarantine hotels, there was then unseemly haste in contracting private security companies to provide the required large number of security guards. Three private companies were appointed, two very well respected large and nationally operated companies (MSS and Wilson Security, both on the government's preferred supplier panel), and Unified Security, a small 'aboriginal owned' and relatively unknown company from New South Wales, that seemed to emerge from nowhere.

If appointing private security to take on first tier responsibilities was not a bad enough error, the Victorian Government then made an even more monumental mistake, the decision to award Unified Security with most of the contracted security work in the quarantine hotels. Not only was this a calamitous decision, but all of the procurement, governance, and probity controls that should have prevented this from occurring where knowingly and deliberately avoided by bureaucrats.

Procurement and probity processes are established to remove personal feelings, personal advantage, bias, and unfounded preference from influencing the expenditure of public money. These same processes are meant to ensure the equitable treatment is afforded to all suppliers, and that products and services are selected to provide the best value for the taxpayer. In other words, the purpose of good probity is to mitigate key risks associated with appointing outsourced providers. Expediency is no excuse for abandoning due diligence, especially for extremely high risk operations. Certainly, when there is an urgent requirement for the purchase of services, the routine lengthy tender process can be avoided, but other controls then come into place to ensure that such a rapid procurement is still conducted appropriately. Unfortunately, in the case of Unified Security it appears that feelings, bias, and personal preference, seemingly driven by political ideology, played a far more important role than proper process. Relying on anecdotal and untested impressions is no substitute for factual evidence and is *prima facie* a profound failure of duty of care.

To appoint a relatively unknown, untested, and non-approved small security contractor for almost any type of work, without a robust procurement process is highly unusual and wholly inadequate. To appoint such a private security firm to work in the high risk environment of the Hotel Quarantine Program, especially given the known issues with the low capability culture endemic within the private security industry, almost beggars belief. To then appoint such a company and not ensure that much needed highly specialised training was provided, to not ensure that strict infection controls were established, and then to fail to establish strict oversight and assurance protocols is not just unfortunate, it appears to lay somewhere between gross negligence and absolute insanity.

Once the decision had been made to use private security for first tier guarding of the quarantine hotels, the subsequent decision to appoint Unified Security[149] is absolutely baffling.

Government breaches its own rules and guidance

At the time that early decisions were made about setting up the quarantine hotels, the Victorian Government already had an established panel of five pre-approved (and pre-evaluated) private security providers that had been established under a whole of government State Purchase Contract - "Security Services Contract" in 2018 (Buying for Victoria, 2020). The purpose of establishing this panel was to address some of the known problems endemic within the security industry, and to provide assurance to government buyers in their procurement processes. The details of the preferred provider panel were freely available online to all government agencies and to the general public.

The existence of the panel provided a de facto exemption from having to go through a lengthy tender process (in effect the selection of panel members was a quasi-tender process). Any or all members of the panel could have been appointed without delay to provide the required services for the Hotel Quarantine Program. These panel suppliers represented some of the largest, best resourced, and most experienced security providers operating nationally

[149] Unified Security Group (Australia) Pty Ltd.

within Australia, and included significant specialist expertise of operating in high infection risk environments such as hospitals. One of the reasons for the existence of such preferred supplier panels is to allow procurement to occur quickly, as was the situation for the Hotel Quarantine Program.

Yet a decision was made to appoint Unified Security, a relatively unknown and unproven small Sydney based company, to undertake the vast bulk of the quarantine work. This was a company that had previously been seen to be unsuitable for providing even general security services to the Victorian Government, when they were refused admission to the State Purchase Contract[150] and membership of the Panel. This is worth repeating, not only did certain bureaucrats deliberately ignore the Panel, but they went out of their way to appoint 'Unified', a company that had been rejected as unsuitable to be a security provider for the Victorian Government!

Flawed and devalued procurement

It is blatantly apparent that the appointment of Unified Security breached the Victorian Government's own procurement and probity rules and advice, during the procurement process undertaken by DJPR. A process that was informal and highly unusual to say the least, even accepting the imperatives imposed by the pandemic and the imposed time constraints.

Like many other failings within the Hotel Quarantine Program, the procurement decisions occurred in a government culture where governance and technical capability had been greatly devalued in recent years. This included the removal of both the Victorian Government's centralised procurement training, and the qualification system for those conducting procurements (Diamante, 2020).

---

150 Coate, 2020a p. 18.

Bad practice built on by more bad practice

Not only was Unified Security appointed, but they were then given the bulk of the security work, worth initially in the region of $30m of public money for three months work[151,152]. Whilst two other companies (that were on the approved provider contract) were also appointed, but collectively offered only a minor proportion of the work and fees.

The Coate Inquiry states that Unified Security was allocated the initial quarantine work on the basis that they were the *first to make a phone call to the responsible* DJPR *executive* on the Saturday morning[153] following the previous day's decision to use private security.

However, this seems to be even less straightforward than the Coate Inquiry implies. It appears that a lot of reliance was placed upon an explanatory email sent by Ms Currie on 30 March justifying the appointment of Unified Security for the bulk of the work, based upon their being the first company to contact Ms Currie at 6.52am on Saturday 28th March (with Wilson not contacting them until 8.00am), with "discussions at 7.00am, as to their capability and capacity"[154]. During the Inquiry it was revealed just how low such capability and capacity was in reality at that time.

Curiously another earlier internal email[155] sent on the Saturday morning at 7.04am from Ms Currie paints a more nuanced picture:

"Morning all - Unified CEO has texted. Will call him shortly to advise that I will get back to him".

In this email, there was no suggestion that discussions about the provision of a contract for the bulk of the security work were to commence with Unified Security.

---

[151] Which probably represents one of the most lucrative government security contracts in Australia' history, and also one of the most informal processes in the history of modern governance practices.

[152] On a $30m initial contract, Unified Security eventually invoiced the Victorian Government for $44m.

[153] Coate, 2020a p. 171.

[154] Exhibit HQI0037c_RP Annexures to Witness Statement of Ms Katrina Currie.

[155] Exhibit HQI0037c_RP Annexures to Witness Statement of Ms Katrina Currie.

Therefore, we are asked to believe that the key selection criteria for the awarding of what eventually became $44m of work to Unified, was actually made on the basis of whichever company was the first to call back a government bureaucrat on a Saturday morning. This sounds more like a radio show phone-in (where the first person to call gets a pair of tickets to the Spice Girls reunion concert), than a major government procurement. The only difference being that when the Victorian Government ran the 'phone competition', the first caller did not have to qualify by answering a quiz question to prove their eligibility. There is obviously less need for prudence and probity when one is just spending tens of millions of tax-payers' dollars.

The DJPR[156] senior executive officer (Ms Currie) involved in the appointment of Unified Security stated to the Inquiry that she did not know that Unified Security was not a member of the State Procurement Contract Panel. In writing this book, it took the author about 11 seconds to find comprehensive details about the State Procurement Contract online and to make a copy of the list of the five approved security companies. Is asking someone to spend 11 seconds validating qualifications in a $60m plus procurement an unreasonable expectation? Furthermore, this same bureaucrat admitted to the Coate Inquiry that "*Prior to my involvement in the hotel quarantine program, I did not have experience contracting for the provision of security services*". Admittedly, senior public servants were under significant time pressures at this time, however the Victorian Purchasing Board had provided official advice to agency procurement teams that during the pandemic the *"State Procurement Contract Panels should continue to be used"*[157]. This was advice that was patently ignored, as DJPR continued with a process that not only seriously breached DJPR's own procurement policies but also consciously and deliberately breached the Department of Treasury and Finance requirements.

Once it started to become more widely known that Unified Security were to be appointed, serious concerns were raised within other government agencies and by the Victorian Trades Hall Council about the unsuitability of this particular company, and communicated to the responsible DJPR bureaucrat. These concerns were met with the all too familiar disregard, and the informal appointment of Unified Security continued. In what has been labelled "one of the worst examples of procurement malpractice in Australia's history" (Rogers, 2020).

---

[156] Department of, Jobs, Precincts, and Regions.
[157] Coate, 2020b, p22.

Why was it so important that Unified be appointed?

How and why Unified Security was initially identified by key decision-makers remains a mystery, although the Inquiry does comment on a positive 'impression' about the company that was held by some bureaucrats. Although it seems that this 'impression' was based more upon on Unified's activities on "inclusive employment" rather than the actual provision of security guarding services[158].

The key differentiator that has been put forward for their selection, and for Ms Currie's[159] strong advocacy[160] for Unified was that they were an "aboriginal owned and controlled" company, and that appointing them met the Victorian Government's social procurement objectives[161]. Certainly, it appears that indigenous employment was a defining priority, perhaps unsurprisingly given Ms Currie' substantive role at the time was *Executive Director Employment and Inclusion*.

However, even this indigenous ownership claim appears to have been a sham structure designed to mislead and make Unified eligible for inclusion in the Hotel Quarantine Program (Ross, 2021a).

Other evidence raises questions about the legitimacy of this explanation, in particular, an email circulated to senior DEDJTR bureaucrats as late as 10.09pm on Friday 27th March, in which two options were proposed for security companies, Securecorp nominated by one bureaucrat and, nominated by Ms Currie - Wilson Security, with absolutely no mention of Unified Security[162]. Although Unified does suddenly make an appearance in an email about 45 minutes later with no explanation given for their unexpected inclusion[163]. During the Inquiry Ms Currie stated that she had selected Unified and Wilsons because they were the first two names on a list[164] of four companies that she

---

[158] Coate, 2020a, p 171.

[159] Ms Currie was the senior bureaucrat within DJPR responsible for directing the security procurement process.

[160] Although in her evidence she tried to deny that this aboriginal status had been a factor in the initial contact with Unified.

[161] Coate, 2020a p. 172

[162] Exhibit HQI0037c_RP Annexures to Witness Statement of Ms Katrina Currie.

[163] Exhibit HQI0037c_RP Annexures to Witness Statement of Ms Katrina Currie.

[164] That was apparently compiled by the employment engagement team reporting to Ms Currie.

had been given[165]. Although Unified's selection was later justified on the grounds that they were an 'aboriginal owned' company. However, it appears that the apparent conflict between these two explanations was not investigated more thoroughly during the Inquiry.

There were also serious integrity issues regarding the Directors of Unified Security existing at the time, that any competent due diligence could have uncovered. Following a notification from the New South Wales Police Security Licensing and Enforcement Directorate (SLED) in *November 2019* that David Milward[166] was not "a suitable close associate", it appears that Unified hid Milward's continuing involvement with the company. Unified Security subsequently informed SLED that Milward was no longer a shareholder, however, in March 2020, just as the Hotel Quarantine Program was being established, all of Unified shares were obtained by a holding company owned by Milward and Luigi Trunzo. A 'change' in ownership that was not notified to SLED. It has also been alleged that Milward and Trunzo operated as shadow directors, receiving over $20m in 'dividends' and loans, as the company began to collapse in 2021, whilst owing over $12m in debts (Ross, 2021b), a considerable amount of which, it has been alleged, was for unpaid sub-contractors working in Victoria and New South Wales.

However, one of DEDJTR senior procurement specialist[167] did raise serious concerns about the appointment of Unified Security, in an email, well before any contracts were signed:

"**Subject:** RE: Security Services Procurement
Need clarity on the rationale for going outside the SPC in this instance. I understand there was an urgency to get things up and running quickly over the weekend but to have a non-approved firm providing security and effectively enforcing government regulation at quarantine sites off the back of some emails and phone calls presents significant risk to individuals involved and the department/Government that is not easily mitigated.
Need to be clear on why this provider was engaged instead of the other SPC providers (noting requests went to Wilson and MSS - who are on the SPC) and whether there is any reason to continue with them (as opposed to switching them out for an SPC provider, for example) in order to assist in determining next steps."[168]

---

165 Inquiry into COVID-19 Hotel Quarantine Program, Transcript of Proceedings Day 8, 27 August 2020.

166 David Milward was one of the owners and Directors of Unified Security.

167 Exhibit HQI0037c_RP Annexures to Witness Statement of Ms Katrina Currie.

168 SPC: State Procurement Contract.

As one of the bureaucrats involved (Ms Currie) stated in an email revealed by the Inquiry, when she justified the appointment of Unified: *"is absolutely in keeping the State Government social procurement objective of utilising an Aboriginal business"*. More than strongly suggesting that social procurement was a far more important priority than ensuring effective public health measures, or looking after the safety and welfare of travellers incarcerated in quarantine.

Thus, it appears that a $44m worth of work was given to an unapproved, largely unknown company, that was arguably the least experienced and least capable compared with any of the security companies that were on the approved supplier risk, and was a company operating with serious integrity issues. Yet despite being the most expensive option, the entire justification for their appointment was that they were 'indigenous owned' and some superficial perceptions of largely uniformed bureaucrats that had no idea of their actual professional security capabilities. This is precisely the issue that a robust procurement process seeks to avoid, a robust process that in the case of the Hotel Quarantine Program was deliberately ignored and set aside.

At a time when identity politics was driving a whole range of decision-making within the Victorian Government, Unified Security ticked the indigenous employment box. A tick that appears to have carried more weight than any rationale and due diligence judgement based on experience, capability, and capacity, or the mitigation of risk, and which went against multiple other sources of advice from both within and outside of Victorian Government agencies. It is ironic that the company chosen for this apparent virtue signalling exercise ended up being the company whose indigenous credentials appeared to be tenuous to say the least.

However, despite the lack of good procurement process, and the appointment of what many regarded as a 'dodgy' company, surely there were some benefits realised for indigenous employment. Well, it seems pretty much no. Unified Security just recruited casuals straight of the street (including advertising on the online Gumtree site), or subcontracted to other non-indigenous security companies. It appears that there was little if any impact on Victorian indigenous employment opportunities, but millions of dollars did flow into a NSW company, and allegedly into the pockets of its two shadow Directors. Even if indigenous employment was the only objective, then it appears that the Victorian Government failed abysmally at achieving even this.

The obvious reason for selecting and appointing Unified Security was........., sorry I can't think of a single valid argument for their appointment, a view that seemed to be shared by several others within the bureaucracy and within the Victorian Trades Hall Council at the time. A reasonable view that was ignored in the rush to appoint Unified as an *"absolutely essential"*, but still officially unexplained, part of the Hotel Quarantine Program.

The questions of conflict of interest and corruption

There has also been some speculation about personal contacts between the owners of the company and unidentified individuals within government that could have influenced the procurement decision. However, such allegations do not appear to have been subject to any rigorous investigation and public scrutiny, and hence remain speculative. Whatever prior relationships may or may not have existed, it is apparent that government officials were easily able to obtain the principal owner's contact details outside of business hours (Credlin, 2020d) to discuss the appointment. It is also interesting that a WhatsAPP messaging group was apparently set up for Unified Security's involvement in the Hotel Quarantine Program at least an hour before they were officially approached via email at 11.33pm on Friday 27th March 2020 (Baker, 2020).

That Unified Security was put forward as one of the preferred providers (despite their manifest unsuitability) is unlikely to have been a result of blatant corruption. There is no evidence suggesting that brown paper bags full of cash were handed over before the decision, or that secret commissions were paid during the contract. It is more plausible that prior relationships and familiarity with the company were highly influential, and equally likely that appointing an 'aboriginal-owned' company provided an irresistible opportunity to grandstand on contributing to the Andrews government's political priorities. It also cannot be ruled out that the desire for virtue signalling by conflicted individuals, which has been prevalent within the Andrews government and bureaucracy over recent years (Cater, 2021b; Rollason, 2021a; Hope 2020, Gottliebsen, 2019; Mulholland, 2017) played a significant role in the decision. It is also possible that there was some political interference in the procurement process.

In the afternoon of Friday 27 March at 12.17pm, around about the time that it appears the decision about private security was made, an internal DJPR email about a cleaning and security workforce was sent:

"Hi there
Unni is going to write to us shortly with potential requirements for a cleaning and security workforce to manage people who might be quarantined in hotel rooms. We might need to act quickly depending on govt policy choices in this space so would be good to think through options. It would be in metro and regions"[169]

This email is interesting on a number of points:

Firstly, it is clear at as early as 12.17pm on the day of the fateful 'private security decision', that the use of private security was being discussed by senior bureaucrats as an apparently accepted fact. Although Ms Currie, during the inquiry, stated this was the Government policy on whether private security would actually be used.

Secondly, that the bureaucracy appeared not to have identified potential contractors at that stage.

Thirdly, that "government *policy* choices" (political interference?) would determine how security services would be procured.

It is a pity that the Coate Inquiry did not more deeply probe the decisions and activities behind this email. The truth may lie in the raft of other emails sent and received by DJPR, but which were redacted at the request of the Department and remain inaccessible for independent or public scrutiny.

A terrible decision becomes a disastrous decision

This grievous non-compliance with government procurement policies was further compounded when Unified's role was substantially increased beyond the two Crown hotels for which they were originally contracted. This reallocation of the bulk of the security contract work seems to have been entirely based on superficial and anecdotal accounts of their 'performance', which were accepted by Victorian government bureaucrats without any form of validation.

[169] Exhibit HQI0037c_RP Annexures to Witness Statement of Ms Katrina Currie.

One of the reasons put forward by DJPR officials for reallocating work to Unified was that one of the other providers (Wilson Security) was perceived as being difficult because they were raising unpalatable issues with the contract managers. However, we now know that these problematic 'issues' were deemed by the Inquiry to have been "valid safety concerns"[170], concerns that any reputable firm that cared about their employees would be expected to raise with their client. Valid concerns, that the government apparently neither wanted to be raised, nor concerns that they were willing to deal with. Accordingly, it appears that Wilson Security was punished for their temerity. Unified, on the other hand, were more than willing to *"do anything asked of it"*[171], apparently without similar concerns for these safety issues.

Interestingly, Alex Kamenev (Deputy Secretary at DJPR) sent an email[172] to Ms Currie on Monday 30 March, providing advice on how Unified Security could be justified for future work, beyond the initial 48 hours for which they were originally approved:

"You can be blunt and say Wilson have proven very difficult to work with and unhelpful, while Unified have been a dream. You should also emphasise, that Unified employ loads of Jobs Victoria clients, so it's actually serving a broader public purpose"

During questioning in the Inquiry[173], Ms Currie admitted that there had been no problems with Wilson Security at that time.

As Counsel Assisting pointed out, Wilson Security had not even started work at a quarantine hotel when the email was sent. Whilst under cross examination by Counsel for Wilson Security, Ms Currie admitted that were *no concerns* with Wilson's performance. It is also doubtful to what extent Unified did *"employ loads of jobs Victoria clients"* at the time, given that nationally they only employed 89 permanent staff, the majority in NSW.

Since Ms Currie admitted under questioning that the statement was not truthful, one therefore should question if the Deputy Secretary's email to Ms Currie constituted instructions to wilfully misrepresent the situation, or if there was a more obscure purpose.

---

170 Coate, 2020a, p171.
171 Coate, 2020a, p171.
172 Exhibit HQI0037c_RP Annexures to Witness Statement of Ms Katrina Currie.
173

Altogether, it seems that extraordinary lengths were taken to justify the appointment and retention of Unified, which with the benefit of hindsight appears to have been a wholly unjustifiable appointment.

Perhaps Unified was the cheapest option?

In many other circumstances when government procurement has gone awry, the potential for cost savings, selecting the cheapest if least competent provider, has often been the major influence on a poor decision. However, in the case of Unified Security, even that becomes the flimsiest of excuses. Unified Security were by far the most expense of the three security firms appointed, a huge financial windfall that does not appear to have been passed on in either higher wages to their employees or increased fees for their sub-contractors. These significantly higher contract costs, and the Victorian government's willingness to pay them, make little sense, since Unified appears to have done none of the value-add activities that the other two contracted private security companies provided in terms of additional training of their employees and instituting their own supplementary infection control measures[174] at their own expense.

Unified Security's owners also had a questionable history. It was public knowledge at the time of their appointment by the Victorian Government, that they had been associated with alleged prior unethical dealings involving bankruptcy and debts in the operation of previous security companies. The two key individuals behind Unified (David Milward and Luigi Trunzo) were linked to the insolvency of "*41 different corporate entities*" in 2016, owing government tax authorities somewhere in the region of $4.5m (Ross, 2021a). These grounds alone should have been sufficient to prevent Unified's involvement in the Hotel Quarantine Program. That the Victorian government's procurement process appears to have not identified this questionable history suggests further gross incompetency in its due diligence (that is, if any actual due diligence was ever undertaken). The appointment and continued contracting of Unified Security makes little rationale sense, in that they:

- Were by far the most expensive of the options available.
- Had the smallest stable permanent workforce.
- Were the least experienced in terms of overall general security expertise, and especially in terms of specialised expertise in health care settings.
- Could claim the least previous or current presence within Victoria.

---

[174] Coate, 2020a, p172.

- Had been refused entry onto Victoria's preferred panel of private security providers.
- Were associated with prior company failures and alleged unethical conduct.
- Were operating under an expired security license.

Despite all of this information being available to decision-makers, Unified were not only appointed, but they were then given more and more work for which they were clearly unsuited and incapable of performing safely. The Brazilian author Paulo Coelho perhaps provides the best summary to describe the situation: *"Ignorance is the absence of knowledge. Stupidity is the presence of knowledge and the refusal to use it"*.

The timing of the appointment decision

Questions have also been raised not only about how Unified Security was appointed, but also about *when* the decision was made to appoint them, and *when* the owners of Unified were told about this decision. The Inquiry concluded, despite the wall of silence, obfuscation, and apparent collective and universal loss of memory, that no Minister or the Premier was involved in the decision-making. However, just because the Inquiry was effectively prevented from uncovering relevant information, an absence of evidence should not be assumed to be evidence of absence of intent or culpability.

Much has been made about a curious email sent from the "Unified boss" (Sakkal, 2021b) to his senior managers on Friday 27th March at 12.30pm[175], demanding that the Commonwealth's online COVID training had to be urgently completed, by 2.30pm that day. This training coincidently was to be completed just *30 minutes before* the Premier made his first public statement about the use of private security, and about 10 hours before United was supposedly first contacted by a government bureaucrat.

Since Unified was not on any preferred supplier list, nor had they any significant presence in Victoria, why would they think it was so urgent to complete what

[175] Which is also curiously close in time to when it appears the actual decision to use private security seems to have been made, senior officials were certainly aware of the private security option shortly after noon on the 27th March, and the VicPol Chief Commissioner communicating the intent to use private security to the AFP commissioner about 50 minutes later.

was to become a mandatory prerequisite for working in the Victorian quarantine hotels? This is particularly puzzling when no other security companies were putting in place similar urgent requests. It is also a curious coincidence that Unified senior management suddenly made the decision to require online training that was aimed at the general public and most certainly not meant for organisations or frontline workers that would be working in high risk environments. An amazing coincidence that this was the very same training that the Victorian Government would require of security contractors later that day.

It is indeed interesting that Ms Currie from DJPR also happened to hold the opinion, around this time, that the Commonwealth's online COVID-19 training would be required for security contractors: *"as a minimum, it would be beneficial if private security guards had completed this training before commencement of duties"*. Ms Currie made this decision without any known experience in public health or infectious disease control, and without apparently seeking the advice of health experts. At the time it was obvious to many with even minimal experience in infectious diseases that this public advice and training was not-fit-for-purpose for staff engaged in high-risk environments[176], and was subsequently determined to be *"clearly misleading"* for quarantine staff[177]. Even outside of the health sector, businesses as diverse as agriculture companies, mining operations, accounting firms, transport companies, retail shops, to cafes and restaurants also realised the inadequacy of this online information, and instead sought additional advice and developed their own training.

It appears rather serendipitous that Unified Security decided that all of their employees should also complete this inappropriate and inadequate training, at precisely the time that the decisions about the use of private security were being made within government. Which scenario is the most plausible, that this was just simple coincidence; that Unified Security had a magical crystal ball; or that someone within government contacted Unified Security about what was happening, hours before the other two security companies were contacted? If this latter scenario occurred, then this appears to directly conflict with the process described by DJPR to the Inquiry, in which it was claimed, outside of an

---

[176] Interestingly most Australian organisations (public and private sectors) I have spoken to about their approaches for their own much 'lower risk' environments had instantly rejected this advice as unsuitable for their purposes and developed their own guidance for their staff.
[177] Coate, 2020a, p. 185.

email being sent out late on the Friday night, that direct contact with Unified Security was not made until the following day, Saturday morning[178].

It is unfortunate indeed that the Inquiry did not seek to explore the reasons behind such apparent serendipity, that two apparently unconnected organisations, came up with the same idea for urgent training, at about the same time. Despite the fact that many other organisations, operating if far lower risk environments, recognised the unsuitability of this training.

A continuing lack of due diligence and proper process

Although emails were sent 'late' on the 27th March[179], the actual engagement of Unified Security was eventually made *informally* via a phone call with a DJPR executive (Ms Currie) on the Saturday morning. This awarding of $44m of work through a single phone call is extraordinary and apparently without precedent in any other state or Commonwealth government entity. The appointment of Unified Security followed a 'process' that seems to have ignored all of the precedents for acceptable procurement and governance practice.

Actual quotes for the private security services were not received until days after the work had already commenced at the quarantine hotels, during the week of the 30th March. The quote from Unified Security being significantly more expensive, despite which Unified were engaged to undertake the bulk of the work[180]. Although, despite receiving higher fees, Unified did not pay its subcontractors or its employees rates above those paid by the other two companies.

A Principal Policy Officer was delegated by Ms Currie to manage the security contracting. This Principal Policy Officer was informed on 30th March, by specialist procurement officers within the Department of Treasury and Finance and from within DJPR itself, that firms on the State Purchasing Contract should be used. Ms Currie's response was to direct the Principal Policy Officer that it was *"necessary to retain Unified"* and that *"exemption (from engaging panel firms) should be sought"*[181]. On 31st March Ms Currie received further advice

178 Coate, 2020a, p. 123.

179 Coate, 2020a, p. 130.

180 Contracts were issued for: Unified Security for $30m (approx. 10 times their previous total annual revenue), Unified eventually submitted invoices to the Government for over $44 million.

181 Coate, 2020a p. 171.

from procurement specialists about the risks involved in the appointment of Unified Security and that the appointment should be reconsidered[182]. Despite advice from within Government and then from Trades Hall Council, the Inquiry found that Ms Currie *advocated* for a contract for Unified Security.

A contract with Unified Security was not entered into until *11 days after they had commenced* duties on site. This should have been more than sufficient time for any half competent person to validate the company's *bona fides* to undertake the work and provide some semblance of probity.

Not only were Unified appointed in the face of advice not to proceed, they were subsequently provided with an increasing proportion of the contracted work, based largely on unvalidated anecdotal accounts of their performance, and their willingness to undertake activities that the other security companies regarded as being unsafe.

There also appears to have been significant unfair *bias against* Wilson Security and substantial inequitable *bias for Unified Security*. During the contract period, allegations were made about inappropriate conduct by security guards of both companies. There was a manifest inconsistency in how these issues were dealt with. Wilson Security was subject to punitive action by the removal of responsibility for some hotels, whilst no action was taken against Unified, but instead they were rewarded by the allocation of additional contract work[183].

Even in the establishment of the contracts, Unified Security was dealt with far more leniently than the other two companies, specifically with regards to the use of subcontractors[184]. Whilst approvals were eventually required for Wilson and MSS contracting arrangements, no such approvals were requested for or provided for the use of subcontractors by Unified[185]. To make matters worse, Unified subcontractors then enter into their own further subcontracting arrangements, to the extent that government officials had absolutely no idea from security companies were actually working with certain quarantine hotels.

These differences in contracts established material advantages to Unified Security that go against established practices for probity, equity, and parity, yet no explanation has been provided for this apparently unequal and unfair treatment.

---

[182] Coate, 2020a p. 172.
[183] Coate, 2020a p. 174.
[184] Coate, 2020a p. 181.
[185] Apart for one subcontractor that was then not used for any work.

The unapproved use of subcontractors

Although Unified had stated to DJPR that they had sufficient capacity to undertake the work[186], they had in fact to rely substantially on a number of small subcontractors and guards recruited through online advertisements on Gumtree, Facebook and Whatsapp[187]. Arrangements which resulted in even more inexperienced and poorly supervised subcontractors and security guards being appointed. This also pretty much ensured that would be increased employment opportunities for indigenous employment.

Whilst the other two security providers, Wilson and MSS, were required to seek approval for the use of contractors, this provision was not applied to Unified Security. This use of unapproved subcontractors introduced uncontrollable and escalating vulnerabilities into the contracting arrangements and contributed to a substantial increase in overall risk exposure for the Hotel Quarantine Program. A risk that was either not recognised or was ignored by the Victorian Government.

Subcontracting is a well-known and common practice in the security industry. The failure to recognise and account for this risk is further evidence of woefully inadequate governance and management of the Program, and raises serious questions about the competence of those officials involved. With the vast majority of the 1754 temporary security guards, employed under the Unified contract, being sourced from other subcontracted security firms, DJPR appeared to have had absolutely no idea of what was occurring from the start. This is despite that one of the mandatory conditions of appointment required prior written approval from DJPR before any subcontractors could be used.

The Coate Inquiry's conclusion about DJPR's mismanagement of the procurement process comes across almost as an under-statement in that it was *"not appropriate or sufficiently rigorous"* (ABC News, 2020b). Whilst such was the professionalism and capability of Unified Security to manage their $44m program of works, that the company apparently ran its Melbourne operations from an apartment in a residential block behind the Blackburn Hotel in Melbourne (3AW, 2021).

Despite all of these factors, Unified Security was eventually given responsibility for the management of security at nine quarantine hotels, including the

[186] Coate, 2020a p. 17
[187] Coate, 2020a p. 195

extremely high risk 'hot' hotel, Rydges, where known infectious cases were transferred, and from where significant community transmission emerged.

The Inquiry concluded that the appointment of Unified Security *"was made in haste and without any risk assessment, led by staff that did not have the requisite experience and knowledge, and without any public health insight, oversight or input"* (Coate, 2020a).

Previous to Victoria's bungled security contracting, In March 2021, following a five-month NSW police investigation into misleading and deceptive conduct, it was announced that Unified Security would lose their licence to operate in that State (Jackson and Ross, 2021). Surprisingly at this time however, and despite the NSW police recommendations, Victoria Police appeared to not have announced any investigation into the company, but instead allowed Unified Security to continue operating on an expired security licence for six months (Houston, 2021a). Considerable negative reporting in the media emerged about the company and its owners, including revelations about previous bankruptcies and owing creditors millions of dollars (Ross, 2021a). Despite these issues and the alleged mismanagement during the hotel quarantine debacle, Victoria Police extended Unified's security licence for a further three years, *without imposing any special conditions or requirements* for that renewal.

On 26 May 2021 Unified Security went into liquidation in the face of a class action lawsuit (ASIC, 2021; Vinall, 2021), and allegedly owing employees and subcontractors millions of dollars (Sky News, 2021d). Fair Work Australia pursued United Security for serious non-compliances, including underpaying its employees in quarantine hotels by almost $1 million. Unfortunately, the company went into liquidation before the monies could be recovered (Fair Work, 2021). This appears to be a case of history repeating itself as Unified Security itself was allegedly established by 'rebirthing' following previous bankruptcies and significant debts.

Not only was the original decision to appoint Unified Security seriously flawed, but decisions were then made to expand their involvement and to continue with their services, regardless of increasing concerns about their capabilities and integrity. The decision to appoint Unified Security was one of the key contributing causes of the public health disaster that was to follow.

Adequacy of directions and instructions

It is a reasonable expectation that the type of security operation put in place for the Hotel Quarantine Program would have, at a minimum, detailed standard operating procedures (for example for working in high risk environments, hygiene and infection control requirements, etc.), including detailed directions for limiting potential exposure outside of work, and detailed duty statements and work instructions. As well adequate personal protective equipment, and specialist training for working in quarantine facility and health settings. One would have also thought that I would have been expected that would have existed even basic risk assessments that the government could have shared with security contractors.

It appears that just before commencing their engagements, the security companies were only given a verbal briefing about the scope of work and required duties, which was provided by the government bureaucrat managing the procurement[188]. Given the nature of the work, the technical requirements, and the extreme risks involved, is it unreasonable to expect that such directions would be given by someone more experienced in security work, or with even a functional understanding of public health and quarantine management?

DJPR undertook the engagement of private security contractors with no clear instructions about the work to be undertaken[189], whilst contractors received little guidance or oversight from any government agency[190]. The expectations of and requirements for security changed significantly during the Hotel Quarantine Program and would have been beyond any initial capability assessments for the contractors, even if such assessments had actually been carried out effectively in the first place. Wilson Security "quite properly" raised industrial safety concerns about guards being directed to undertake additional non-security duties that materially increased their infection risk, by exposing them to direct contact with infected 'guests'.

DJPR regarded the raising of these concerns as Wilson Security being "difficult"[191], and dealt with the company punitively. Conversely, Unified Security was more willing to undertake these high risk activities, in fact to undertake any activity asked of it (without apparent regard for the need for

---

188 Coate, 2020a p. 171.
189 Coate, 2020a p. 175.
190 Coate, 2020a p. 176.
191 Coate, 2020a p. 177.

additional risk mitigation or security guard safety), obviously for a price[192]. In addition to government directions directly increasing the risk of eventual community transmission, this also revealed a very real ignorance on the part of DJPR about managing the risks of the Hotel Quarantine Program, and a functional lack of understanding of infection control measures.

Two of the security contractors, Wilson Security and MSS, appear to have recognised the Victorian Government's gross inadequacies, and invested in additional specific program-related training, including infection control measures, for their staff. Unified Security did not invest in such training, and allegedly failed to provide sufficient basic personal protective equipment for their employees and subcontractors.

It appears from the available information that those government officials issuing directions to security contractors had neither the relevant experience or the competence to do so, and that this was compounded by the absence of any real risk assessment, re-evaluation, or effective monitoring. This was especially the case when 'fresh air breaks' were introduced for the quarantined travellers, when the suitability of using private security for supervision of these 'breaks', should have been an obvious concern. Although concerns about what was happening were raised by Victoria Police[193], the risk appears to have again been ignored by those in charge.

Part of the reason for such risk being ignored may have been the absence of clear responsibilities in setting up the Hotel Quarantine Program. Individual officials may have believed that someone else had responsibility for certain activities, when in fact no one did. Even at a departmental level, no agency saw themselves as being in charge. This represents a cascading failure of even the most basic governance from the very top decision-makers down.

---

[192] A price that appears to have been in the region of $14m, invoiced in addition to the agreed contract of $30m.

[193] Coate, 2020a p. 178.

Security contractors as a source of community transmission

It quickly became apparent that the re-introduction of COVID-19 back into the Victorian community from April 2020 and the subsequent deaths of 801 people, was a result of transmission via security guards infected whilst working in quarantine hotels, especially the high risk Rydges 'hot hotel'. The nature of the work, close proximity to infected persons, lack of training, lack of experience, inadequate procedures, and the lack of proper direction about personal protective equipment made infection of one or more security guards an almost certainty. That such infection could (and did occur) should have come as no surprise. Yet the risk of such an event leading to community transmission appears not to have been seriously considered by those 'in charge' of the Program.

Private security was one of the most vulnerable populations that could have been selected to work in the environment of a quarantine hotel, to the extent that it was almost guaranteed that community transmission would ensue. Much of the casualised security workforce are young and socially active, meaning that they were more likely to be asymptomatic but infectious; were less likely to seek testing (until directed) whilst infectious; less likely to socially distance outside of work; and more likely to have multiple contacts in multiple locations. Given the nature of the industry, many security guards come from low socioeconomic backgrounds and live in high density housing further increasing the potential for community transmission. Given their generally low pay, many security guards also work in multiple jobs (such as taxi drivers, food delivery drivers, supermarket workers, hospitality, etc.). These security guards are also more likely to continue to work when unwell and symptomatic, having limited or no access to sick leave or other sickness benefits. This, along with associated fatigue from working multiple jobs, further increased the potential for non-compliance, infection, and for community transmission to occur.

The significant power imbalances between guards and employers (and between the head contractor and its subcontractors) along with cultural issues also meant that guards were far more likely to work in environments that were unsafe, and perform duties that they were not competent to undertake, thereby exposing themselves to even higher levels of unacceptable risk. With the gross imbalance of power making the vast majority of guards too fearful of retribution to raise any concerns about safety.

The risk of using private security in this context was further amplified by the appalling management and work practices within the quarantine hotels. With at least 14 security guards eventually testing positive, the potential for infection was exacerbated by holding shift changeover meetings with up to 70 security guards crammed into a single room, and allowing guards to carpool (Consultancy, 2020). The risk of infection and transmission was further amplified by other officially mandated work practices which included security guards, nurses, and various DHHS staff required to work across multiple quarantine hotel sites[194].

Whilst these factors certainly amplified the risk of community transmission of COVID-19, they also increased the difficulty of contact tracing (exponentially increasing the number of contacts). Again, the nature of the casual employment in the industry, resulted in the employment of many security guards from non-English speaking backgrounds. Which in turn resulted in cultural and language issues that created "distrust and caution about government services"[195] and a reluctance to deal honestly with contract tracers. Such avoidance of honest disclosure should not have been unexpected, and continued to occur in subsequent hotel quarantine, border control, and self-isolation breaches.

Any half competent assessment of risk should have recognised the elevated risk for security guards to become infected and become sources for community transmission of COVID-19. A key question is, was there a failure to recognise this risk or was the risk recognised but ignored by decision-makers?

---

194 A lesson that appears not to have been learned following the Inquiry. During subsequent quarantine failures, community outbreaks, and lockdowns in Victoria this behaviour appears to have persisted with some health workers continuing to work at multiple sites, including in federally controlled aged care facilities (ABC News 2021a; Bucci, 2021a; Clarke et al 2021a; Davey and Rashwani, 2021; Sakkal, 2021a; Sakkal and Ilanbey, 2021a; Smith 2021; Zagon et al, 2021; Johnson and Turner Cohen, 2020). These practices continued despite Premier Dan Andrews' assurances that the issue had been dealt with as far back as October 2020 (ABC, 2020).

195 Coate, 2020a p. 197.

The approach to managing risk

The Victorian Government should have recognised the inherent vulnerabilities within the security industry and within their own contracting arrangements. The government should have recognised the extreme risk that private security guards could become infected with COVID-19 as a result of their exposure to infected individuals in the quarantine hotels. The government should have recognised the extreme risk of infected security guards becoming major sources for subsequent community transmission.

Rather than fulfilling their responsibility to manage these risks, the Victorian Government attempted to unfairly transfer the risk wholly and entirely onto the private contractors through its contractual arrangements[196], a move that in itself may have been a serious breach of the Occupational Health and Safety Act. Not only did the State (through DJPR) inappropriately try such a transfer, but it also failed to put in place any adequate oversight to ensure that these contractors were managing the risks.

It is a very clear concept within risk management that risk cannot be effectively wholly transferred to a third party. Rather, risk can only be shared with others, a proportion of risk will always be retained (Standards Australia, 2018) and must be dealt with. The Government appears to have failed to recognise their ongoing responsibilities for this risk, representing either incompetence or negligent abandonment of those responsibilities for protecting the health and lives of the public. By the very act of concentrating potential, suspect, and known COVID-19 cases into hotel quarantine, the Andrews government clearly took on responsibility for ensuring the safety of these arrangements. The government further exacerbated the risk by placing uninfected travellers (the majority of those placed into quarantine) into close proximity with those infected, but with adequately ensuring the safety of the travellers.

In fact, the DHHS, the very agency tasked with public health and ensuring community safety, not only apparently failed to fulfil its clear responsibility, but it also tried (unsuccessfully) to deny that any such responsibility existed[197].

To compound the egregious failings in risk management around the establishment of the Program and the appointment and (mis)management of security contractors, the Victorian Government continued to operate with an

---

[196] Coate, 2020a p.182.
[197] Coate, 2020a pp. 184-185.

unbelievable disregard for manifest emerging risk in the Program. The initial appointment of private security contractors was entirely based upon the premise that security guards would only be used to provide static guarding. This quickly changed to a more active role in which they had a greatly increased exposure to quarantined travellers, included those infected with COVID-19 virus. A change in role for private security that completely changed the risk landscape and should have imposed critical additional controls. In the complete absence of any meaningful risk assessment, with confusion and systematic dysfunction running rampant, and common sense apparently going missing, no one looked at the need for improvement in the arrangements. This complete failure to consider risk led directly to private security guards becoming infected and introducing the virus into the Victorian community and thus generating the devastating second pandemic wave.

Ultimately, it appears that the selection of CBD hotels and the appointment of manifestly unsuitable private security was made because they were expedient and aligned with Labor government ideology. Not because they in anyway represented an effective quarantine solution or offered effective protection of public health.

Training of security guards

There was an assumption, within the Victorian bureaucracy, early in the Program, that the Commonwealth Government's online COVID awareness material (provided for the general public) fulfilled some unspecified requirement for the training of security guards at quarantine hotels. This assumption appears to be yet another disastrous error that led ultimately to the deaths of 801 people. The Commonwealth's awareness material was provided to the public as a means of helping everyday businesses and community organisations to put in place some simple and very basic measures to help reduce exposure to, and transmission of COVID 19. The limitations of this training were very obvious from the start and many organisations, including ordinary high street businesses, introduced arrangements beyond those covered by this online awareness content. Independent experts have subsequently confirmed the gross inadequacies of this online 'training'. especially for the activities undertaken in the quarantine hotels (Grayson, 2020).

These limitations seem to have escaped the attention of certain government officials. However, Wilson Security and MSS appear to have recognised these limitations and provided, at the companies' own expense, their employees with additional training in infection control along with significant quantities of personal protective equipment, as well as implementing a range of new of policies, procedures, and guidance material. This would be a reasonable expectation of any competent and responsible contractor. Unified Security stated that they provided some onsite induction training and basic standard operating procedures, however the adequacy of their approach is highly questionable, both in comparison to the response of the other security firms and in light of the significantly higher risk profile of Unified Security operations. The Inquiry highlighted that Unified Security had a far greater reliance (compared to the other two security companies) on DHHS providing specific training to their employees. However, this training would not materialise at any time during the first phases of the Program.

The Victorian Government's role in providing (or rather not providing) adequate training is a major issue. There was an expectation that the DHHS would provide specific training, including in infection control. This expectation was not met, and the only training provided to security personnel by the Victorian Government was 15 minutes of *diversity training*, although this did meet the Government's ideological desires.

The contracts established by the Victorian Government required that the individual security companies work out for themselves what personal protective equipment and specialist training would be required "*consistent with public health standards*". However, despite this requirement, such Standards were not identified or provided by any Victorian government officials, probably because they did not actually exist at the time[198]. ***Six weeks*** after Unified Security commenced their duties, these Standards were eventually provided with government guidance on when personal protective equipment was to be used. It would be over ***8 weeks*** into the Hotel Quarantine Program[199] , before Wilson Security and MSS were provided with the same guidance.

This subsequent advice provided by DHHS on the use of personal protective equipment was insufficient, and contradicted industry advice and the contractual requirements (which was better practice advice to wear personal protective equipment at all times), thus creating further confusion for security guards. The rationale for DHHS providing advice not to wear masks in the quarantine hotels remains unclear, but was similar (for many months) with their own public advice ***against*** the need to wear masks for personal protection.

---

[198] Coate, 2020a p. 186.
[199] Coate, 2020a p. 188.

Advice which ran contrary to multiple other sources of expert advice, including the World Health Organisation (WHO). Ironically, a matter of a few weeks later, anybody in public *not* wearing a mask would be fined or arrested by Victoria Police.

The Inquiry concluded that the practices of security guards at the Stamford Hotel (managed by MSS) and at the Rydges 'hot hotel' (managed by Unified Security) fell short of the necessary standards to prevent infection. That this could occur should have been recognised as a highly likely situation. After all it was well known at the time that a significant proportion of the security industry workforce had English as a second language, along with generally low education levels, including poor "levels of language, literacy, and numeracy skills"[200]. This combined with the effects of a highly casualised, part-time, and largely insecure workforce further compounded the risk of using private security, a risk that Government did little to address.

Management of the security contracts

The Inquiry found that the management of the security contracts by DJPR was seriously deficient[201], relying on staff that had no experience in or understanding of the unique requirements of a quarantine program. Whilst those senior bureaucrats responsible for overall management, did not even visit the quarantine hotels.

Such specialist knowledge and expertise should have been available from within DHHS, the agency which should have been better placed to manage the security contracts. In practice what occurred was a fragmenting of responsibilities between two government departments, with a lack of clarity about who was responsible for the Hotel Quarantine Program itself. A situation that could only occur in the absence of good leadership, or under the influence of particularly toxic leadership.

---

[200] Coate, 2020a p. 196

[201] Coate, 2020a p. 189.

Conclusions about the management of security

It was stated early on in this book that positing counterfactuals would be avoided. However, it is well beyond the balance of probabilities that the failures of DJPR to *clearly* specify training and personal protective equipment in the contractual requirements, the failure of DHHS to provide expected training and appropriate guidance, and the failure of some security operations to address known capability gaps, that directly contributed to the failure of the quarantine program. Those government officials that advocated for and drove the appointment of an inadequately qualified security contractor, and those responsible for the deficient contract management, supervision, and monitoring of the security providers also contributed to this eventual failure.

The decision to use CBD hotels as quarantine facilities

The decision to use CBD hotels as quarantine facilities did not receive anywhere as much media attention as some of the other decisions in the pandemic management failure. It was only a year or so after the establishment of the Hotel Quarantine Program that the true inadequacies of using hotels as quarantine facilities were disclosed publicly, and action started to be taken to develop more suitable purpose-built facilities.

The decision to use CBD hotels as quarantine facilities was a crucial contributing factor that greatly amplified the likelihood and magnitude of serious breaches and outbreaks occurring. Given the importance of this decision, it remains unclear to what extent a robust assessment of risk was actually undertaken during discussions on setting up the Program. It has even been suggested that economic considerations for the use of CBD hotels had more influence than public health and public safety risk management on the decision-making.

That there was more than sufficient time for the Victorian Government to consider the risks associated with the Hotel Quarantine Program is evident by the fact that that Premier himself has admitted to $80 million being allocated by his Cabinet's Expenditure Review Committee (which the Premier chairs) for the procurement of hotel rooms as early 20 March 2020 (a full week before the Hotel Quarantine Program started). Although initially slated for "emergency accommodation" and workers, this became part of the thinking for establishing the eventual quarantine program[202].

The risks of using CBD hotels for the quarantine of potentially infected individuals should have been obvious to someone with even high school understanding of infectious diseases, or even a basic knowledge of European and colonial history. The successes and failures of previous large-scale epidemics and pandemics are well documented in the medical and scientific literature, and have been written about at length in many popular books. Even a visit to a high street book shop would probably provide a useful history of how past attempts at quarantine have worked and failed[203]. History shows that whether it is influenza, SARS, MERS-COV[204], bubonic plague, Ebola, yellow fever, tuberculosis, or cholera, all quarantine systems carry a high risk of a breach (Guerrieri, 2020; Markel, 2020; Snow, 2020; Cunha, 2014; Drews, 2013; Tognotti, 2013; Porter, 1997). The vulnerabilities of quarantine programs are manifest and obvious, and historically are usually the result of both policy and infection management failures (Kim et al, 2016).

Whilst the need for quarantine is essential, to expect that quarantine arrangements will not be breached is naïve at best, and just plain negligent in many situations. The COVID-19 pandemic occurred with a rich set of historical experiences of different approaches to quarantine (Cliff and Smallman-Raynor, 2013; Mandavilli, 2003) over many years. As the long history of quarantine attempts across the world shows, infected individuals will frequently seek to avoid or break out of the 'cordon sanitaire', whilst those working in the quarantine system will probably be exposed and become infected. The current COVID-19 pandemic continues this history. In fact, there is a whole area of epidemiology about predicting quarantine failure rates (Day, 2004), although it appears that no effective modelling was undertaken and incorporated into decision-making for the Victorian Hotel Quarantine Program.

That infected individuals (staff or 'guests') would leave the quarantine hotels and enter the general community was not only predictable, but it was also a certainty. Whilst largely successful in limiting an initial re-introduction and community transmission of the disease, quarantine programs in different

[202] Coate Inquiry, p 109.

[203] In the midst of the pandemic, and in one of the lulls between lockdowns, the author visited a bookshop in a regional country town and purchased a copy of Frank M. Snowden's excellent book "Epidemics and Society". I am sure that just reading this bestselling paperback would have improved the bureaucrats' understanding of what had to be done to better manage the response to the pandemic.

[204] Middle East respiratory coronavirus.

jurisdictions have experienced breaches during the pandemic (Grout et al, 2021). The key differences between Victoria and these other jurisdictions have been the more limited nature of the breaches and the greater speed and effectiveness of the other States and Territories' subsequent containment responses, compared to Victoria's faltering efforts.

All governments within Australia should have had a great deal of understanding and capability around quarantining, long before the pandemic occurred. It's not like the whole idea of quarantine for incoming international arrivals was a new thing for Australia. The nation has had a history of over 150 years of running quarantine operations to try to prevent diseases like plague, smallpox, and Spanish influenza from entering the country (Parks Victoria, 2021; Qstation, 2018). Dedicated quarantine facilities in several locations on the mainland were in use up to 1984.

The decision to use hotels

The use of hotels as quarantine facilities introduced exceptionally high levels of infection exposure, transmission, and outbreak risk (Cheng et al, 2021; Weeramanthri, 2021a; 2021b, 2021c). However, given the extreme time constraints placed upon States to 'stand to' quarantine arrangements, using hotels presented an easy and pragmatic choice. The decision to use hotels as quarantine facilities cannot perhaps really be criticised itself, that is if there was an absence of feasible alternatives. However, some influenza pandemic planning over the last few decades has considered the use of university student accommodation (since universities were expected to be closed down during the pandemic), old military bases (several of which would have been available), or temporary mobile accommodation (on standby for natural disasters). All of which would have provided facilities that were easier to control, were not located in high density city centres, and where the ventilation problems (ubiquitous in a hotel building) would be much lower.

The extent to which accommodation alternatives were realistically considered is unknown, but no evidence of a robust assessment being conducted has yet surfaced. Similarly, there is no evidence that government decision-makers had adequately assessed, considered, or even understood the extreme levels of risk involved in use of CBD located hotels. Such an understanding should have led to well-developed risk mitigations being put in place, involving the highest levels of governance, leadership, and supervision; lessons learned and knowledge management; consultation and communications; capability development; surveillance, monitoring and situational awareness and reporting; infection control and other protective measures. That these critical mitigations were either not in place or were inadequate is now a matter of public record. For any jurisdiction to not have in place such mitigations, suggests that either risks were not considered, or that advice on those risks was wilfully ignored in the pursuit of other competing priorities. If either of these situations occurred, then this suggests that one or more of those involved were indeed grossly negligent.

Even if the Victorian Government was totally incapable of performing an adequate assessment of risk, there was still sufficient historical precedent and guidance available about the infection and transmission risk in using hotels. There was also a range of guidance, openly available on the internet, about managing respiratory diseases specifically in hotel settings and based upon the experience of the 2003 SARS pandemic, as well as the 2009 H1N1 influenza pandemic (Hung, 2018; CDC 2003b; HK Government, 2003). That hotels could become a major point in establishing a large-scale community outbreak was not something new, it was something that should have been well known to those making decisions in the Victorian Government. Although it now seems to be something that the Victorian Government simply ignored.

The decision to quarantine in the Melbourne CBD

The use of quarantine hotels in the Melbourne CBD, however, raises additional issues. The same DHHS Deputy Secretary (an economist – Melissa Skilbeck), that allegedly sidelined the Chief Health Officer, Professor Sutton (Cunningham et al, 2020), was the same person that made the decision about using hotels located in the Melbourne CBD, against what seems to have been the Premier's preference for using airport hotels (Fowler, 2020). Apparently, a key issue involved the denial of the Premier's request to accommodate 80 COVID-19 positive passengers from a cruise ship (the 'Greg Mortimer') away from the CBD (AAP, 2020). Instead, these infected passengers were placed in the Rydges Hotel in the Melbourne CBD. That the use of non-CBD hotels was a feasible alternate was later demonstrated with the move to the Holiday Inn at Melbourne Airport, in the aftermath of the devastating second wave of the pandemic. Not wanting to get into counter-factuals, but Skilbeck's refusal to allow the quarantine of Covid infected travellers away from the CBD would have substantially increased the risk of difficult to control community transmission once quarantine breaches occurred.

It is interesting that an economist would apparently advocate for a policy direction that broke a fundamental economic principle of effective policy: the Tinbergen Rule, named after one of the first Nobel laureates for economics[205] in 1969. The Tinbergen Rule states that to successfully achieve different (independent) policy targets, then an equal number of policy instruments must be used (OECD, 2021; Carillo et al, 2017; Clemens and Ippolito, 2017; Howlett, 2017; Howlett et al, 2015; Yuan and Miller 2013; Knudson, 2008; Schaefer and Willardsen K. 2020; Tinbergen, 1952), and if there are fewer policy tools than targets, then those policy targets will not achieved.

In other words, if multiple diverse objectives are trying to be achieved, then different individual policies or strategies need to be developed to achieve each of those objectives. If you try to achieve two or more policy outcomes (for example, (i) prevent community outbreaks through quarantine of travellers and (ii) also generate economic benefit, but are only deploying a single policy instrument (the Hotel Quarantine Program), then it is likely that neither outcome will be achieved effectively. It is also arguable if 'public health' was even understood as a key objective by some of the senior decision-makers involved in the Program[206]. Where the major focus seems to have been on achieving 'detention' and 'jobs', rather than preventing community transmission of COVID-19.

There are numerous examples of policy failures that flouted the Tinbergen rule, especially where two very different policy targets were pursued simultaneously with the same instrument. For example:

- The Rudd Government's 'pink batts' home insulation scheme, where 'economic' and 'green' policy targets where conflated, and where health and safety priorities were ignored.
- The second Iraq war, where regime change was allegedly conflated with an objective of increasing the global standing of the USA (Butt, 2019).
- Australia's COVID-19 vaccine strategy, which tried to combine a public health target with the economic policy target of increased jobs through local manufacture of the vaccine (Harvey et al, 2021).
- Using banking regulation to also pursue climate change objectives (Weidman, 2021).

---

[205] Officially known called the "Sveriges Riksbank Prize in Economic Sciences in Memory of Alfred Nobel"

[206] Coates, 2020a, pp. 297-298.

- Proposing height regulations in post-earthquake Christchurch (New Zealand) to try to improve building safety, and also pursuing green policy targets (Crampton, 2019), which eventually had to be abandoned.

The Coate Inquiry identified that the Premier viewed the Hotel Quarantine Program as fulfilling two purposes (i.e., two conflicting policy objectives): detaining travellers and boosting jobs for the hotel sector, and that these two objectives were built into the design of the Program. The Inquiry concluded that this dual focus diverted attention away from what should have been the primary purpose of the Program: to contain any potential outbreak of disease, and prevent it from getting out of a hotel and into the community. Such a distraction ultimately resulted in dysfunctional management and inadequate quarantine practices on the ground, and created for Operation Soteria[207], what the Coate Inquiry concluded was a *"catastrophe waiting to happen"*[208].

In the case of Operation Soteria, however, the Victorian Government did not just break the Tinbergen rule by pursing two different policy objectives, but instead went for the trifecta: 'detain travellers', 'provide an economic stimulus for the CBD hotel sector', and virtue signal diversity and inclusion by appointing an unqualified 'aboriginal owned' security firm (Sloan, 2021). A gamble that failed catastrophically.

Yet the decision to use CBD hotels as quarantine facilities and in particular to use such hotels to isolate known positive cases conflicted with a number of basic infectious diseases control principles. The use of CBD located quarantine facilities (whether they were hotels or not) introduced a number of new risks, substantially amplifying the overall risk profile for the Hotel Quarantine Program. The proximity of commercial facilities (such as café venues and shops) increased the likelihood that isolated travellers would seek to breach their quarantine, as well as that (potentially infected) staff would use such facilities.

The lack of affordable nearby parking would encourage quarantine staff to use densely packed public transport, or carpool to commute to and from work. With Melbourne CBD at the centre of the city's transport network and with a large daily commuting population, any transmission of virus within the CBD could be rapidly disseminated throughout Melbourne. With such an amplified level of risk, the need for effective risk mitigation was at a much higher level than for

[207] The operational name for the Hotel Quarantine Program.
[208] Coate, 2020a, p. 301.

any other type of quarantine arrangements that could be established at any other location.

That effective risk mitigations were not established is now evident from the various quarantine failures, community outbreaks and lockdowns, as well as from a number of inquiries, reviews, and other disclosures. This was another one of the many failures in Operation Soteria and is one of the two critical proximal causal factors[209] in the subsequent community outbreaks and 801 deaths.

A similar debacle with hotel cleaning

To compound the problems with the private security arrangements and the use of hotels in the Melbourne CBD, the Victorian Government approached the cleaning of quarantine hotels with a markedly similar cavalier attitude. Hotel operators were initially expected to undertake the cleaning of hotel rooms, without any detailed guidance on infection control or specialised cleaning regimes being provided by government. Individual hotels had to organise their own individual subcontracting arrangements with various private cleaning companies. Cleaning was only undertaken after 'guests' had departed their rooms at the end of quarantine. No cleaning was provided during the 14 day quarantine period, creating hygiene and sanitary problems for those forcibly detained. The Inquiry told the story of one 'guest' that requested a toilet brush and cleaner, apparently giving up after making three separate requests and being provided with dishwashing liquid, antiseptic wipes, and hair conditioner, and then being told that cleaning supplies had run out.

Contracted cleaners undertook this hazardous work without any training or advice on infection control or personal protection provided by DHHS or DJPR, and without any monitoring from government to ensure that cleaning was undertaken to an adequate standard. Whilst some basic training was provided to cleaners by some of the hotels, the appropriateness and adequacy of this training was not looked at by the government[210].

DJPR was responsible for the procurement of specialised commercial cleaning services for hotel rooms where a confirmed positive COVID-19 case had stayed. This was a condition that had been put in place at the time of the initial set up of the Program. As part of this procurement, these specialist cleaning

---

[209] The other critical causal factor being associated with the failure of Victoria's test and trace program.

[210] Coate, 2020a p.227

contractors, that would be working in high risk contaminated hotel rooms, were to use the cleaning protocol described in a general document for the public[211]: *"Cleaning and disinfecting to reduce COVID-19 transmission – Tips for non-healthcare settings, March 2020"*. Hardly the sort of advice for cleaners working in an environment where they would almost certainly be exposed to high levels of virus. Fit for purpose advice was not provided to specialist cleaning services until 16 June 2020, well after the outbreaks from quarantine hotels had occurred.

The Coate Inquiry found that DHSS' failure to provide specific advice on cleaning quarantine hotels was because of a "scarcity" of infection and prevention control expertise in the Department. A situation that had to be resolved eventually by hiring external consultants[212].

During the Inquiry DJPR and DHSS both tried to deny that they were responsible for overseeing and supervising cleaning, each blaming the other.

Even when the government started to procure specialised cleaning services, it was hardly a model approach. DJPR's attempts to procure these cleaning services for the hotels proceeded very slowly, with requests for quotes for services not even starting until the second week of April 2020[213]. Prior to the outbreak of COVID-19 at the Rydges Hotel, the government had only managed to procure the services of a single cleaning company, IKON[214].

Not only did Victorian Government inaction unnecessarily expose contract cleaning staff to infection, it also potentially exposed other travellers that subsequently occupied improperly cleaned rooms.

---

[211] And written for a reading level of Year 12.
[212] Coate, 2020a p.230.
[213] Coate, 2020a p. 227.
[214] Coate, 2020a p. 228.

On the nature of decision-making

Reversibility of decision-making

It is apparent that the conditions typified by the Hotel Quarantine Program were accompanied by high uncertainty, high volatility, novelty, and complexity, and presented a number of wicked problems. That key decision-makers failed to recognise the nature of the situation and were ill-prepared to manage an effective response is now obvious. It appears that this failure to understand the emerging conditions as well as government's own inadequacies led senior decision-makers to rely on old familiar routine decision-making processes. Decision-making processes that were wholly inadequate for the task at hand and for what was to come.

From what has been publicly revealed, it is a reasonable assumption that government decision-making was largely advocacy based with little, if any, evidence that 'inquiry-based decision-making' was used for any of the key decisions. This was a wholly inappropriate and unsatisfactory approach for the type of situation being faced and is indicative of either massive ignorance or crass stupidity. Further, it is obvious than many of the decisions being made were highly irreversible (or difficult to reverse) and required a different approach to routine decision-making habits.

Decision-making and communication

The extent to which individual senior public servants, or Ministers and their staff were complicit in these decision-making failures remains uncertain. If true, the claimed lack of Ministerial involvement in key decision-making relating to private security and to the operation of the Hotel Quarantine Program (and the expenditure of substantial amounts of public money) is more than puzzling. For a government (and in particular for Premier Daniel Andrews) that has a long time reputation for control and micromanagement of the bureaucracy, not to be directly involved in the minutiae of such a high profile program is exceptionally out of character.

If Ministers were not intimately involved in critical oversight and decision-making at a time of such State and national emergency, then this is a much greater monumental governmental failing than Ministers simply making bad decisions. That whoever did make the critical decisions, did so either in ignorance or disregard of the manifest risk further compounds this failing.

It is apparent that there were serious failures in communication and information provision from the first decision-making about the Hotel Quarantine Program, during the procurement and contracting process, and through to the operations within the quarantine hotels and beyond. Sure signs of a government and bureaucracy in disarray. Ministers were allegedly not informed of key decisions and issues by those senior public servants making operational decisions. However, it also appears that those same Ministers did not actively seek out this information or attempt to fully understand what was occurring. Whilst this represents a further significant governmental failing, it has fortuitously for some Ministers allowed 'plausible deniability' over their involvement.

Necessary information was either unavailable, inaccessible, misunderstood, inadequate, or ignored. Whilst there are multiple examples of this occurring, the Inquiry provides a particular example that affected how infection control was approached. A DHHS senior medical advisor believed fomites (potentially contaminated surfaces and objects – including hands) did not constitute a significant source for transmission of the COVID-19 virus. This opinion conflicted both with the understanding of some other medical officers within the Department and with the WHO guidance available at the time, which emphasised the role of fomites and stressed the "utmost importance of environmental cleaning and disinfection, among other infection prevention measures"[215] . The senior medical advisor later admitted that although he had access to the WHO guidance at the time, this had not affected the advice he provided. Such confusion was prevalent in many other aspects of the Hotel Quarantine Program, no doubt contributing to the unfolding disaster.

Whilst DJPR was eventually responsible for managing the cleaning contracts for the quarantine hotels, DHHS was responsible for providing advice on required cleaning protocols. Although copies of general (public) advice and advice for general medical practitioners was provided in late March and early April. It was not until 17 June that DJPR was provided with specific advice for cleaning in quarantine hotels, ***some 82 days after the Program commenced,*** despite repeated escalations to DHHS[216]. It was further revealed that the DHHS did not proactively adopt an oversight or implementation role with respect to infection prevention control cleaning, despite expectations that it would do so. With the

---

[215] Coate, 2020a p. 225.
[216] Coate, 2020a p. 229.

result that the required rigorous monitoring and control did not occur in what were "self-evidently dangerous spaces"[217].

Inadequacies in the Victorian Government's establishment of cleaning arrangements for quarantine hotel facilities was further compounded by the attempts to wholly transfer the risks to hotel operators and contractors. These actions, accompanied by a lack of any adequate guidance, introduced further substantial vulnerabilities that were either unrecognised or ignored, and that contributed to a further escalation in the risk profile for those facilities, materially amplifying the likelihood of transmission and community outbreaks.

The Inquiry Final Report did not assign blame to individuals, but regarded the key causal factors to be systemic failings. However, such failings must ultimately arise because of the decisions made by those in positions of authority, and effects of these decisions perpetuate because of their promotion by or acquiescence of others in positions of authority. Organisations do not make decisions, decisions do not just spontaneously arise independently. Ultimately, a single person or a select small group of people has to make those decisions. Whilst some such decisions will have occurred during the time of the Hotel Quarantine Program, many influential decisions will also have occurred in the weeks and months (and even years) before the Program was set up. In that respect then, the Hotel Quarantine Program was a systemic disaster, due to failed administrative, technical, and governance systems, occurring because of several years of compounding poor decisions and errors. This calls into question the diligence, relevant experience, and the competence of those individuals making these key decisions, as well as the prevailing culture that influenced those decisions. These matters were not fully explored by the Inquiry and remain as issues that require further investigation and as questions that still need to be answered.

Whilst individual and team capability, along with institutional culture, all had causal and contributing influences on the Hotel Quarantine Program disaster, they also had similar effects on the circumstances leading to subsequent public health failures once community transmission of COVID-19 commenced.

[217] Coate, 2020a p. 231.

Information and sensemaking

Both Operation Soteria and the subsequent (post- Coate Inquiry) revamped Hotel Quarantine Program have been the subject of frequent revelations of attempts at secrecy and preventing information getting into the public domain (Taylor, 2020b). These attempts to control information even extended to not sharing critical information with other agencies and stakeholders involved in the Program. This culture of secrecy, which was exposed during the initial failure of the Hotel Quarantine Program in the first half of 2020, appears to have continued following attempted revamps of the Program well into 2021. Information leaks exposed a number of secret reports about continuing control failures and mismanagement within the Hotel Quarantine Program (Editorial, 2021a; Fowler, 2021a; Hannan and Johnston, 2021a; Tuffield, 2021c). It appears that not only were lessons not learned, but their existence in some cases may have been actively and purposefully supressed.

Even where information was obviously shared, there is little evidence that this effectively informed subsequent collective sensemaking and decision-making (such as at the 27th March 2020 SCC meeting). Previous studies have shown that simply exchanging factual information does not effectively establish either a common operating picture or support decision-making during a crisis (Treurniet and Wolbers, 2021). The different individuals involved in decision-making will often access different aspects of the available information[218], will have very different personal interpretations of that information, and will assign different weightings and importance to that information according to their own beliefs and interests. As a crisis progresses, this discontinuity and misalignment of understanding can increase (Wolbers et al, 2018), requiring that specific and concerted efforts are made to maintain common shared sensemaking. The emphasis in not on trying to develop a complete common operational picture, but is rather on maintaining a current shared situational awareness that continues to adapt as the situation evolves.

Throughout the pandemic, and the Victorian Government's incapability to manage subsequent outbreaks effectively, we have seen very little evidence of robust fact-informed decision-making based on meaningful shared sensemaking. Clarity and transparency in decision-making seems to have increasingly become alien concepts in Victoria.

---

218 Known as the "variable disjunction of information" which results in an inability to develop an effective perspective on a complex situation (Turner, 1976).

Part 3

Then failure after the quarantine breaches

8
In the aftermath of failure – yet more failure

In the aftermath of the gross breaches and failures of hotel quarantine, community transmission of COVID-19 emerged in multiple locations throughout metropolitan Melbourne over the succeeding days and weeks. Some of the Victorian Government's control responses, such as lockdowns, travel restrictions, and curfews have come in for substantial criticism, particularly where those measures were not supported by requests from police or based on the advice of public health experts. However, the imposition of unprecedented draconian restrictions of human rights during the second pandemic wave helped to eventually reduce community transmission, albeit after several months. Although whether more effective control could have been imposed (without such restrictions) by a better resourced public health service remains open for debate.

The situation in the immediate aftermath of the hotel quarantine breaches however was a different story, with multiple avoidable failures contributing to the second wave with an eventual 20,000 plus positive cases and 801 deaths. That a few quarantine breaches could result in such a rapidly expanding outbreak is both a result of the unmanaged risks within the Program itself (discussed above in Part 2), abject failures in situational awareness at the time of the breaches and subsequently, and the compounding failures in the trace and test program managed by the DHHS.

Risk management failures

Even a superficial consideration would be expected to identify a high risk (with an almost certain likelihood) of confirmed positive cases occurring when travellers are arriving from countries with high rates of COVID-19 community transmission. Given that such a high risk should reasonably be expected, would it also not also be reasonable that some planning and processes would be in place to deal with such positive cases when they were identified.

However, it appears that the first positive case in hotel quarantine caught everyone unawares, with no agreed response in place, and emails flying between senior staff trying to play catch up. For example, an email on the 31 March 2020 (4 days into the Program) from the Deputy Health Commander (a

DELWP[219] Parks Victoria fire officer) to the senior executive responsible in DJPR: *"whilst this scenario was nearly always guaranteed to occur, the realm of emergency management and priorities, until the case was confirmed today, a process was never created"* (Eagle, 2020).

Effective risk management requires that relevant subject matter experts are involved. Whilst experts in forests and jobs may be excellent in their own domains, did they have the right expertise to be making decisions on what were complex matters of public health?

Situational awareness failures

The Hotel Quarantine Program itself was characterised by systemic failures in situational awareness in different areas of the Victorian Government, and at multiple levels of leadership. If the evidence presented to the Inquiry is to be believed, and in the midst of a range of apparent collective memory failures that occurred, then:

- The Premier and responsible Ministers had no situational awareness of key decisions being made and their impacts on managing the pandemic, nor did they actively seek to improve their situational awareness through several critical periods of the pandemic. It is interesting that a Premier and Ministers known for their intense involvement (even micromanagement) in the daily workings of other major initiatives, could be so 'hands-off' at a time of State and national crisis.
- Key decision-makers (senior bureaucrats) had little situational awareness about issues they were making decisions on; about the responsibilities and actions of other senior decision-makers; about their legislative obligations; about their governance responsibilities; about pre-existing preparedness arrangements; about critical arrangements that had been put in place; about what was actually happening within the quarantine hotels, about resourcing and capability gaps, about how their own staff were performing (and in many case how they were not performing), and about what was happening with community transmission.
- Even when the first positive cases were occurring, key decision-makers were not being notified about these occurrences, and were subsequently not provided with sufficient information to build any reasonable situational awareness (Eagle, 2020).

---

[219] Department of Environment, Lands, Water and Planning.

- There was an almost universal absence of effective appreciation of risk, particularly informed by what should have been an ongoing changing situational awareness.

Accountability and responsibility failures

Who was in control?

Under the Victoria's emergency management arrangements, the DHHS – 'Health' should have been 'in charge' of the Hotel Quarantine Program as the designated 'Control Agency". However, 'Health' has consistently denied that it controlled the operation of the hotels, and that this part of the operation was under the control of DJPR. A responsibility that DJPR has consistently tried to deny. Although, in the lead up to and immediately following the quarantine failures, DJPR - 'Jobs' appears to have had little issue with these responsibilities and accountabilities being assigned to them. It further seems that having these responsibilities did not become an issue until blame (for the disaster) started to try and find a home. 'Jobs' then started to transfer blame to 'Health', saying that it had no expertise in infection control and that they relied on 'Health' for direction. Despite not receiving this direction, 'Jobs' appeared to be quite happy with managing the high-profile Hotel Quarantine Program whilst it still appeared to be a success and congratulations were being thrown around.

However, if the senior bureaucrats of both of these Victorian Government departments believed that the key responsibilities belonged to the other department, then this represented a most egregious dysfunction from the top of the hierarchy that could only ever result in dysfunction and failure on the front-line. Accordingly, with no clarity about which agency was in control, and with the infection control directions conflicting and changing frequently, confusion reigned supreme. The management of infected travellers proved to be wholly inadequate, and attempts at any meaningful infection control quickly descended into chaos. The whole process of providing infection control advice was described as *"ad hoc, fragmented and reactive"*[220]. That such inadequate infection control was allowed to persist is inexcusable. It is not as if the Victorian Government had to undertake a lot of work to get this information out in the form of practical directions. The National Health and Medical Research Council had produced detailed guidance on infection control just the year before, that

[220] Coate Inquiry, 2020a, p. 310.

could have been simply provided to those working in the Program (NHMRC, 2019).

This failure to establish adequate infection control arrangements was then further compounded by the absence of any meaningful monitoring and oversight. Victoria's public health command was not even aware of any infection control issues until after the outbreaks and community transmissions had occurred.

Was the Premier 'in charge'?

Premier Daniel Andrews stated on several occasions, that he was accountable and responsible for the Hotel Quarantine Program, but as the Coate Inquiry proceeded, he appeared to try to distance himself from any such responsibility or accountability (Hannan, 2020; Smith, 2020; Wooten, 2020).

From the very start, Daniel Andrews sought to establish his own personal involvement in establishing the Hotel Quarantine Program whilst it looked as though it was going to be successful. On 12 May 2020, as the burgeoning 2nd wave was under way in the aftermath of quarantine failures[221], Daniel Andrews made a statement to Victoria's Public Accounts and Estimates Committee in which he laid claim for his government's starring role: "*under a plan put forward by Victoria at the national cabinet to move to a compulsory hotel quarantine model, which was very quickly adopted around that national cabinet table by all States and Territories. I think it has served us really well*" (PAEC, 2020). Whilst emails released by the Inquiry indicated that the Chief Health Officer, Brett Sutton had played an early key role in promoting the use of hotels as quarantine facilities (O'Brien, 2021b). It is interesting that the nation's peak intergovernmental health body, the Australian Health Protection Principal Committee (AHPPC) of which Dr Sutton was a member, did not endorse hotel quarantine as proposed, and to the contrary advised (on 27 March 2020) that quarantine should only be used for "high risk cases"[222].

The WorkSafe investigation into health and safety compliance breaches within the Hotel Quarantine Program concluded the that 'Health (then DHHS now DoH[223]) was directly responsible, resulting in their prosecution for 58 breaches

---

221 And with no public knowledge of the Program's failure and role in causing the second wave.

222 Coate Inquiry, 2020a pp. 107-108.

223 Department of Health.

of the OHS Act[224], [225]. During much of the pandemic the Premier had 'Health' reporting directly to him, receiving regular reports from senior DHHS bureaucrats. Health and safety law clearly carries the expectation that those in a position of directing management (which the Premier clearly was), have an obligation to take reasonable care in their decisions and actions. They have to make themselves aware of health and safety performance controlled by that management (although Ministers are not regarded as an 'officer' with obligations under a range of different legislation). The questions then become:

- What level of understanding did the Premier have regarding the failed management of the Hotel Quarantine Program and the high levels of unmanaged safety-related risk?
- When did he become aware of these issues?
- What actions did he take based on this information?
- What level of understanding should the Premier have reasonably pursued, and what actions should he have taken?

The failure of trace and test

Further lack of awareness

The identification of potentially exposed individuals and determination of their infectious status are essential in containing any outbreak. This is absolutely dependent upon both receiving and providing information that is accurate and timely. In these primary requirements, DHHS tracing efforts, following the outbreaks from quarantine hotels, failed repeatedly. Whilst the use of private security seriously complicated tracing[226], other factors played equally important roles in the failure.

The probability that quarantine breaches would occur was high, and given the possible nature of those breaches, the probability of community transmission was an equally high risk. Any appreciation of such a risk should have seen a prepared and effective trace and test capability in place from the very start. This requirement for tracing capability even formed part of the advice on quarantine

[224] At the time of writing this book, the case is to still to be resolved in the courts.
[225] WorkSafe, 2021. Since these matters remain sub judice at the time of writing this book, no discussion is entered to into regarding any of the charges.
[226] The Inquiry found that using police instead of private security in the quarantine hotels would have substantially lowered the problems encountered in tracking and testing (Coate, 2020a p. 206).

arrangements provided to the National Cabinet[227]. However, in Victoria this was not the case. As with the other failures in the Hotel Quarantine Program, the causal factors leading to the trace and test program failure preceded the pandemic by several years of neglect. In the face of inadequate resourcing, loss of capability, and inadequate leadership, such failure was entirely predictable.

Problems with contact tracing are not new and should have been well known from other jurisdictions' experiences with a number of different disease outbreaks. Even earlier during the COVID-19 pandemic, the experiences of NSW, as a result of the Ruby Princess cruise ship quarantine breaches[228], aptly demonstrated how problematic contact tracing could be if insufficient attention was given to it. The Victorian Government's performance following the Hotel Quarantine breaches show that lessons were not even learned from the earlier public housing towers outbreaks of COVID-19 that had occurred in Melbourne[229] (Woodley, 2020b; Liotta, 2020).

Capability – a victim of long-term neglect

Victoria's contact tracing arrangements were severely criticised during that earlier public housing outbreak (see below), including criticism from the Australian Government (Coorey and Durkin, 2020a: 2020b), and concerns about Victoria's slowness in sharing its data with other jurisdictions. These criticisms were highly alarming, especially since they contradicted the now obviously false) assertions from Premier Daniel Andrews and from the Victorian Government about how well the system was working.

The scale of this apparent official misrepresentation finally came to light when the Chief Medical Officer (Brett Sutton) later gave an indication of the true extent of failures in the Program in a briefing to medical practitioners (Faruqi, 2020). In the same briefing he also outlined other systemic problems with Victoria's pandemic response, including a failing pathology service that was a "*hotchpotch of public and private pathology providers that are not able to be stewarded centrally*". Again, this should not have been news to anyone involved in the health sector in Victoria. Issues regarding government health capability and a heavy reliance on private pathology services has been subject to significant discussion and concern over previous years (Dyrenfurth, 2021; Gibson et al, 2020; Public Pathology Australia, 2020a; MSAV, 2018; Knibbs,

---

227 Coate, 2020a p. 108.

228 That had occurred prior to the commencement of the hotel quarantine program.

229 Discussed in more detail in Chapter 11.

2017; Dahm, 2016; Anon., 2015). However, the Victorian Government appears repeatedly to have ignored these issues and concerns.

It has been alleged that serious COVID-19 testing delays had arisen, at least in part, because of decisions to outsource testing to some private sector providers[230], that had a reduced capability due to cost cutting measures and commercial pressures (Gibson et al, 2020). This resulted in huge testing delays, with some asymptomatic COVID-19 infected patients taking up to *12 days* to obtain results. This failing system was not something that suddenly collapsed under the demands of the pandemic, but appears to have been a progressive deterioration in pathology services that had been occurring over several years. A failing system that was especially problematic in regional Victoria. However, despite the warnings, these significant problems had not been addressed by the Victorian Government as the outbreaks from quarantine hotels spread into the community.

The level of the privatisation and outsourcing of the public health response to the pandemic within Victoria was extraordinary compared with the other jurisdictions within Australia, with some 85 private contracts issued to a value of over $116 million in the initial periods of the pandemic. Of this about half of the outsourcing spend was on contact tracing. In contrast, other States, such as NSW did not extensively outsource, but used public servants (whom would otherwise have been paid to sit at home, as was the continuing situation in Victoria) from other areas of government to provide the surge capacity. This also included using members of the Australian Defence Force to provide additional capacity, a solution that Victoria seems to have rejected for a long time.

A range of problems are often experienced with new outsourcing arrangements (inappropriate/inadequate capabilities; poorly specified or misunderstood delivery requirements; unrealistic expectations, etc.). These sorts of issues are generally well known and understood, and effective outsourcing arrangements take account and put in place additional measures to both prevent and deal with such problems should they arise. However, the Victorian Government seems to have been caught by surprise yet again when these same sort of issues arose in their outsourced pandemic response. The Victorian Government seemed to have believed that could simply outsource all of the responsibilities

[230] Even the national peak body for public pathology has been highly critical of decisions to rely so heavily upon private laboratories during the pandemic (Public Pathology Australia, 2020b).

and the risks associated with the pandemic response, without putting in place sufficient direction, supervision, monitoring, or assurance.

A common theme throughout the first year or more of the Victorian Government's pandemic response appears to have been a fundamental lack of understanding about and disregard for the need to manage risk. This abject attention towards risk seems to have continued into the Victoria's outsourcing arrangements, including its outsourcing of contact tracing. Again, the Victorian Government appears to have believed that it could transfer all responsibility and risk to private companies, and in doing so, seems to have ignored one of the most basic tenets of risk management, that risk cannot be fully transferred. Whether it accepted it or not, the Victorian Government would always retain some responsibility for the risk associated with a sub-optimal contact tracing service. This somewhat alien concept for the Victorian Government would come back and bite it, as the contact tracing system faltered then failed under relatively low numbers of positive COVID-19 cases in the community. A failure that arose from long term government neglect of its public health responsibilities.

Responsibility for the chronic long-term under-resourcing of public health capability generally and of contact tracing capability in particular, ultimately rests with the central leadership of the Andrews government. However, Victoria's DHHS leadership shared some responsibility. Over several years DHHS had been progressively deskilling and under-resourcing its expert workforce. Whist at the same time, significant time and budget was being poured into pursuing various 'woke' initiatives, including regular "gender pronoun days".

For a government department that did not have the budget to properly fund effective public health delivery, they still found the staff and resources to put together ideological propaganda campaigns[231]. This included buying stick on gender neutral badges, producing videos to encourage employees to use "they" instead of "he or she", and holding "They Days" (Gidley, 2018; Morecombe, 2018) when staff are instructed to not use 'gendered' pronouns on the first Wednesday of every month. Prior to the onset of the pandemic, and whilst public health capability continued to fall behind that of the rest of Australia, unknown amounts of DHHS budget were diverted in the pursuit of further virtue signalling – such as seeking a bronze employee diversity award for LGBTI inclusion initiatives and gender fluid/non-binary/intersex relabelling of toilet facilities (Urban 2018). This is not an issue of the right or wrong of such

[231] This is not an attack on the need for inclusivity and individual rights, but is raising the issue of inappropriate prioritisation and a government entity losing sight of its prime purpose.

initiatives, they may have been very worthwhile endeavours in their own right and in a well-resourced and high performing organisation. But in the broader operational picture of a government department that could not even adequately deliver basic services for the people of Victoria, these were little more than ideological vanity projects.

Problems with Victoria's DHHS capability go back several years, and were not just funding related, but included significant long term cultural and leadership issues. The outcomes of which have seen many frontline workers, including general practitioners, become isolated and disenfranchised (Woodley, 2020a), as well as the departure of capable departmental employees in the face of a continuing toxic work culture. Poor leadership and the accompanying cultural decline played a significant role in the Department's deteriorating capability, where transparency and health priorities became increasingly ignored. For those good people left behind, their jobs just continued to get harder.

Failing technology

It had been recognised for some time before the pandemic that processes and technology to support public health in Victoria were not fit-for-purpose. Even when the capability gaps, especially for contact tracing, became apparent during the pandemic, it still took DHHS bureaucrats several months after the outbreaks had occurred before they travelled to NSW to review that State's more advanced and effective arrangements for tracing and tracking. Whilst NSW was using electronic databases to map and trace contacts, Victoria was still relying on pen, paper, and fax machines. Even when it became absolutely clear that existing arrangements and systems were failing, it still took a considerable time for the Victorian Government to rectify the problems (Baxendale, 2020d).

For example, QR code contact tracing was not approved for use until 28 November 2020 (Weekly Source, 2020), and was problematic in its roll out and subsequent use, with multiple different types of readers being used. IT experts were highly critical of the flawed QR code design, and its unnecessary complexity, slowness, and frequent failures to scan properly, compared to systems being used elsewhere in Australia (Mannix, 2021). An issue highlighted once individuals were able to travel interstate and experience these other more reliable QR code tracking systems.

Some of these other jurisdictions offered to share their technology with Victoria at no cost. However, true to form, the Victorian Government refused and instead decided to spend yet more of the taxpayers' money on trying to 'reinvent the wheel' by developing its own system. The Victorian Government's rationale for taking its own design approach was that their system would provide additional cyber security for the collected data. A commendable aim, although in retrospect this now appears to be more spin than substance. It was subsequently revealed that other government agencies and private companies could apply to get access to this QR data (see below).

Through the first half of 2021, the use of QR code check-ins within Victoria appeared to have dropped off due to poor user experiences, and the multitude of different systems for reading the codes (Beers, 2021). Problems with the technology were compounded by poor government guidance and the resulting confusion about how and where QR code checks were to be used. This confusion led to residents of apartment blocks being required to use the system for entering their own homes and body corporates levying exorbitant fees for putting the QR codes in place (Anon, 2021; Dean, 2021; Tuffield, 2021b).

This chaos carried on for months, with venues using a wide variety of different systems (pen and paper, the venue's own systems, or a government app), that had encouraged an increasingly widespread avoidance of 'check ins. The Victorian Government's inability for many months to put in place a single centralised and reliable QR code check in system was highly criticised in the face of repeated contact tracing failures. Excessively slow tracing and notifications, (in some cases taking over 6 days to list primary contact sites) were compounded by unexposed venues being wrongly identified as high-risk primary contact sites (Flower, 2021b)m whilst actual high risk sites remained unidentified. It was not until late April 2021, that the Victorian Government establish the mandatory use of the single Service Victoria app (Murray-Atfield, 2021a). These problems still continued following the roll-out of the new app. Victoria's problematic QR code system and its teetering contact tracing arrangements were quickly blamed[232] as the leading contributor to uncontrolled community transmission and Victoria having to enter yet another lockdown (its fourth) in mid 2021 (Clarke and Rooney, 2021; Coorey 2021, Flower, 2021b; Sky News, 2021c).

[232] Including by federal authorities (Coorey, 2021).

QR data – the cover up

The Victorian Government's problems with effectively using QR data that was collected, were added to with increasing concerns about the privacy of that data yet again. The government assertions (this time about protecting the public's privacy rights) again proved to be misleading, when it appeared that the government allegedly lied to the Victorian people and had tried to cover up[233] how the QR system could be abused.

In late December 2021 it was revealed that a *secret* court case had been held to decide on whether WorkSafe Victoria could access QR data in its investigations following a refusal by the Department of Health to provide this access. WorkSafe had tried over several months to access the QR data (for purposes unrelated to contact tracing), threatening criminal penalties if the data were not handed over, the Department of Health argued that its refusal was based upon "public interest immunity". That is, if the data was handed over it would undermine public confidence in using the QR contact tracing system. In other words, if people in Victoria knew how easy it was for the data to be used by the Victorian Government and its agencies for purposes other than contact tracing, then they would stop using it.

The issue came to the Supreme Court in June 2021, but the case and the decision was never publicly disclosed because the Victorian Government obtained a suppression order to prevent any disclosure of the proceedings for *five years (Murray-Atfield, 2021b)*. The decision of the Court, which was leaked in the media in late December 2021, was that the QR data could not be afforded absolute protection, and that any third party (police, WorkSafe, other government agencies, or even private companies) could seek access to the data. Ultimately, if such access was sought and refused, it would then be a matter for the Courts to decide.

It subsequently revealed that Victoria Police had also made attempts to gain access to individuals' QR data in pursuit of criminal investigations completely unrelated to anything to do with the pandemic. In some other jurisdictions, such as Western Australia, police were granted access to QR tracing for their investigations into relatively trivial criminal matters, including a bar brawl. Due to public concerns about invasions of privacy, Western Australia along with some other jurisdictions introduced emergency legislation to prevent this non-

---

[233] And appeared to be just the latest, at that time, in a history of cover ups (Gottliebsen, 2020a).

COVID related access from occurring again[234]. However, the Victorian Government consistently refused to put such limitations in place (Galloway, 2021; Piovesan, 2021a; Sadler, 2021).

The Victorian Government knew that QR tracing data could be accessed for non-tracing purposes, but continued to assure the people of Victoria (through various mechanisms, including on the government's coronavirus website) that the QR data would only be used for contact tracing purposes, specifically: *"Your check-in details are only used or shared for contact tracing purposes if there is a suspected or confirmed COVID-19 case at a venue you have visited"*[235]. The website page links to another document on *"How we use COVID 19 Check in information"* which again confirms that data will only be used for contact tracing, and also states *"We have designed this feature to protect your privacy"* and *"If we get asked to share check-in data for purposes other than contact tracing, then our general position is to say 'no', except where an individual asks For their own data. This includes requests from law enforcement agencies"* [236].

Subsequent checks were made on government websites following the revelations of the alleged cover up in late December 2021, and it appears that all references to these false assurances had been deleted. Government censors apparently forgot about the archived websites accessible through the Wayback Machine, and their earlier misinformation could be easily brough back to the surface.

It seems that the Victorian Government's major concern has not been about the integrity and security of the QR tracing data (the official spin about protecting privacy), but rather that they wished to cover up that their repeated public assurances about QR data integrity (that continued for months after the Supreme Court decision) were false representations to the Victorian people. Given the recent establishment of a de facto intelligence agency reporting to the Premier, it remains unclear to what extent political staff may be able to access historical QR data, or could be granted access in the future should the QR system be reinstated.

---

[234] The WA Government introduced "emergency legislation" some six months after WA Police started to use QR code data for investigating trivial crimes.

[235] Accessed through Wayback Machine stored archive of the Service Victoria website information about the tracing app, archived on 9 December 2021:
https://web.archive.org/web/20211209065825/https://www.coronavirus.vic.gov.au/checking-in-qr-codes.

[236] Accessed via the Wayback Machine stored archive from 24 November 2021:
https://web.archive.org/web/20211115105244mp_/https://service.vic.gov.au/check-in-privacy.

In the aftermath of these disclosures, any expectation that Labor government Ministers might apologise would prove to be extremely naïve. The Acting Premier (Jacinta Allan) tried to defend the cover-up by arguing that by deliberately misinforming the Victorian public that the government was preventing a 'scare campaign" (Murray-Atfield, 2021b; Bond, 2021). This is the same type of excuse that totalitarian governments[237] across the world have used to justify their abuses against their citizens. Although I have to admit that Jacinta Allen did make a good point, the thought of an unaccountable government purposely accessing private data to keep track of its citizen's private lives is admittedly 'scary'!

As William Pitt the Younger (Britain's youngest ever 'Prime Minister') said *"Necessity is the plea for every infringement of human freedom. It is the argument of tyrants; it is the creed of slaves[238]."*

This is not the first time that such coverups have been alleged, with the Andrews government being implicated in establishing what has been described as the "cover up state" because of a number of apparent attempts to prevent public disclosure of serious issues (Wilkie, 2021; Slezak, 2021; Smethurst, 2021b; Woods, 2021; McKenzie, 2021; Anderson, 2018), and continuing right up to the publication of this book, with the alleged Commonwealth Games cancellation cover-up.

Structural issues

Compounding the serious DHHS budget cuts that had left contact tracing capability dangerously under resourced (Victoria had to rely on contact tracers from interstate), Victoria's system had also been centralised which rendered it even more ineffective. In comparison, NSW capability was largely decentralised and embedded within local area health districts, providing a capability already within the affected local communities (Bennett, 2020). This NSW decentralised approach for tracing was important, not only providing a far more rapid response and more trusting relationships with the community, but also provided vital local knowledge and ground sense about the information being provided. All of which was largely absent from Victoria's efforts during most of the outbreak.

---

[237] Especially those masquerading under the façade of democracy.

[238] In this context Pitt was using the word 'slaves' to denote where the people blindly follow unreasonable orders because it comes from the government under the demand of 'necessity'.

Contact tracing – a litany of errors

It was apparent that the contact tracing arrangements within Victoria were under extreme stress, with the state's failing performance even visible in reports to the National Cabinet. Victoria was trying to develop its tracing capability as the outbreak was racing away, akin to trying to construct an aircraft in mid-flight. In later outbreaks Victoria's capability (such as shown in the Kilmore exposures) apparently improved dramatically, but it took a long time to get there, and was still subject to severe criticism with subsequent breaches in 2020 and 2021[239] (Cunningham and Sakkal,2021; Longbottom, 2021; Paynter, 2021a; Smethurst and Sakkal, 2021, Duckett, 2020; Triple M, 2020).

In October 2020, the Liberals, with the help of independents managed to force through a motion for a Parliamentary Inquiry into the contact tracing disasters. An inquiry that the Andrews government unsurprisingly tried to prevent (Baxendale, 2020d). Some of the key failures identified in this Parliamentary Inquiry (Parliament of Victoria, 2020) included:

- The unreasonably long time taken by the Government to put in place wastewater surveillance of COVID-19 virus, until after the second wave of infections had occurred.
- Extreme reliance on outdated, labour intensive, and ineffective manual data entry processes. These processes were wholly inadequate to deal with the increasing number of cases and the system was quickly overwhelmed.
- The introduction of serious data errors because of a manual processing system under stress.
- The eventual "misguided" purchase of an expensive analytics platform that was not fit-for-purpose, and which was subsequently abandoned[240].
- The Government was "significantly unprepared" to obtain and use data to understand its trace and testing performance until months after the outbreak (not until ten months into the pandemic in October 2020).

---

[239]Contact tracing problems remained throughout the subsequent pandemic lockdowns and state-wide lock downs, in the aftermath of further apparent problems with the government's contact tracing capability. The system was so overwhelmed, that the government put out a call for help from nursing, medical and public health students to assist in contact tracing (amazingly at a time when most would be on compulsory clinical placements or preparing for their upcoming exams, and so would be expected to be unavailable)

[240] A more effective system used by multiple other jurisdictions was originally offered to the Victorian Government in March 2020, but the approach was rejected in favour of a wholly unsuitable IBM system (Kwan, 2020), which proved to be another waste of taxpayers' money.

- The centralised health system proved to be ineffective for local operations and directly *"contributed to confusion and delays in contact tracing and test result management"*.
- The failure of the Government to act on multiple earlier reports about under-resourcing in public health.
- A lack of Government commitment and inadequate investment in pandemic preparedness that resulted in contact tracing *"being driven by a reactive crisis response leading to poor decision-making and unnecessary delays"*.
- Insufficient transparency about, and unwillingness to take responsibility for the failings.
- Unclear communication and conflicting advice from Federal and Victorian Government agencies that hindered access to testing services.
- A lack of communication and consultation with general practitioners, in what amounted to their effective exclusion from contact tracing and testing.
- The absence of clear guidance, in particular for small businesses[241].

The Victorian Government appeared to have wilfully ignored the manifest critical problems inherent within their contact tracing approach. Despite a range of warnings that the contact tracing arrangements could not cope with an escalation in cases, the government refused to deal with the problems. This lack of action directly contributed to what amounted to a limited number of local clusters getting out of control, resulting in the second pandemic wave, and contributed to the number of deaths that occurred (AAP, 2020;).

Omicron emerges and stretches an already stretched system

Although Victoria's Hotel Quarantine Program was an unmitigated disaster and the subsequent trace and test regime would have been laughable in less traumatic and tragic circumstances, the rest of Victoria's fragile health systems managed to struggle through. Admittedly, during the first few COVID-19 waves, the 'shaky' health system only had to deal with what were relatively tiny case

[241] There were multiple complaints that businesses that had been exposed to both known and potential positive cases were not notified by DHHS for several days, whilst a growing number of business were provided with no advice or their requests for advice were ignored by government agencies.

numbers compared to those being faced in many other countries overseas, and the severe restrictions that were put in place helped to hide the extent of Victoria's fragile health system. However, these chronic problems within the health system could only be hidden for so long.

In November 2021 a new variant of SARS-CoV-2 emerged, initially detected in southern Africa. This variant, Omicron, although causing a less severe illness than early variants of the virus, its rate of spread was much more rapid (Mallapaty, 2022), and was quickly transmitted around the world becoming the dominant strain. The emergence of Omicron laid bare once and for all the fragility and incapability of Victoria health system to cope with anything but a relatively small number of COVID19 cases.

In early 2022, with the increasing transmission of the Omicron variant of SARS-CoV-2, Victoria saw steadily increasing numbers of positive COVID-19 cases and hospitalisations[242], with acute health resources being put under substantial strain. Remember, the Victorian government had been given 2 years to prepare for this.

The extent of the true weakness in Victoria's health services were finally exposed. Ambulance Victoria had to announce 'CODE RED' situations on several occasions when its capacity was overwhelmed (Dow, 2022b; Hales, 2022a; Morgan, 2022; Juanola and Morgan, 2022; Tahir, 2022), and it was unable to respond to many of the calls for assistance. Already under-resourced and under-equipped before the pandemic, even more paramedics and ambulances were taken out of the system, long queues of vehicles ramped up outside hospitals, waiting hours to drop off patients. Additional volunteer resources such as the SES[243], Lifesaving Victoria, and paramedic students had to step up to try and fill shortfalls in capability. In these situations, COVID-19 was merely the trigger that caused an already fragile and under-resourced system to collapse. Even weeks before the surge in COVID-19 cases, Ambulance Victoria specialist MICA crews were unable to attend a number of serious emergencies because of substantial shortfalls in specialist capacity, affecting about a third of Melbourne (impacting an area of over 3,000km^2).

The tracing system, already creaking, was quickly overwhelmed resulting in close contacts not being informed or followed up, or high risk premises not being notified. Despite all of these problems, the public was still being

---

[242] The majority of which were patients admitted with other conditions that coincidently were infected with COVID-19.

[243] SES= State Emergency Service, a volunteer organisation.

encouraged to use a sign-in QR tracking app that the government *had already secretly abandoned months earlier* (Waters, 2022).

Despite the readily available experiences of the UK over several previous months during late 2021, there again appears to have been little effective planning and preparedness for what was always going to be the inevitable and very predictable massive increase in cases within Victoria. Even if senior leadership within Victoria were completely unaware of what was happening elsewhere in the world, what was happening in early 2022 with the pandemic has been foreseeable since its start. Irrespective of the emergence of Omicron or any other variant, the government knew from its very first lockdown that eventually society would have to open up, and that it was more than likely that COVID-19 would remain a serious health problem for years to come. When Victorian society eventually did open up, it was entirely predictable that the health system would be faced with a significant surge in infections, and increased patient numbers requiring both acute and longer-term care.

Why then was Victorian preparedness still in such a lamentable state, when it had two years advance warning of what would happen once Victoria went to a freer society. Over twenty years ago, Victorian preparedness for an influenza pandemic was based upon the potential for significant disruption to essential services (especially the sudden unavailability of health staff) and planning considered a range of mechanisms for dealing with such capacity losses. There was also a lot of thinking about how a return to post-pandemic normality might be achieved and planned for. What had happened within Victoria that had so adversely impaired the State's resilience?

As 2022 progressed, the situation appeared to be worsening for the under resourced health system in Victoria. The number of avoidable deaths of Victorian citizens was increasing because of the multiple occasions on which Ambulance Victoria were unable to attend different medical emergencies The triple zero emergency call system collapsed with multiple urgent calls for help going unanswered. Yes, COVID-19 did put strain on the health system, but this was but a proverbial 'straw on the camel's back' of a system that had been in decline for almost a decade. The pandemic has merely served to highlight a chronically failing system.

The Victorian Government tried to lay all of the blame for the failure of its health services onto the 'unexpected' emergence of the Omicron variant. This again needs to be seen as more smoke and mirrors. Within the first weeks of the pandemic, new variants of the SARS-CoV-2 virus started to emerge. The prospect of new variants was never unexpected, it is what these viruses do, they mutate. The emergence of new variants which would result in different patterns of disease was always pretty much a certainty. Omicron was a fairly gentle reminder of this, there was (and still is) the potential for another new variant that is more transmissible, causes a much more severe disease, and for which current vaccines offer little or no protection. The Victorian Government had almost two years after the COVID-19 first appeared to get its house in order and fix the health system, and get ready for an upsurge in cases. That was two years, during which the government got regular reminders of the emergence of new SARS-CoV-2 variants (Alpha, Beta, Delta, Gamma, Epsilon, Eta, Iota, Kappa, Zeta, Mu, etc.) all before Omicron was detected (CDC, 2022). Yet the Premier Dan Andrews and his government were caught floundering again.

Ignoring the psychological impacts

The Victorian Government has been subject to severe criticism, from many quarters, for their mismanagement of the Hotel Quarantine Program, and for their subsequent dismal response. A key issue, which is often given less attention in an ocean of major failings, is the extent to which the government made an already terrible situation even worse by their failure to adequately consider the psychological impacts of their decisions. Both for people detained in the quarantine hotels and for those forcibly prevented from leaving their homes.

It appears that there was little to no detailed consideration of the psychological and wellbeing impacts during the initial 'planning' for the Hotel Quarantine Program, or for the Victorian population before they were forced into isolation (a situation that was already evident following the Flemington public housing towers fiasco). When psychological wellbeing was eventually considered, the measures that were rushed into place were so ill-conceived that they amplified (rather than diminished) psychological harm and actively contributed to increasing the risk of transmission and for a community outbreak. The Coate Inquiry concluded that expert advice should have been sought, but that those involved in managing the Program failed to seek such advice[244]. Consideration of the health and wellbeing of those being detained was sacrificed for a *"disproportionate focus on logistics"*[245]. This is hardly surprising when those bureaucrats making decisions about the Program were comfortable with

---

[244] Coate Inquiry, 2020a, p. 33-35
[245] Coate Inquiry, 2020a, p. 34.

dealing with simple administrative issues, but seemingly had no expertise or apparently even a fundamental understanding about health and complexity.

It is an absolute requirement that the public health benefits of imposing quarantine and isolation on a mass population needs to be carefully weighed against the negative impacts of doing so (Smith et al, 2019). There is little evidence that has entered the public domain that this issue was subject to even a basic informed risk assessment by anyone within the Victorian Government.

That imposed quarantine and isolation can and will result in acute stress, and severe psychological and emotional trauma is not something that just became apparent with the advent of the COVID-19 pandemic. There is a long historical experience of these effects from the multiple occasions on which these measures have been enforced, including for SARS, MERS, Ebola, influenza, etc. (Brooks et al, 2019). The need to include the management of mental health impacts into quarantine and isolation planning has been enshrined for decades in the scientific and medical literature, and in generally accepted practices, including the need to consider adverse impacts on health care workers (Huremović, 2019; Dailey and Kaplan, 2014; Shultz et al, 2014; Schiltz, 2007; Douglas et al, 2009; Johal, 2009; Perrin et al, 2009; Chen et al, 2007; DiGiovanni et al, 2004; Maunder et al, 2003).

A range of factors have been associated with the increased risk of adverse psychological impacts, including the duration of quarantine/isolation (where effects increased significantly after a period of 10 days confinement); the fear of infection whilst quarantined; the adequacy and clarity of information provided on entry into quarantine, the transparency of authorities; and the availability of amenities and supplies, especially the delivery and quality of food. Unsurprisingly, these factors seem to have been of low priority for those in charge of hotel quarantine during the early days, and frequently became issues of concerns for the remainder of the Program.

With so much good practice information easily available from reputable sources, how could the government have got so much wrong for so long?

Continuing problems: incompetence or ignorance?

The apparent inability of the Victorian Government to understand the nature of risk, to think strategically, and to properly make decisions about uncertainty was not just limited to the conduct of the Hotel Quarantine Program. Many other aspects of dealing with the pandemic's impacts have also been subject to severe criticism for poor foresight, planning and implementation, and for serious shortcomings in outcomes. The Victorian Government's initial strategy was one of complete prevention of entry of the disease into Victoria. When realisation dawned that this was never going to be practical it was back to the drawing board, with a new strategy for slowing down the impacts of the pandemic on already fragile public and acute health systems. The entire State went into the most draconian limitations of individual freedom within Australia seen up to that time.

With the curve apparently flattening during April and May, a small (but growing number) of community cases saw the burgeoning 2nd wave emerge as a result of the catastrophic failure of the Hotel Quarantine Program, with even more draconian restrictions being enforced to flatten the curve again. The Premier, Daniel Andrews, made promises to improve health capability including the establishment of a further 4000 hospital beds to deal with any future outbreaks. A promise which remained unfulfilled through the third, fourth, fifth and sixth pandemic waves.

All consideration of a proportional response to the pandemic (such as the flattening of the curve, to allow health capabilities to manage the inevitable increased numbers of ill people once restrictions were eased) seemed to have been abandoned in the belief that zero cases should be the new target. Accordingly, lockdowns and other restrictions continued to be imposed upon millions of Victorians for what were a handful of cases. With such small numbers of cases, an effective public health system should have avoided the need for those continuing lockdowns. That successive severe lockdowns occurred is not just indicative of a failed public health system, it is also indicative of the Victorian Government's complete lack of confidence in that system.

Eventually there seemed to be an acceptance, within the Victorian Government, that instead of the thinking that drove the lockdown mentality, Victoria would need to open up and that the de facto mandated vaccination would be the best approach to allow an easing of restrictions. Through the latter part of 2021 and into 2022, the emergence of new SARS-CoV-2 variants (the Delta and Omicron variants) seemed to come as a complete surprise to the government. This was accompanied by the now usual panicked response, despite the fact that new variants had been emerging since the earliest days of the pandemic. Again, the Victorian Government appears to have lacked any real effective foresighting and planning.

With restrictions relaxing in many parts of Australia over the 2021/2022 summer, the New Year of 2022 saw a health system in crisis mode. Increasing numbers of doctors, nurses, paramedics, and support staff became infected or went into isolation; as supply chains collapsed; retail outlets closed down; and supermarkets had to reintroduce rationing as shelves were emptied once again.

Should it have been any real surprise that the number of community infections would increase suddenly and dramatically once restrictions were eased and large numbers of people travelled over the Christmas period and families reunited? With any significant increase in community transmission, the requirement for close contacts to test and isolate would obviously increase. How unreasonable was it to assume that large numbers of infected people would be removed from the workforce for a week or more at a time. Was it a really huge leap in logic to consider that a significant number of these isolating individuals would be essential workers, and that essential services would be disrupted as a result? Yet where was the detailed planning, preparedness, and contingencies from the Victorian Government for such a situation? Real life, and the predictable continuation of the pandemic again seemed to be wholly unexpected by the government.

Twenty years ago, this author was involved in running workshops (within Victoria and for other Australian and international jurisdictions) to help build pandemic plans that could deal with such disruptions. Why two decades later had did this very situation come as such a surprise to those decision-makers in authority within Victoria?

Despite the very predictable disruption to supply networks and the now familiar overwhelming of the health system, the government was again 'caught with its trousers down'. The situation also appears to have caught the State's testing regime unprepared. In the lead up to and following Christmas 2021, queues at testing centres often exceeded eight hour wait times, rapid antigen tests completely sold out in retail outlets across the State, and the PCR testing system in laboratories started to collapse in early January. Many thousands of tests were not completed, with patent samples having to be thrown away because they could not be tested in time, and results went missing or went unreported. On 15 January 2022 it was revealed that around 100,000 tests from the previous week were abandoned, which had left potentially infected people waiting in vain for test results that would never come (Seyfort, 2022a). That's over 100,000 Victorians waiting for COVID test results, many of them waiting in self isolation or about to travel interstate, that would never receive their results. To make matters worse, the first time that many of these people knew they would not receive their results was when they saw the media reports in the following weeks. Just when you thought that things could not be mismanaged more, the Victorian Government again exceeded expectations.

With this predictable exponentially increasing number of infected Victorians, was it not also very predictable that there would be a massive demand for COVID-19 testing?

It soon emerged that Federal and State governments (including Victoria) were warned by independent health experts almost a year previously to expect that testing sites would be overwhelmed once restrictions eased, and the inevitable widespread community transmission would follow. The Communicable Disease Network of Australia and the Public Health Laboratory Network undertook joint modelling of different transmission scenarios and provided this "testing framework strategy" information to the various governments (Martin, 2022). It soon became very apparent that the Victorian Government's risk management was still lamentable in a large number of areas. However, even when presented with what amounted to a free detailed risk assessment and strategic approach from independent expert bodies, the government could apparently still not incorporate it into its decision-making. Even then the Victorian Government was provided with a 'second chance' to get it right, 6 months before this testing debacle occurred, when an emergency health doctor raised fresh warnings about the potential for rapid antigen test kit shortages (Mimis, 2022). But in what was now typical behaviour, the government allegedly ignored these warning and rejected offers of assistance from the private sector.

The Victorian Government seems to have been unprepared and was taken by surprise yet again once these 'new' variants started to cause an increase in local case numbers. One argument that has been raised in defence of the Victorian Government's inaction has been the 'unpredicted' emergence of the highly infectious Omicron variant of SARS-CoV-2. However, this seems to have been yet another 'smoke and mirror's distraction by the government, given that specific warnings about an upsurge in infections were available from other countries where Omicron had begun circulating months before it became an issue within Australia.

Yes, without doubt the Omicron variant proved to be far more infectious than previous variants. A number of mutations on its spike proteins allowed the virus to evade the host's immune response (Haseltine, 2022; Meng et al, 2022; Callaway and Ledford, 2021; Chen et al, 2021; Garrett et al, 2021; Marks, 2021), including the ability to evade immunity from multiple dosed vaccination.

Omicron caused a significantly less severe disease in vaccinated individuals compared with other known variants. However, lower lethality did not mean a reduced impact on population health (Kavanagh, 2022b), Omicron's higher transmissibility meant that more people got sicker over a shorter time period. Combined with small numbers of unvaccinated individuals within the Victorian population, this resulted in an increased number of individuals with serious illness requiring medical assistance. The increased stress on Victoria's already fragile health system was therefore understandable. However, did this provide the Victorian Government with anything resembling a valid excuse for the collapse of the health system and for the deaths of over twenty people, in the first half of 2022 alone, that were prevented from receiving urgent medical attention?

The emergence of Omicron was never a surprise to government decision makers. There were ample warnings specifically about Omicron and what its impacts would be, long before this variant started to cause disease within Australia. Health professionals across the word had long recognised the evolutionary capability of SARS-CoV-2, and of coronaviruses generally (Marks, 2021; Reardon 2021; Forni, 2017; Li, 2016; Kan et al, 2005; Song, 2005; Bush 2004; CSMEC, 2004; Holmes and Rambaut, 2004). It is one of the reasons that a great deal of money had been invested internationally in research since the SARS pandemic in 2003.

The potential emergence of new and more 'dangerous' variants of SARS-CoV-2 was discussed widely in the scientific literature and by the media since the early days of the pandemic. The SARS-CoV-2 virus has been continuously mutating since it was characterised in the first couple of months of 2020 (Chen et al, 2020a; Wang et al, 2020a; 2020b), and it was shown very early in the pandemic that some mutations could expand across the world very rapidly. It was also known from the very start that some mutations had the potential to substantially increase infectivity of the virus, whilst other mutations could increase its lethality. It had also been discussed extensively, for at least the previous twelve months before this latest collapse of the testing system, that vaccines may not be effective against new mutations (Head and van Elsand, 2021).

Some of the basic tenets of a pandemic are that numbers of infected persons can rise rapidly and require urgent medical support, and that rates of morbidity and mortality can change, as a result of emergence of new variants. Should either infectivity or lethality change significantly (one or the other change was always going to happen at some stage) then this would increase the strain on the health system, by increasing the overall number of infected individuals (and thereby increasing the number becoming seriously ill and requiring hospitalisation. Understanding and managing such potential stressors are just part of fundamental pandemic planning and preparedness. Why then was Victoria so poorly prepared for the almost certain emergence of new variants such as Omicron?

The Victorian Government's disastrous mismanagement of the Hotel Quarantine Program and the findings of the subsequent Coate Inquiry should have at least had the positive outcomes that lessons would have been learned and that Ministerial and bureaucratic decision-making would become more informed and effective. However, the continuing bungles through 2021 and into 2022 showed that even into the third year of the pandemic, it was still 'business as usual' for the Victorian Government. With almost every key challenge it had faced, there was little evidence of good foresight, planning or preparedness. The Victorian Government's approach consistently appeared to be a sudden realisation of reality (once the horse had bolted) and a snap gut reaction, rather than a well thought out strategy that considered different plausible scenarios ahead of time.

It would, however, be unfair to think that the Victorian Government was just sitting on its hands doing nothing. We know from repeated media reports about different leaked secret reports, that the government was very well aware of what was happening, why it was happening, and how likely it was that the situation would deteriorate in the future. It just appeared, with a State election looming in 2022, that the Andrews government just didn't want the voting public to know about how parlous Victoria's capabilities really were.

Again, despite the government blaming COVID and patient numbers for the problems with the health system, media leaks about another report provides insight into the real reason for some of these failures. This revelation clearly showed that one of the reasons for ambulances failing to get to emergency medical incidents on time was because of simple understaffing at the Emergency Services Telecommunications Authority (ESTA), running Victoria's triple zero emergency call system (Dow and Eddie, 2022; Seyfort, 2022b). Even though the Secretary of the Victorian Ambulance Union has previously warned about the problems in the system were a result of "inefficient use of resources", (Geraets and Dow, 2022).

This was a result of chronic understaffing that had little to do with the pandemic, but was a problem stretching back years earlier. A continuing problem that in 2021 and 2022 resulted in over 100,000 calls for emergency help being delayed or going unanswered, including for 357 patients in cardiac arrest, and was estimated to have caused avoidable serious harm to at least 1,000 patients (Dow and Eddie, 2022). Staffing levels at ESTA (and almost everywhere else in the health system) were not the only problem, as critical technology also failed in May 2022, plunging the state into another Code Red for the ambulance service. Emergency call takers, unable to match resources to calls for help, were forced to use pen and paper (Geraets and Dow, 2022). The government eventually forced to pay attention, after at least 18 people died, started to address ESTA's capability problems, in the middle of 2022.

Part 4

interconnecting causal, contributing, and influencing factors

9
A convoluted mess of interacting and interdependent failures.

Organisational culture

The poor organisational culture within some of the Victorian agencies involved in the Hotel Quarantine Program (and those involved in the subsequent pandemic response) was almost certainly a major contributor to the catastrophic failure of the Program and the mismanagement of the second pandemic wave.

There is a continuing history of toxic culture being present in many Victorian Government agencies, including in Corrections Victoria (Moore, 2021; Cluff, 2019a), Victoria Police (Hill, 2019; Le Grand and Cooper, 2019), Ambulance Victoria (O'Sullivan, 2020; Tuohy, 2020), Coroners Court (Neilson, 2020) some hospitals (Judd, 2017), Victorian Auditor General's Office (Edwards, 2015a), Emergency Management Victoria (Anon., 2019; Whalquist, 2018), Fire Rescue Victoria (Smith, 2021; McGinn, 2019b), and others.

Multiple reports and incidents suggest that the health sector within Victoria, and the DHHS in particular, was suffering chronic toxicity over several years (Field, 2019; HACSU, 2019; IBAC, 2017; VAGO, 2016), with over 182 bullying and harassment allegations made in just two years within the DHHS (Easton, 2017). As recently as 2019, DHHS was prosecuted by WorkSafe Victoria for alleged discrimination against a worker that had raised health and safety concerns within the Department (WorkSafe, 2019).

There are suggestions that increasing work demands caused by funding cuts had been a significant causal factor, whilst DHHS 'leadership' was specifically criticised (VAGO, 2016). Poor collaboration between individual fiefdoms within and between agencies was also evident (VAGO, 2016a), most probably as a direct outcome of ineffective and toxic leadership.

Cultural toxicity within DHHS and the wider government

It is plausible that such a toxic culture within the DHHS (and in other Victorian Government agencies) would have profound effects on the way that staff were recruited and promoted, on how decisions were made, on how and to whom information was provided, and on the way in which staff undertook their duties. For example, some of these cultural problems manifested in alleged tense antagonistic relationships, a lack of cooperation, and even hostility (according to anecdotal accounts of some former insiders) between the Chief Health Officer and his team, and the Department's emergency management team.

Some of the devastating effects of toxicity within DHHS seems to have established a culture of denial, a lack of transparency, and the desire for secrecy that became apparent during the pandemic. These effects became especially evident during the gross mismanagement of the lockdown of the public housing towers in Melbourne during July 2020, which garnered worldwide attention and condemnation for human rights breaches (Albeck-Ripka, 2020; BBC, 2020b).

The public housing towers debacle

In late June and early July 2020, the SARS-CoV-2 virus began circulating in a high-density public housing estate of nine residential tower blocks in Flemington in Melbourne's inner west. The 3000 occupants of these tower blocks were living in overcrowded accommodation and represented some of the most disadvantaged communities within the State, being mainly immigrants and refugees many with little if any English language skills (Pockett, 2020). It was just the sort of high-density communities that many of the private security guards, working in the Hotel Quarantine Program, could have called home.

What was to happen on this housing estate would be reported around the world and would gather widespread condemnation of the Victorian Government. As hundreds of armed police swarmed outside the high-rise buildings, residents found themselves suddenly forcibly detained inside their homes, without any prior warning. A result of the Victorian Government struggling to try and contain a burgeoning second wave of the pandemic following infection control failures at two of the quarantine hotels.

Another flawed decision?

Following the detection of a number of positive COVID-19 cases within the public housing towers, on Saturday 4 July 2020 at 11am, a group of senior government bureaucrats made the decision to initiate a mandatory lockdown. They started planning for the logistics, support, and engagement that would be required in the lead up to the lockdown intended to come into place at midnight the next day – Sunday. Giving them, or so they believed at the time, some 36 hours to prepare. However, some five hours later that same Saturday at 4.08pm, Premier Daniel Andrews publicly announced an immediate lockdown. The suddenness of this lockdown was not based upon the advice of senior health officials. To the contrary it appears that the Acting Chief Health Officer was given only fifteen minutes to read the necessary documents before *being directed to sign the public health order* (Ombudsman, 2020).
The Ombudsman, in her investigation into the lockdown concluded that this decision and direction came from a Cabinet meeting, chaired by the Premier that had been held earlier that afternoon[246]. Certainly, the decision to use police to enforce the detention of residents came directly from the Premier's Office[247]. It appears the Victoria Police and DHHS staff were provided with as little as 90 minutes warning about the lockdown operation, whilst local council authorities were provided with no warning at all (Simons, 2020). The first time that any of the residents became aware of the lockdown was when hundreds of uniformed police arrived and surrounded the towers to prevent anyone from leaving. Leaving residents terrified, as scenes reminiscent of Nazi and Stalinist eras unfolded, a developing situation on the ground that must have reminded some of the refugee residents of the totalitarian regimes from which they had fled.

The following days of the Towers' lockdown were described as 'chaotic'. With residents forcibly detained inside their homes without food, medication, or other essential items. To compound the initial shock and distress, the residents were provided with little in the way of information about what was happening. At one stage temporary fencing was erected to surround the tower blocks to help armed police enforce the detention. It was some days before residents were even allowed outside of their overcrowded accommodation to gain access to fresh air and exercise.

Eventually, some food began to arrive from outside for the beleaguered residents. Given the government's previous planning failures, it was not

---

[246] Ombudsman, 2020, p. 4-5.
[247] Ombudsman, 2020, p. 117.

surprising that much of the food provided was out of date, semi-thawed, (and for a community represented by a significant proportion of Muslims), non-halal and included pork sausage rolls (Boseley, 2020; Eddie et al, 2020; Kolovos, 2020e). The government had to rely on food being donated, but even then, they had great difficulties in in getting it to the 3000 residents, significant delays resulting in spoilage and waste of unknown quantities of this food (Hall and Eddie, 2020).

The Ombudsman concluded in her investigation that the lockdown was unlawful and represented a clear breach of the residents' human rights. It was also apparent that by this time (early July) that the government already had serious concerns about the use of private security in enforcing restrictions in the quarantine hotels[248], with the Premier's Office issuing instructions that police and not private security had to be used at the tower blocks.

Other documents that were uncovered by the Ombudsman's investigation appeared to have justified the sudden lockdown on the grounds that the *"towers were a hotbed of criminality"*[249], which was contrary to the known facts. The decision to immediately lockdown the towers is in stark contrast to the early warnings and the eight hours that was provided to neighbouring residential properties to prepare for the lockdown. That the occupants of the housing towers were singled out for 'special treatment' is unarguable. Given the large proportion of non-Europeans in the housing towers (McGhee, 2020; Om, 2020;), that the Andrews government was not more widely condemned for stereotypical racism now seems extraordinary.

Following the release of the Ombudsman's report condemning the Victorian Government's decisions and actions, it came as little surprise that the government still refused to apologise for their abuse of human rights (Boseley, 2020). Even 12 months later, the government continued in their failure to recognise the difference between the necessity of a lockdown, and the manner in which such a lockdown is conducted (Yussuf, 2021).

Despite the DHHS appearing to have had little actual involvement in the timing of the lockdown decision, it appears that they were complicit in the culture of secrecy and denial that affected other public housing-related COVID-19 issues (Bevege, 2020) in addition to the operational chaos that ensued around the Flemington lockdown. As serious issues began to emerge, the DHHS response was to avoid admitting to the problems, and then doing little to address them

---

248 Ombudsman, 2020, p. 118

249 Ombudsman, 2020 p. 5.

(Simons, 2020a; 2020b). The Flemington residential lockdown was not an isolated problematic incident. Similar cultural issues contributed to the cloak of secrecy that tried to prevent any public disclosure of data on quarantine hotel infections and the origins of the second wave outbreaks (Sakkal, 2020b). Such denial of responsibility and secrecy was to become commonplace within the Hotel Quarantine Program, and into the subsequent revamped system.

Media revelations continued to expose continuing toxicity and secrecy that extended beyond DHHS, including apparent attempts to cover up multiple subsequent infection control breaches, and the emergence of the hotel nebuliser scandal.

Operational reset, cultural malaise – "the neubuliser man"

Following the release of the Coate Inquiry Final Report in late 2020, and in the face of the Inquiry's findings of failures and mismanagement, the Hotel Quarantine Program was 'reset'. This saw the establishment of COVID-19 Quarantine Victoria (CQV) a new agency tasked with overseeing the revised 'accommodation program' (VicGov, 2021; Andrews, 2020a; Thorne, 2020). This new initiative at last recognised the unsuitability of using CBD based hotels and instead saw a movement out of the high-risk CBD locations and into the Holiday Inn at Melbourne Airport for incoming overseas traveller accommodation.

However, this new reset was soon beset with a litany of failures of its own, with the ultimate failure being another quarantine breach, and escape and transmission of COVID-19 into the community, which sent Victoria into its third lockdown. The Victorian Government directly blamed this latest breach upon a returned male traveller who was using an "unapproved" nebuliser to treat an asthma condition. The male traveller in question and his family had tested negative on entering quarantine, but tested positive later in their quarantine period. The traveller subsequently became seriously ill with COVID, and was admitted into intensive care. With no immediate means of defending himself, he fell victim to the government's unfounded claims that his use of the nebuliser had created virus laden aerosols which had then escaped and infected others in the Holiday Inn. The Victorian Government thought that it had found an ideal scapegoat.

As officials continued to unfairly blame the "nebuliser man", he tried to defend himself from his hospital bed, disputing the government's story. The nebuliser man's account ran somewhat contrary to the government's own narrative. He claimed that that the use of the nebuliser had been approved by quarantine staff and that they had also offered to provide additional Ventolin for the device. Government bureaucrats continued to scapegoat the "nebuliser man" over coming weeks (Cunningham and Mannix, 2021; Lackey and Parsons, 2021; Lathouris, 2021; Sky News, 2021c), despite published scientific evidence showing this route was highly unlikely (Cazzola et al, 2021). Other research. published several years before, presented evidence from the previous SARS coronavirus outbreak showing that the use of nebulisers did not pose an increased risk of widespread transmission (Tran et al, 2012; Wan et al, 2004). Evidence that government bureaucrats seemed to have conveniently ignored in their blame game.

The extent to which this scapegoating was unwarranted and egregious finally came to light when the content of another government secret report and the staging of an alleged cover-up was leaked to The Australian Newspaper (Credlin, 2021; Editorial, 2021a; McPhee and Coe, 2021; Varga, 2021b). It emerged that the government had conducted a covert investigation into this latest outbreak, producing a secret report that actually exonerated the 'nebuliser man. The Government, in receipt of this secret report, continued for another two months to publicly blame the 'nebuliser man' for starting the third pandemic wave. The 'nebuliser man' would probably have remained the official cause had the report and cover-up not been leaked to the media (Hannan and Johnston, 2021a; Mitchell, 2021; Noah 2021).

Rather than blaming the 'nebuliser man', this report provided evidence that the new outbreak arose from yet more bureaucratic bungling. Victorian Government quarantine officials had been using harmful procedures for testing 'guests' that massively increased the transmission risk within the hotel. According to the secret report, the primary cause of the quarantine failure was believed to have been caused by officials inappropriately swabbing an infected female traveller for an extended period of time in an open doorway inside the Holiday Inn. This allowed an aerosol of the virus to travel down the corridor and pool outside the "nebuliser man's" hotel room door. From where he and his family became infected once their door was opened (Hannan and Johnston, 2021a). Rather than being the culprit, the "nebuliser man" was another victim of government incompetence and cover-up. What sort of culture was prevailing within the government, and CQV in particular, that influenced officials to think that such secrecy, cover-up, and denial was acceptable behaviour?

CQV's problems continued through 2021, with a number of senior staff being stood down or dismissed over various mismanagement and misconduct issues. One individual, the overall head of infection control (Matiu Bush) had allegedly refused to follow testing and infection control directions on at least two occasions, which did not appear to result in any disciplinary action, and Bush continued in his role. As in other cases, Bush was only stood down several months later, but only after incident reports into his behaviour were leaked to the media (Davey, 2021; Hannah and Johnston, 2021b; Rollason, 2021b). Bush subsequently resigned whilst he was under investigation into further allegations over the hiring of two gym workers (from a fitness business Bush was also allegedly promoting) for senior positions at quarantine hotels (Hannan and Johnston, 2021c; 2021d).

Another senior CQV bureaucrat (the Infection Prevention and Control director) also resigned following counselling over an infection control breach at one of the quarantine hotels (Hannan and Johnston, 2021b). These were obviously not isolated issues within CQV as in late April 2021, just a few weeks after Bush was stood down, another two senior infection control managers were sacked following 52 reportable incidents that had occurred in their first four weeks on the job (Cunningham, 2021; Fowler et al, 2021b).

More attempts at change

Due to continuing problems with the Hotel Quarantine Program, it was again 'revamped' in March 2021 following the earlier February quarantine failures, community transmissions, and the third lockdown (Sakkal and Ilanbey, 2021b). Entering a fourth lockdown in late May 2021, following another quarantine failure and subsequent community transmission, again it appeared that contact tracing could not match the speed of the outbreak and was quickly overwhelmed (Trioli, 2021; VOA News, 2021). With allegedly flawed health advice, and an apparent lack of government confidence in its own public health arrangements to contain an outbreak, a transition into another lockdown was inevitable (Bramston, 2021; Editorial, 2021b).

DHHS was the subject of significant criticism throughout the COVID-19 pandemic, although criticism of ineptitude was not new to the department and long predated the pandemic. DHHS has been criticised for its lack lustre performance on a range of major initiatives before the pandemic, including significant failings with its $45 million homelessness program (Skatssoon, 2019). Whilst ineffective leadership and decision-making are highly probable causes of such failings, breakdowns in communications within DHHS and with other agencies also appears to have been a major contributing factor. Problematic organisational culture and poor leadership have both been implicated as drivers of such poor communications, although the real extent to which culture influenced the substantial breakdowns in DHHS communications is likely to remain unknown. Certainly, problematic organisational culture within DHHS was identified as being at the heart of the hotel quarantine failure (Sakkal, 2020c) and the contact tracing operations (Asher, 2020). At the heart of its cultural problems, DHHS has long been regarded as defensive and unwilling to acknowledge errors[250], traits that were demonstrated on multiple occasions throughout the pandemic. However, these problems were not just unique to DHSS, or just restricted to a few agencies within the Victorian Government.

This cultural lack of communication not only occurred within and between different areas and agencies, but it also extended into those private contactors involved in the Hotel Quarantine Program. The breakdown in communications with private security operators (and later with contracted medical providers) had obvious direct consequences for the subsequent outbreaks of disease. However, given the apparent toxic culture and attendant communication breakdowns, the eventual extent of these outbreaks could plausibly have been much worse, and could have involved multiple other routes of exposure than just security guards. We will probably never know the extent of cultural issues and systemic communication failures that occurred over the first two years or so of the pandemic. However, those cases that have come to light show staggering individual and institutional ineptitude in dealing with these matters.

Amongst the myriad of other failures that occurred, the case of a private cleaning company 'Ikon' is especially prominent and worrying. Ikon was contracted to clean hotel rooms using fairly standard routine cleaning regimes. However, they were not informed that their work in the Rydges Hotel was in a designated 'hot hotel' for COVID-19 infected individuals (Kolovos, 2020c). Accordingly, they did not recognise the need to establish any additional arrangements or precautions to deal with these conditions, exposing themselves and others to unprecedented levels of exposure to COVID-19 and levels of risk of additional quarantine breaches. The really incredible thing is that cleaning staff were not implicated in quarantine breaches or as a major source of community transmission .

Whilst this problematic culture was evident within DHHS through the first half of 2020, a culture of secrecy and denial appears to have permeated other areas of the later pandemic response including the reset Hotel Quarantine Program[251] (Sakkal, 2020a), and well into the 3rd and 4th pandemic waves (Dexter and

---

[250] Parliament of Victoria (2020), pp. 94-97.

[251] Run by a new agency - COVID-19 Quarantine Victoria (CQV) under Corrections Victoria, the agency responsible for running the prison system.

Fowler, 2021; Editorial, 2021a; 2021b; Hannan and Johnston, 2021b) and possibly even later. The Victorian Government's attempts at secrecy and alleged cover-ups[252] were derailed by leaks that revealed multiple potentially deadly breaches of quarantine and infection control rules by front-line and senior government officials working in the refreshed reset Hotel Quarantine Program (Editorial, 2021a; Sakkal, 2020a).

These leaks included allegations that a toxic workplace culture was created by a fear of public disclosure, had resulted in a loss of transparency about decision-making. This prevailing secrecy has apparently allowed senior bureaucrats' attempts to 'crush' any dissent, and to take retribution against staff that dared to question or stand up to this toxic culture. Following Corrections Victoria's takeover of the Program, there was substantial turnover of staff due to "poor workplace culture" (Sakkal, 2020a), including several senior roles. It was also claimed that many of the staff that decided to remain with the agency were increasingly ignored by management. This significant loss of expertise and 'corporate' memory further increased the already extreme risk exposure faced by the agency. Especially that earlier lessons learned (from multiple previous failures) would be lost and that the recent history of disasters would be repeated.

The attempts to maintain secrecy over hotel quarantine bungles also extended as far as the Premier's own office. In one particular instance the Premier was allegedly "livid" that the Chief Health Officer had provided a report (on the quarantine hotel origins of the burgeoning 2nd wave outbreak) to other senior staff within the pandemic response, instead of keeping the report secret to only the Premier's Chief of Staff (Le Grand, 2020b).

Leadership of the pandemic response

A great deal of the pandemic response within Victoria, and especially with regards to the Hotel Quarantine Program, has been characterised by an absence of consistent effective leadership by the government, and its various agencies and bureaucracies (Karpin, 2020). This is not a new concept for the Victorian Government, failures in leadership, decision-making, breakdowns in interagency coordination and communications were critical contributing factors in Victoria's last major mass fatality disaster, the 2009 Black Saturday

[252] With staff allegedly being ordered to NOT submit reports about breaches.

bushfires (Teague 2010), and probably a 'root cause' of many of the other Victorian Government policy and program failures since that time.

Whilst vital lessons were identified from the 2009 disaster, those lessons appear not to have been learned, or to have been forgotten in the lead up to and during the COVID-19 pandemic. Many of the failings that have happened in Victoria's pandemic response were predictable, and indeed had been predicted by many former public servants that had departed from what they perceived to be an increasingly dysfunctional system. Indeed, the defining characteristics of the Victorian Government's leadership during the pandemic response were the public portrayal of internecine bickering and transferring of blame, a lack of cooperation and transparency, a common denial of any form of individual or collective responsibility for errors, and an overall absence of accountability.

As the outbreaks from hotel quarantine continued to expand through the Victorian community, public health leadership within the State failed according to multiple sources (Le Grand, 2020b), with allegations that the leadership *"either didn't accept or were unwilling to admit they had serious problems and were reluctant to ask for help"*.

Health leadership

The leadership of the health response has come in for particular criticism, with claims that the Chief Health Officer (Brett Sutton) was actively excluded from the control and key decision-making of Operation Soteria[253]. A Public Health Command was established early on in the pandemic, but was given no actual operational leadership or oversight role, being relegated to the writing of policies for other non-experts to implement and lead (Sutton, 2020). Certainly, the structure that was established placed the Chief Health Office and Public Health Commander away from the main 'health control' leadership (see Figure 8) for some time as the outbreaks developed into a widespread pandemic.

[253] Operation Soteria: the Hotel Quarantine Program.

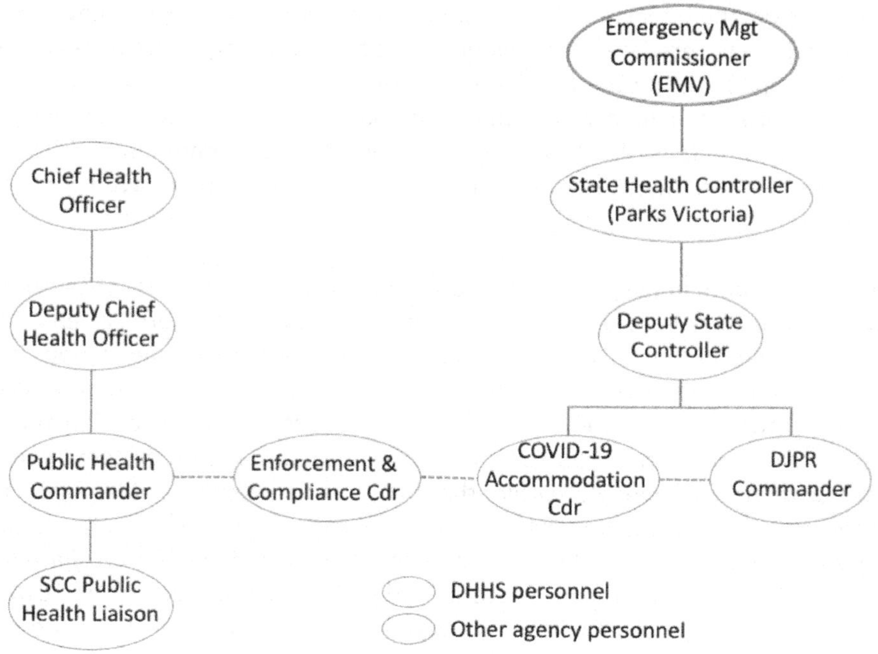

Figure 8[254]: governance structure[255] for Operation Soteria – hotel quarantine
(Cdr = Commander)

These arrangements appear to be inconsistent with the AIIMS[256] structure, especially the dilution of 'unity of command', and are inconsistent with the State arrangements and responsibilities for a control agency (ABC, 2020). This reflects evidence provided by the Chief Health Officer to the Inquiry, when he raised his own personal concerns about how the leadership of the pandemic response had been set up[257]. Dr Sutton appears to have been personally concerned that he had not been appointed as the State Controller (as expected under preparedness and pandemic plan arrangements, including the State Health Emergency Response Plan), but instead had been sidelined by two "DHHS bureaucrats" (one being a former police senior sergeant) appointed to

254 Based upon Eagle, 2020 and Crisp, 2020.

255 This structure was in place until mid-April 2020, at which time a 'dotted line' connected the State Health Controller and the Chief Health Officer.

256 AIIMS: Australian Inter-service Incident Management System, a nationally accepted approach designed for complex emergences and disasters, especially providing a control, command, and coordination structure for multi-agency responses.

257 Coate 2020a, pp. 272, 274-275, 292-295.

the role from the Department's emergency management area. There have been rumours, that predate the pandemic, of a long-term break-down in relationships between the DHHS emergency management area and the Chief Health Officer's portfolio. Anecdotal stories had been circulating for some time that these two areas of DHHS allegedly would not even communicate directly with each other, any questions or information having to be relayed through another party.

During the Coate Inquiry, the DHHS had withheld several emails that they were later forced to release after they were discovered during a forensic audit. It should be noted that this only occurred after The Age newspaper found that certain emails had been deliberately withheld from the Inquiry. These emails provided further evidence supporting the rumours about the dysfunctional relationships between Dr Sutton's public health team and other "emergency management colleagues", within the DHHS and Emergency Management Victoria (Baker et al, 2020). These emails reveal a "turf war" about who should have been in charge of the Program. In these emails Professor Euan Wallace (as the then CEO of Safer Care Victoria, later to be appointed as the DHHS Secretary) communicated with Dr Sutton regarding the rumours about internal tensions with the Department, and serious concerns about the governance of the Program.

Dr Sutton's responses show that the Program was set up by Emergency Management Victoria without the approval and without seeking advice from any of the key expert health roles that should normally have been consulted: the Chief Health Officer, Deputy Chief Health Officer or Deputy Public Health Commander. Victorian control of the COVID-19 pandemic, the largest public health crisis to face the state in over a hundred years[258], was therefore under an ad hoc organisation run by former police, firefighters, and other bureaucrats (with no medical expertise), and with the apparent deliberate *exclusion of public health experts.* Dr Sutton's emails reveal that the Program was wholly disconnected from the management of a public health emergency and instead was being conducted as a purely logistical operation.

It later became evident that the decision not to appoint Professor Sutton to the controlling role was made by the DHHS Deputy Secretary, Melissa Skilbeck, an economist responsible for both the Chief Health Officer, public health, and emergency management areas within the Department (Cunningham et al, 2020).

---

[258] Since the 1918/19 'Spanish lady' influenza pandemic.

State leadership

At two weeks into the Hotel Quarantine Program, senior health officials were openly calling into question the Program's leadership and management, including that there was *still no unified plan in place*, as well as an *absence of appropriate policies or processes* for managing the Program. These officials raised matters about substantial risks and were demanding an urgent review into the handling of the Program (Varga, 2020). This seems to have been a call for action that was roundly ignored by those actually making the top decisions. These leadership problems were greatly exacerbated by a general lack of clarity about what agency and which individuals were in overall charge of the Program. There was no transparent overall authority, and since neither DJPR or DHHS (or rather the relevant senior bureaucrats and Ministers) viewed themselves as in charge and accountable, then no one took overall responsibility for ensuring that the Program was being governed and managed appropriately. As the Coate Inquiry concluded, these were just some of the *"systemic governmental failings"*[259]

It is unclear why, during the peak of a disastrous health emergency, that the government appointed an individual with no health background or significant interagency disaster management expertise into the State Controller- Health/ Health Commander role. Whilst as the second pandemic wave expanded, the State Controller role was filled variously by *"a middle-ranking health bureaucrat, a forest firefighter, a career policewoman, and a State Emergency Service executive, none of whom have a medical background"* (Le Grand, 2020a). Similarly, during this time, the Deputy Health Commanders were a series of Deputy Chief Fire Officers from the agency responsible for managing Crown land (DELWP[260]).

It was not until July 2020 that the DHHS Secretary (Kym Peake) took over the role of State Controller. It is interesting that the two top decision-makers on pandemic matters within the DHHS at the time had no medical or public health experience, the Secretary had law and arts degrees and the Deputy Secretary was an economist. Whilst at the same time senior health officials, including the Chief Health Officer were being sidelined (Kolovos, 2020b). It does appear that at some stage Professor Sutton was appointed as State Controller, although *nobody actually told him that this had occurred*, so it was hardly surprising that he did not immediately undertake his responsibilities.

---

[259] Coate Inquiry, 2020a p. 202

[260] Department of Environment, Lands, Water and Planning.

It is perhaps a reflection of the lack of infectious disease control experience within the senior ranks of the State's incident management team that a coordinated and effective pandemic response was not evident in the lead up to and for the entirety of the hotel quarantine failure and second wave outbreak. A "Victorian Action Plan for COVID-19 Pandemic" was reported as still in *draft form and unpublished* in mid-August 2020, whilst an internet search in January 2021 (a year after the pandemic started) could find no evidence for the publication of a finalised document with that title.

Whilst there are valid neuropsychological reasons why decision-making degrades under conditions of extreme stress and uncertainty, it must be remembered that much of the poor decision-making that contributed to the quarantine failure was made under very different and much calmer conditions. These were critical decisions made in the months and years before the actual pandemic even surfaced. Whilst during the pandemic, many decisions appear to have been driven more by ideology, dysfunctional culture, low competence, and hubris, than by the needs of a rapidily and complex evolving pandemic situation.

Muddy waters

The Coate Inquiry revealed that not only was there a great deal of confusion about which agency was in overall charge of the Hotel Quarantine Program, but also that the management structures and processes put in place for both the Program and for the overall response to the pandemic were a complete mess. It may even be an overstatement to have thought of them as either management or control structures at all. Roles and responsibilities were unclear, confused, and fractured. This confusion was added to by parallel roles and structures resulting in potential duplication of effort and conflict, whist other much needed responsibilities were not assigned to the relevant positions within the structure. Concerns were raised by some senior bureaucrats about the control and management arrangements for the Program and at least in some quarters, there were worries that these would *"be a risk to the health and safety of detainees"*[261]. A prophetic concern that seems to have been ignored by more senior leadership.

It is also concerning that at a time when woke agenda seemed to drive everything within the Victorian Government, especially concerns about how

[261] Coate Inquiry, 2020a p. 301.

certain language could be harmful, create prejudice, and cause offence, that the government persisted with using the term '*detainees*'. Most definitions of 'detainee' are based on the concept of unwilling imprisonment, especially for political reasons. The widespread use of 'detainee' would almost certainly have unconsciously influenced perceptions and behaviours of officials towards those being held in quarantine. That Victorian Government bureaucrats even thought that using the term 'detainee' was acceptable is telling of their attitude towards returning travellers and helps to explain the subsequent dehumanisation and abuses that occurred.

Other arrangements

The Inquiry and some sections of the media have made a great deal about Dr Sutton misleading the Inquiry over when he knew about private security arrangements. Whilst he certainly received emails informing him about the arrangements, given the work demands at the time it was not unreasonable that the significance of these emails did not resonate. However, the significant focus on this matter has, perhaps, been yet another misdirection. Especially since it appears that Dr Sutton (or other medical experts) had no material role in the decision-making process about the use, set up, or operational management of the CBD hotels; no role in the decision to use private security; no role in the procurement of private security or of the selection of Unified Security; and no role in the day-to-day management of security contractors. It appears that the more conspiratorial minded began to perceive the attempted setup of a scapegoat during the process of the Inquiry. This may yet prove to be prescient.

WorkSafe investigation and prosecution

WorkSafe Victoria has never been shy regarding publicity about its investigations and prosecutions into alleged breaches of the occupational health and safety law, with multiple public announcements made each year (just a few recent examples include: Editorial, 2021; Piovesan, 2021b; Steibel, 2021; Vince, 2021; WorkSafe Victoria, 2021a; 2021b; 2021c; 2021d, 2021e, 2021f; Godde, 2020; Harcourt et al, 2020; Cluff, 2019b; Whyte et al, 2017; Harris, 2017). WorksSafe has often publicly announced an investigation is being undertaken within a very short time of an incident is occurring, often within *24 hours* of an incident occurring, and long before any such investigation is near completion.

It is therefore very interesting WorkSafe Victoria was silent about potential health and safety breaches associated with the pandemic response, taking nearly four months to decide it would investigate what had been described as Australia's single largest mass casualty event (SEA, 2021b). Once the investigation commenced, WorkSafe then failed to meet its six-month obligatory timeline for completing an investigation and making a decision on the need to prosecute. A search of the internet has failed to find any case where WorkSafe Victoria took this long on a decision to prosecute a private company or an individual[262].

It was not until November 2021 (some 18 months after the alleged breaches occurred) that WorkSafe decided to prosecute[263], and then only the Department of Health (no other departments and no individuals – Ministers or bureaucrats were to be prosecuted). This decision to prosecute was finally made after over a year's worth of complaints about WorkSafe's apparent inaction regarding this matter.

There were calls for several bureaucrats and the Premier to be investigated and prosecuted for breaches under Victoria's OHS Act. This decision to not investigate individuals and the apparently unreasonable delays in the process naturally led to speculation about a possible coverup (Philips, 2021) and that there may have been political pressure on WorkSafe to turn a blind eye (Gottliebsen, 2020b). There was also speculation about the nature of the relationship between Premier Daniel Andrews and WorkSafe's CEO Colin Radford (also a former chief of staff to a Labor Minister), and whether this could have influenced WorkSafe.

Dissatisfied with what they saw as a lack of justice, Self Employed Australia made a mandamus application[264] Victorian Supreme Court to try to force WorkSafe to prosecute "27 individuals and entities" (including the Premier) involved in the Hotel Quarantine Program for health and safety breaches (Houston, 2021b; SEA, 2021). In December 2022 the Court dismissed the application on a technicality of expired time for the application (Supreme Court of Victoria, 2022). Unfortunate, especially since WorkSafe had failed to meet its

[262] With the exception of the prosecution of St Basil's nursing home in July 2022, the location of several residents' deaths in the aftermath of the Hotel Quarantine Failure (WorkSafe, 2022).

[263] WorkSafe Victoria, 2021.

[264] A writ of mandamus is an application to the Court for it to order the government to perform a duty that is owed that the government owes to the public.

required timelines to complete the investigation, with no apparent consequences.

In some cases, the prosecution of a government department (rather than the prosecution of individuals) by WorkSafe could plausibly be seen as a smoke and mirrors exercise. Hypothetically, if a government 'Department' is found guilty (or pleads guilty) and if the maximum penalties are applied (which in the case of the prosecution of the Department of Health the media has reported could be up to about $95 million), then what parties are really being punished. The 'Department' pays its $95 million fine, which goes into consolidated revenue managed by Treasury. The Department now faces a shortfall in its budget for that year of $95 million, does it defund its essential services to the people of the State? In that scenario, the only people to be punished are those members of the public that need those essential service.

Alternatively, the 'Department' can ask for a special appropriation of $95 million from Treasury, which would be paid from consolidated revenue (which just happens to have had an unexpected windfall of $95 million paid into it from a rather large fine). Thus, the money is simply transferred from one part of government to another until it is paid back into the 'Department's' coffers. The only net effect of this will be the hundreds of thousands of dollars spent on a WorkSafe investigation and prosecution, and on defence lawyers hired by the 'Department'. As well as a few hundreds of thousands of dollars expended by public servants as they push around the paperwork to move $95 million from the 'Department', giving it a short holiday in Spring Street, before returning it back to the 'Department'. The overall result of this hypothetical scenario is that tax-payers' money is again wasted.

Going back to the real world, the final question is: what actionable learnings will emerge from the actual prosecution? The previous incarnation of the Department of Health was prosecuted by WorkSafe for other offences on multiple occasions, and problems with the leadership, governance, and culture of the Health Department persisted for years, how much has really changed as a result?

Given that the WorkSafe prosecution is still before the Court, this book will not discuss any of the specific charges made against the now Department of Health, and any discussion in this book should not be viewed as relating to these matters before the Court.

Ideology

Ideology is a central tenet of politics and of government, it is what drives and differentiates the different political parties. However, when ideology drives government priorities against the societal good, or perverts expected standards of good governance and decision-making then it is harmful to the community as a whole (Belido et al, 2021).

It is entirely plausible that the Andrews government's ideological bent may have played an influential role in how the pandemic was approached and managed. In particular, its ideology appears to have set in place processes that have resulted in a long-term degradation of expert capability within the State. It is also important to remember that self-serving ideology alone does not automatically lead to governmental failure and corruption[265], where both lack of government capacity and government accountability can also play major roles (Hollyer and Wantechekon, 2014). Even where governments are widely perceived to be 'corrupt' they can still retain their popularity and attract voter support (Cordero and Blais, 2017)

A range of assertions have been made that the Andrews government has been more concerned with ideology, particularly with its identity politics, than with good government. For example, substantial resources were being directed towards 'woke' projects (such as "sexism in fairytales") whilst Victoria's public health capability was left under-resourced and over-worked (Sheridan, 2020). Yet the Victorian Government seems to have even failed to achieve some of the absolute basic diversity and human rights obligations whilst pushing its own diversity virtue signalling. During the pandemic, the government on a number of occasions completely abandoned any semblance of reality and practicality when they had to deal with actual serious diversity and inclusion issues affecting the general public.

In the Victorian Government's interactions with real linguistically, ethnically, and culturally diverse communities, for example: in the lockdown of the Flemington public housing towers; contact tracing within migrant and refugee communities; dealing with ethnically diverse security guards and their families, in each and every case the government failed abysmally[266]. Although the Victorian Government has had a long history of implementing its ideology through promoting 'micro-issues', when it came to actually addressing real

---

265 Corruption as an abuse of the political system

266 Parliament of Victoria, pp 114-124.

people's needs at a time of crisis, the government seemed to have had no idea what to do. Their experience in virtue signalling was of little use when their actions often only succeeded in disenfranchising and marginalising the very people that needed their help.

Even when the Victorian Government attempted to meet its own diversity and inclusion obligations, these were apparently approached with a mix of incompetence and a fundamental lack of understanding. There seems to have been an overriding (and misinformed belief) that engagement with a diverse community could be achieved simply by relying on providing documents translated into multiple different languages. This appears to have completely ignored the real issues in dealing with such communities, especially in trying to conduct contact tracing over the phone; the lack of coordination between government and external multicultural organisations; providing COVID-19 test results in English language text messages that could not understood by recipients; etc.

The biggest criticism about the Victorian Government's handling of diverse communities was that they did not understand the real problems that needed to be solved. The issue was not about translating pamphlets, but was rather about how to deal with individuals and communities that had a fundamentally different understanding about how government and health systems operated, and did not really understand what compliance actually meant (Bennett, 2020). The issue was also about the government failing to understand how to deal with communities that had a deep-seated distrust of authority (many were refugees from failed or oppressive regimes). On top of all of this, the government took next to no account of people's fear of and stigma associated with catching COVID-19, and what would happen if they individually tested positive (Victorian Multicultural Commission, 2020). Spending significant time and resources on pushing a diversity ideology onto educated and privileged public servants obviously did little to prepare them for dealing with diversity problems in the real world.

Government ideology has also been implicated in a continuing loss of expertise and capability from the public service and a degraded leadership within departments and other agencies (McArthur, 2020). For example, when a government has been shown the extent to which its public service is under skilled and under resourced in both routine and crisis situations, it might reasonably be expected to do something meaningful about it. Like rebuilding real leadership and reforming its aged care, police, public health, human services, procurement, program management, governance, crisis and emergency management capability. Instead, during the height of the pandemic the Victorian Government continued to pursue its own ideological priorities, such as advertising for a "Director Inclusion and Intersectionality", with a salary of about $250,000 plus super (d'Abrera, 2020b).

Whilst the DHHS might have been expected to be taking notice of the calls to improve and have a priority on addressing a chronically under-resourced public health service, it instead continued to drive ideology by mandating that all of its employees use only gender-neutral pronouns on the first Wednesday of every month. Such issues have been recognised at a national level with even the current Labor Prime Minister (whilst in opposition) quoted as saying "the endless culture wars are undermining national discussion" and "you're either a cultural elite, or you're cancelled" (Albanese, 2020).

This is not to say that elements of this ideology are wrong, but it does question the priorities of a dysfunctional and failing government department, where petty rivalries and ideological misalignment potentially contributed to hundreds of Victorian citizens dying.

Within the wider pandemic response, what has been described as the Andrews government's "social experiment" appears to have led directly to the appointment of a security company on the basis of 'social inclusion politics' and not on its capability to undertake the work. The appointment of underqualified applicants to often senior positions within the Victorian public service appears to be a recurring theme. In addition to various media assertions, informal conversations with various executive headhunters have revealed multiple appointments where their preferred candidate was replaced by someone not even on their shortlist because this particular person "ticked the ideology boxes". The question needs to be asked, to what extent did such ideology of identity politics contribute to the lack of leadership and competency within those agencies involved in the Hotel Quarantine Program?

That individuals were put in positions of responsibility for which they were ill-suited is obvious. That they apparently approached these responsibilities with good intent and to the best of their abilities (as the Inquiry found) is no excuse. Many senior bureaucrats were not capable of undertaking the jobs they had to do, and 801 people died as a result. This is not to say that they are personally to blame, although the extent to which some individuals may have knowingly acted in conflict of interest or wilful negligence was not determined by the Inquiry. The 'system' placed them in positions in a manner that made success unlikely. Some, if not many of those involved may not have even realised how unsuited they were to their position and duties.

However, it does appear that some individuals may have knowingly and deliberately acted in a manner that was not in the interest of the public good. That such individual fault could exist was supported by the plethora of media reports suggesting that there were attempts to prevent disclosure of advice and decision-making processes, as well as alleged cover ups. Attempts to hide errors and continuing problems in the management of the Hotel Quarantine Program continued through its various guises. The potential for wilful negligence and abandonment of duty of care needs a level of independent investigation that the Coate Inquiry was unable or unwilling to undertake.

Culpability and accountability

The Coate Inquiry very surprisingly concluded that no individuals were to blame for the catastrophic failure of the Hotel Quarantine Program. Surprisingly, because it was apparent from the evidence that many named individuals did not think through issues adequately, frequently made appallingly poor decisions, and on a number of occasions appeared to have wilfully disregarded meaningful advice when it did not align with their own agenda. Certain individuals were involved in developing and implementing 'plans' in areas where they had no prior experience or competence, and in doing so they failed to consider the risks that their decisions and actions were creating. In a number of circumstances, some senior leaders displayed appallingly toxic behaviours. Any one of these failings could be grounds for dismissal in other jurisdictions or in private companies but seemed to be some form of protected behaviour within the Victorian Government.

One Minister and three senior public servants were allowed to resign when their involvement in the Program was revealed by media investigations and by the Coate Inquiry. Yet those few individuals that were actually publicly dismissed appear to have been fairly junior public servants.

Any analysis of possible culpability in the events leading up to the 801 deaths is outside of the scope of this book. With the high degree of obfuscation and misleading (deliberate or unintentional?) representations, along with key evidence not being made available publicly, it is not possible to simply draw conclusions on culpability. The Hotel Quarantine Program has been characterised by the Premier and a whole range of Ministers and bureaucrats seeking to distance themselves from any accountability or responsibility for the ultimately fatal decisions and actions that were undertaken. At the same time, the Victorian's Government's inability or unwillingness to hold key decision-makers to account appears unprecedented in Australia's history. The remainder of senior bureaucrats that were involved in the Program retained their positions through much of the remaining pandemic period, a few eventually quietly 'disappearing into the night'.

Interestingly, the Premier remained relatively tight lipped about the 'quality and capability' of his senior bureaucrats. Especially so given his previous swift retribution on those that have embarrassed him in the past. For example, in 2015 a public scandal emerged about continuing water contamination at the CFA's[267] training centre at Fiskville in Victoria. Following inaction by various governments and ignoring warnings for over thirty years, various investigations conducted under the Baillieu Liberal government in 2012 confirmed that the facility was heavily contaminated (Joy, 2012). This confirmed that that some firefighting chemicals used in training were toxic and had caused a number of cancers in firefighters as well as contaminating neighbouring private land.

The revelations also included allegations that some senior bureaucrats knew about the health and safety risks, but ignored them. After apparently addressing the issues following the investigations, the facility was declared safe and allowed to continue operating under monitoring by WorkSafe Victoria. However, it later transpired that the facility was still not safe, and questions were raised about whether the required testing at the site had even been conducted (PoV, 2016; Savage, 2015). This public revelation in 2015, under the Labor government, led to the rapid dismissal of WorkSafe's Chair and CEO (Donaldson, 2015). At the time Premier Dan Andrews stated: *"I will not be lied to, and I will not accept incompetence"* (Whittaker, 2015).

How different the Premier's furious reaction to incompetence was in 2015 compared to his 'silence' about incompetence in the much larger disaster in 2020 during the Hotel Quarantine Program. Was this a reflection of his own different levels of knowledge and involvement between these two terrible failures of government?

Despite the compelling evidence of health and safety breaches at the Fiskville facility, WorkSafe decided not to prosecute senior officials because of its inability to gather sufficient evidence and the time taken to undertake the investigation, which exceeded the statutory limits (Edwards, 2015b). As with the Hotel Quarantine Program investigation, it took pressure from external parties (in the case of Fiskville, pressure from the United Firefighter Union) before WorkSafe launched an investigation into another government agency.

---

[267] Country Fire Authority.

Psychology or wilful intent?

To what extent did the failures of the Hotel Quarantine Program result from 'good decisions gone bad', or simply from poor decision-making due to inadequacies in those people making the decisions?

In the vast majority of disasters, individuals do not deliberately go out of their way to make bad decisions, wilfully and negligently take actions, or set out to misinform and lie. However, that well intentioned health policy decisions can result in manifest policy failures is a reasonably common occurrence (Sterman, 2006). For example, budgetary decisions limiting access to expensive medication has led to increased overall health costs; promoting the use of low tar and low nicotine cigarettes has increased the exposure of smokers to dangerous carcinogens that were present in those type of cigarettes; improved effectiveness of anti-retrovirus drugs resulted in an increase in high risk behaviours of some of those infected with HIV.

Most decision-makers face their challenges with good intent and a desire to do the best that they can. They make decisions on the information available at the time and often take actions (based on their experience) that have worked well in the past. However, at some point in time they rely on inadequate information, make inappropriate decisions, and take actions ill-suited for the evolving situation. This commonly occurs because those individuals do not recognise that their own understanding and capabilities are no longer sufficient for the requirements of the evolving situation. The consistent failure to revise and update conclusions in a timely manner seems to have been a common phenomenon throughout the pandemic (Schippers and Rus, 2021). As the situation spirals increasingly out of control, such individuals often retreat further back into their 'comfort zones' and continue to rely on their already outdated situational awareness, formed habits, and familiar (but inadequate) scripts. Along with a growing self-denial, they commonly try to hide their errors and seek to blame others (Shepherd, 2021; Roulet and Pichler, 2020; Fast, 2020;). This was undoubtedly the situation for a good proportion of decision-makers involved in the Hotel Quarantine Program.

In the early stages of the Program, a number of players seem to have thought that they had done an excellent job, given the hubris and self-congratulation that was evident. When it became apparent that the 'wheels were falling off the bus', instead of admitting errors, promoting transparent decision-making, and seeking help, some of these officials instead retreated into a 'deny and defend' posture.

People do react differently in a crisis, and training and experience (which seems to have been missing for a number of the key decision-makers during the COVID-19 pandemic) can help to avoid or manage some of the common psychological effects that occur (CERC 2019). Under high stress, individuals try to simplify the messages they are receiving. For example, cognitive biases filter out 'unacceptable' information, and focus attention on information that support the beliefs already held by the individual. An individual will often actively seek out information that further confirms these beliefs, whilst ignoring or disregarding any conflicting information, so called 'confirmation bias' (Strasshelm, 2019; Parkhurst, 2019; Parkhurst, 2019). Such beliefs become erroneously reinforced and become even more difficult to change, allowing self-denial to proliferate. (Heller and Darling, 2011; Sweeney, 2003).

Sometimes, the content and meaning of information can be significantly misinterpreted, working memory capacity limits the amount of information that can be held and processed, and memory formation can be significantly impaired. The more complex, uncertain, and unfamiliar the situation, the more these effects will be amplified.

Less commonly, but not unknown, some individuals are misdirected in their decisions and action by personal objectives that are antagonistic to the public good. They are directed by the self-centred need for more power, to boost their status, advance their personal causes, acquire other rewards, or diminish the standing of others. In doing so they achieve their personal objectives, whilst their professional duties become, at best, of secondary importance. For some this selfish pursuit can be largely unconscious and remain unrecognised for some time, for others it is a very deliberate and calculating strategy.

Some of these individuals are influenced and encouraged by long term factors such as prevailing cultures, professional pressures, and toxic relationships, and are subject to a gradual degradation in their 'moral compass'. Others, from the very start, only want to pursue their own objectives, and follow group and organisational objectives only whilst these objectives support their own sense of entitlement and fulfilment. During a crisis, some individuals also gain a highly elevated sense of personal privilege and an inflated need to be in control, which can manifest in rule breaking and ignoring directions from others. Again, a practice that was seen on multiple occasions during the Hotel Quarantine Program.

Organisational toxicity

To what extent did toxic culture and toxic individuals play a decisive role in the failure of the Hotel Quarantine Program?

It has been recognised for many years that organisational culture has powerful effects on individual and team psychology and performance (Körner et al, 2015; Mohelska and Sokolova, 2015; Taştan and Türker, 2014; Carlström and Ekman, 2012; Tsai, 2011; Lucas and Kline, 2008; Smollan, 2008; Milne, 2007; Alas and Vardi, 2004; Martins and Terblanche, 2003; Gray, 1998).

Culture becomes a particular concerning issue when it becomes 'toxic'. Such toxic cultures are characterised by fear (staff are too frightened to speak up or contest 'stupid' decisions); poor communication becomes the norm; meaningless policies and rules become more important than good decisions[268]. Although noncompliance and rule breaking can become acceptable with senior leadership when it is expedient to do so. Toxic cultures also mean that individuals have little control over their own work; job titles and status are valued more than competence and performance; interaction diminishes and divisiveness increases between different groups; collaboration diminishes in the face of self-interest and self-protection; toxic individuals are rarely challenged and are allowed (even encouraged) to prosper (Başkan, 2020; Ryan, 2016; Aubrey, 2012; Appelbaum and Roy-Girard, 2012). Toxic cultures impose additional adverse psychological effects that further impair critical thinking and decision-making.

Such toxic cultures usually arise as a result of inadequacies in leadership, from the very top, down and through the organisation. That toxic cultures were (and probably still are) widespread across many Victorian Government agencies is apparent from the various reports and media articles that have been published. This should not be that surprising since it is also well known that such toxicity is far more prevalent in public sector organisations compared with the private sector (Hodgins et al, 2014; Salin, 2008). Notwithstanding the higher frequency of toxicity in government agencies, why are such toxic cultures so apparently widespread in Victoria Government agencies? Again, the lack of transparency makes this a difficult question to answer, but it is a reasonable assumption that a critical causal factor is the failure of senior leadership. Ideological alignment (box ticking), unfair political and personal patronage, and poor recruitment practices mean that poorly skilled and inadequate senior staff will be appointed

[268] Typical of so called 'functional stupidity'.

and promoted in government agencies. Once a poor leader is in position, their decisions and behaviour promote a spreading toxic culture, by establishing a poor 'cultural tone', ignoring or failing to address toxic behaviours in others, and by encouraging and promoting other toxic individuals to more senior and influential positions. Thus, toxic behaviours become increasingly normalised within the workplace.

Yet some senior public servants may not be the source of apparently rampant toxic cultures within Victorian Government agencies. There have been allegations about toxicity, intimidation, and bullying within the Labor party and its elected members in government, including Daniel Andrews himself (Powell, 2023; Durkin, 2022; Hales, 2022b; Huitson, 2022; Murray-Atfield, 2022).

Most readers would quite reasonably believe that individuals that would engage in gross wilful negligence and pursue self-interests should be comparatively rare, especially in senior positions. However, the research paints a rather different picture, and such deliberate negative activity may be much more common than we generally think. Senior leaders are frequently associated with both organisational toxicity and 'dark leadership' (Harris and Jones, 2018; Camm, 2014; Slattery, 2009; Padilla et al, 2007; Lipman, Blumen, 2005), and strongly associated with a range of negative traits (Kiehl, 2018; Gillespie, 2017; Burns, 2017; Burgo 2015; Ghaemi, 2011; Ronson, 2011; Babiak and Hare, 2007) including:

- Low or absent empathy.
- High levels of narcissism, along with high levels of grandiosity and superficiality.
- No conscience in their dealings, particular the ease with which they exploit others.
- Low or absent feelings of guilt and remorse.
- Inability to accept responsibility for their own actions, often shown by an absolute willingness to blame others for their own failings.
- No hesitation in claiming the successes of others as their own.
- High levels of impulsivity and irresponsibility.
- Frequently disloyal, even to those with which they share apparently close relationships.

Concerns about the harm caused by toxic cultures, and the need for a positive organisational culture led some senior bureaucrats within Victoria to try to do something about it. The result was the publication of a nice glossy sourcebook, aimed at public sector leaders (State Services Authority, 2013). How this document was received and used leads us to further questions:

- How many elected and bureaucratic leaders actually read this guidance document about toxic cultures?
- Out of the few leaders that probably did read the material, how many actually understood and accepted the content?
- From that even smaller group, how many leaders tried to implement the recommended measures?

From the apparent wide prevalence and persistence of toxic culture from with the corridors of Labor power itself[269], and through many government department and agencies, it would appear that few leaders have taken positive step to remove toxic cultures and deal with toxic individuals.

In informal conversations with many current and former public servants within Victoria, both prior to and during the pandemic, a common theme emerged. Almost every single person had appalling 'horror stories' of toxic culture and mistreatment by toxic leaders that pursued their own advancement over the 'corporate good'. This should not be news to senior leadership in the State. IBAC has identified numerous examples of toxic cultures and behaviours, quoting a number of affected public servants (IBAC, 2021b):

---

[269] In February 2022, a female Victorian Labor MP (Kaushaliya Vaghela) made allegations of systematic bullying from within Premier Daniel Andrews' Private Office, stretching back to before the pandemic in 2019. On top of the bullying allegations, Ms Vaghela also claimed that the bullying started because she had left the hard left socialist faction within the Victorian Labor Party, and that her calls for help from the Private Office were ignored. Premier Daniel Andrews subsequently dismissed these claims as a "fantasy" (Daly and Clure, 2022; Godde, 2022; Talbot, 2022; Woods, 2022). Ms Vagahela also alleged that Premier Daniel Andrews and the Minister for Women (Gabrielle Williiams) had also engaged in bullying against her. Opposition attempts to have the matter discussed in the Victorian Parliament were "silenced" by the Labor majority (Kealy, 2022). Allegations that subsequently prompted an investigation by WorkSafe Victoria following a complaint made by the Liberal opposition (Talbot, 2022). Ms Vaghela famously crossed the floor to vote with the Opposition on an investigation into alleged Labor Party corruption in the 'red shirts' scandal misuse of $400,000 of public funds (Eddie, 2022; Ilanbey, 2022). Just a month later, the federal Labor Party was rocked by allegations of bullying of one of its female Senators by the Party's hard left wing (Clarke and Zaczek, 2022; Coorey, 2022; Mahoney, 2022).

- *"Everyone is too scared to challenge issues for fear of reprimand/reprisals".*
- *"There is nepotism and obvious favouritism of individuals who are known bullies".*
- *"I would feel anxious about complaining unless really blatant and witnessed, especially with probable loss of VPS jobs - people talk about "keeping their head down"".*
- *"A general reluctance to report for fear of repercussions and a lack of faith in the process".*

The psychopathic leader?

A number of studies have associated toxic leadership with the dark triad (Figure 9), a "dark personalities" model of subclinical "socially aversive traits" (Paulhus, 2014). This constellation of abnormal traits contributes to an overall tendency towards callous manipulation and self-advancement that are the most common characteristics of toxic leaders (Kornilova and Krasavtseva, 2017; Figueredo et al, 2015; Hams and Spain, 2015; Schyns, 2015; Furnham, et al, 2013; Paulhus and Williams, 2002). The dark triad consists of narcissism (overwhelming sense of entitlement, self-importance, and the need for excessive admiration); Machiavellianism (selfish and self-serving); and psychopathy (superficial charm[270], dishonesty, manipulative, abusive supervision, lack of guilt, and lack of empathy). Toxic leaders often establish an unquestioning following, especially of loyal lieutenants, that become captured by their superficial charm and charisma. This followership buys in to the toxic leaders "grand vision", which eventually is revealed to be a "grand illusion" divorced from reality, (Lipman-Blumen, 2005) by those that did not drink the 'kool-aid"[271].

However, the 'loyal followers' can continue to support the toxic leader for years, disregarding all of the evidence of poor leadership, right up to the time that the toxic leader abandons them because they have ceased to be of use. Cynically many of the 'loyal lieutenants' continue to idealise and publicly promote the toxic leader, even though they are fully aware of the inadequacies and failing of 'their leader'. Again, because such promotion continues to serve these lieutenants' self-interests.

---

[270] Psychopathic individuals are also often regarded as charismatic at least until their other psychopathic traits become more recognisable.

[271] A metaphor for following a leader or ideology in a cult-like manner.

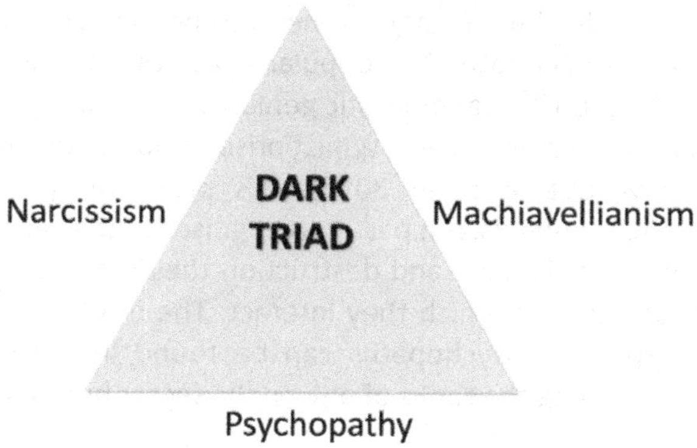

Figure 9: the Dark Triad

It is galling to think that anyone in a senior leadership position in any organisation during the pandemic would deliberately act in a way that ultimately rendered that organisation's efforts largely ineffective. To what extent toxic leadership could have contributed to these failings in the Hotel Quarantine Program, and in the pandemic response more generally, requires plausible inferences to be made from the available information. That toxic leadership is present within government agencies is not only plausible, it is probabilistically near certain, with multiple studies looking at toxicity in public sector leadership within many different jurisdictions (Franken and Plimmer, 2019, Kline, 2019; Lucas, 2019; Williams, 2019; Dobbs and Do, 2018; JDD, 2018; Omar et al, 2017; Ronnie, 2017).

That toxic cultures existed within Victorian Government agencies is a matter of fact. That serious problems associated with leadership and organisational culture were identified by the Coate Inquiry and in subsequent revelations by the media, is also a matter of fact. The Coate Inquiry did not, however, reach any conclusions about specific toxic individuals.

Many people will easily recognise narcissistic and Machiavellian traits in their bosses and in public figures. But is suggesting that 'psychopaths' may hold positions of authority and power within public institutions stretching plausibility too far? It is an interesting exercise to reflect back to the Coate Inquiry, and to other public appearances of the various players, and then think about the extent to which some of these individuals have exhibited the various traits associated with the dark triad.

To what extent might psychopathy have been a contributing factor to such toxic culture and toxic leadership? Firstly, we need to be very clear about what we mean by the term 'psychopath'. The popular image of a scalpel wielding serial killer or 'Hannibal Lector'[272] cannibalistic genius, could not be further from the reality of the corporate psychopath. Whilst prison populations hold a very high proportion of psychopaths (over 30%), it is probable that a majority of psychopaths are not criminals, but pass unrecognised in the general population. That is apart from the damage and destruction they can cause to the people and the organisations with which they interact. The more successful of these non-criminal (corporate) psychopaths can be found in both private sector leadership and ascending the ranks of any public sector bureaucracy.

In reality, the corporate psychopath is likely to be a high achiever in their chosen field, to have no criminal record, but to be ruthless and amoral. The prevalence of psychopaths in professional positions is likely to be much higher than in the general population, (probably somewhere in the region of 6% of all employees) and a number of studies have shown that corporate psychopaths are far more concentrated in the senior ranks of an organisation (Boddy et al, 2021; Klarskov Jeppersen and Leder, 2016; Boddy et al, 2015; Boddy, 2013; Gudmunsson and Southery, 2011; Babiak et al, 2010; Clarke, 2005). Indeed, some psychopathic traits may be more common among senior leaders than in criminals with mental disorders (Kosonen, 2014; Board and Fritzon, 2005). As high as one in five senior managers could have psychopathic traits (Brookes and Fritzon[273], 2016). This is hardly surprising when one considers that the key psychopathic traits are usually those same traits that see individuals promoted over more empathetic and organisationally focussed team players.

Typically, these successful corporate psychopaths show behaviours such as doing whatever it takes to 'win', regardless of the impacts on other people and the longer term costs to the organisation (and without remorse); taking credit for other's work; pathological lying; misusing and blaming others; highly manipulative and controlling; rushing into critical decisions without consulting others; and portraying a polished and charming public (illusory) image. However, despite these toxic traits, the majority of corporate psychopaths do not show certain traits commonly associated with criminal psychopaths such as antisocial behaviour, physical violence (although corporate psychopaths are

---

272 Dr Hannibal Lector is the fictional forensic psychiatrist turned serial killer in a series of Robert Harris novels and Hollywood movies.

273 Note that the Brookes and Fritzon paper was subsequently retracted due to an issue of apparent unintentional and unattributed use of paraphrased sentences in the body of the text. This retraction did not reflect on the validity of the findings.

often associated with bullying and sexual harassment). Instead, corporate psychopaths maintain an outward appearance of balanced mental health. These psychopaths can remain hidden in plain sight for considerable periods of time, hiding behind a mask[274] of normality or 'attractiveness', known as a 'psychopathic fiction' (Babiak and O'Toole, 2012), and often achieve a cult-like status. Whilst incapable of experiencing normal emotions such as empathy, remorse or guilt, they are capable of simulating these emotions as part of their facade, successfully deceiving both followers and casual observers.

Not surprisingly, chief executive officers and public servants represent two of the top ten professions for non-criminal psychopaths (Dutton, 2012) There are indications that the numbers of corporate psychopaths within the public sector may be increasing (Grimmelikhuijsen et al, 2017; Boddy 2016; Fennimore and Sementelli, 2016) and there have been calls for the screening of public servants for psychopathic traits (Boddy, 2015). Even though a majority of politicians and senior bureaucrats would not be meet the definition of a psychopath, many still exhibit one or more psychopathic traits. Concerning behaviours that contribute to toxic leadership and ultimately toxic workplace cultures.

The political sphere is not without its fair proportion of psychopaths, and not just limited to the likes of Stalin, Hitler, Pol Pot, Mao, or Che Guevara. Many iconic political leaders have demonstrated typical psychopathic traits, including US Presidents Theodore Roosevelt, John F. Kennedy, and Lyndon B Johnson (Smith et al, 2014). Such psychopathic traits have been regarded as indicators of success in high political office, and it is certainly plausible that a significant proportion of successful politicians would score highly on either or both of the narcissistic disorder assessment and psychopathic assessment (Hughes, 2019; Nai and Toros, 2019; Taylor, 2021; 2019; Eddy, 2019; Erikson, 2018; and Anestis, 2018; Elder, 2017; Hill, 2016; Whitehead, 2016; Carswell, 2013; Nuwer, 2012; Silver 2012).

Many organisations have an extremely short-term performance focus and provide incentives and rewards for individuals that achieve short-term organisational objectives, irrespective of the long term harm that may be created (Bircham and Connolly, 2013). It is in such organisations that corporate psychopaths thrive, and ultimately cause much destructive harm, creating a "morally bankrupt" organisation leading to its demise, should the psychopathic leaders remain in situ (Boddy, 2011; 2010).

---

[274] Successful corporate psychopaths are able to maintain multiple such 'masks' simultaneously.

Organisational programs that aim to change and improve leadership behaviours are often counterproductive where corporate psychopaths are concerned. It is almost impossible to change toxic thinking that is 'hard-wired' into their brains with such 're-education' attempts, whilst at the same time these programs teach corporate psychopaths new skills that they can then exploit to their own advantage.

Throughout the pandemic we have seen a whole range of behaviours in different elected officials and senior bureaucrats that include many of the traits associated with toxic leaders, and in some cases traits found in psychopaths. Within Victoria, over recent years, there have been multiple examples of toxic cultures in different agencies. The Coate Inquiry and the media have exposed situations within the Hotel Quarantine Program that are either evidence or highly indicative of organisational, cultural and leadership toxicity, and of potential psychopathy. That organisational culture plays a major influential role in how decisions are made, the extent to which information sharing and transparency occurs, how trust within and between different groups is built, and how people work and cooperate, is supported by decades of independent research. This now leaves us with two key questions about the Victorian Hotel Quarantine Program, that the reader needs to think about:

- To what extent did toxic culture within key Victorian Government agencies influence the unfolding disaster that was the Hotel Quarantine Program from March 2020 onwards?
- To what extent could inept, inadequate toxic leadership, or psychopaths in senior roles have contributed to the overall mismanagement of the Program?

This book has reviewed a range of plausible interrelated and non-linear causal pathways, with underpinning conditions being traced back over the months and years preceding the pandemic. Many of these factors will have not just created the conditions that adversely affected situational awareness and decision-making of 'normal actors' involved in the response to COVID-19 within Victoria. These factors will also have established favourable conditions that would have allowed any corporate psychopaths present to flourish and achieve positions of authority. These causal pathways (Figure 15) therefore help to both explain any unintentional errors or deliberate malfeasance that contributed to this Victoria disaster.

Part 5

Bringing together the themes

10
Bringing it together

A network of causal and influencing factors

There were multiple direct causes and other contributing factors that contributed to the Victorian Hotel Quarantine failures. The gross mismanagement of hotel quarantine, the subsequent massive community outbreak, the failure of the trace and test program, and over 800 deaths all represent a complex network of interrelations that go back months and even years before the first suspected cases of COVID-19 occurred in Wuhan, China.

The various preceding chapters of this book have explored the evidence uncovered by the Coate Inquiry the results of various media reporting, and investigations regarding the establishment and management of the Hotel Quarantine Program, and subsequent failures in pandemic response. To put this evidence into context and provide a meaningful analysis it has also been necessary to look back at the history of the Andrews' Labor Government and its predecessors to determine the extent to which earlier policy decisions may have influenced decisions relating to the pandemic.

As a result of the obfuscation and evasiveness of various witnesses to the Coate Inquiry, and the failure of the Inquiry to delve sufficiently into these pre-existing factors, we can only develop plausible explanations and inferences as to what really happened and why. It is acknowledged that new evidence may emerge over coming years that could either validate or invalidate some of these assumptions and inferences about the events and decisions that occurred and their interrelationships.

By the very nature of the prevailing circumstances, this analysis has to some extent depended upon reasonable supposition and subjectivity. It is possible that any single piece of evidence could be interpreted with a different conclusion. However, when the sum of the evidence is considered, it paints a damning picture of dysfunctional government, failed leadership, disastrous decision-making, and incompetence at the highest levels.

The analysis throughout this book argues that, although serious mistakes were made by the Victorian Government early in 2020 (and continued through the pandemic), the origins of these mistakes had their foundations in the months and years preceding the very start of the pandemic. The mismanagement of the Hotel Quarantine Program and the test and contact tracing system were very much the unavoidable outcomes of a complex interplay of misplaced government ideology, inappropriate priorities, inadequate resourcing, and ineffective leadership that has typified so much of the Andrews government's efforts.

Much has been made, by the Coate Inquiry and the media, of the seriously flawed decision making around the use of private security and the appointment of an unqualified and incapable private security company. However, it is just not possible to say that if police were used instead of private security at the quarantine hotels, or if Unified Security had not appointed, then the disaster of the second wave would not have been occurred. Key aspects of the Victorian Government were so dysfunctional and poorly led that even if the police, army, or some other specially trained teams were used, then it is more than probable that a similar catastrophic outcome would still have occurred. There was so much fragility and so many vulnerabilities in the whole system of hotel quarantine, public health, contact tracing and testing, and centralised leadership, that multiple critical and existential failures would in all likelihood still have eventuated. The bad decision to use private security compounded by the bad decision to appoint Unified Security just made the disaster unfold sooner than it might have otherwise.

However, instead of guessing what might have been, it is far more useful to try and determine why these failures occurred. Lessons need to be learned so that systemic problems within the systems of government and the bureaucracy within Victoria can be more effectively addressed.

Complex relationships

Throughout this book a complex web of interdependencies of various causal, contributing, and influencing factors has been progressively revealed. A great deal of effort has been made to base this mapping on indisputable evidence obtained from the Coate Inquiry and from the investigations and reports of various journalists. However, this has not always been possible. The pandemic period in Victoria was characterised by government misdirection, secrecy, obfuscation, denial, collective memory loss, bullying, and blame shifting. This by its very nature keeps many of the facts hidden from public view and requires that inference and supposition are necessary to put forward a reasonable explanation of what could have happened in Victoria.

The central tenet of this book has been to present evidence and argument creating a framework that allows the reader to make their own judgements about what happened as the Victorian Government struggled to manage the Hotel Quarantine Program and the wider pandemic response. In presenting the framework, evidence, inferences, and suppositions there may some errors of fact, analysis, and conclusion which come to light when (or if) additional evidence is made public. For these errors, if they exist, I apologise in advance. The truth of what really happened in Victoria under the stewardship of the Andrews' Labor Government may never be properly known unless the culture of secrecy is finally pushed aside by a fully independent investigation with coercive powers, such as a Royal Commission. Until that time, I provide the following summaries and conclusions by way of helping the reader to answer some of the remaining questions.

How are the various causal factors interlinked?

It would be nigh on impossible to develop a causal relationship map that shows all of the poor decisions, destructive ideologies and beliefs, collective and individual failings, degraded ethics, conflicts of interest, inadequate knowledge, and lack of capabilities that resulted in the disaster that was to follow. However, Figure 15 has attempted to make a best endeavour to provide a detailed view of what appears to have occurred over the last few years leading up to the Victorian disaster. This is, by its very nature, a very complicated picture. To help the reader more quickly grasp some of the key themes, a simpler overview is provided (Figure 10), and which is discussed in more detail below.

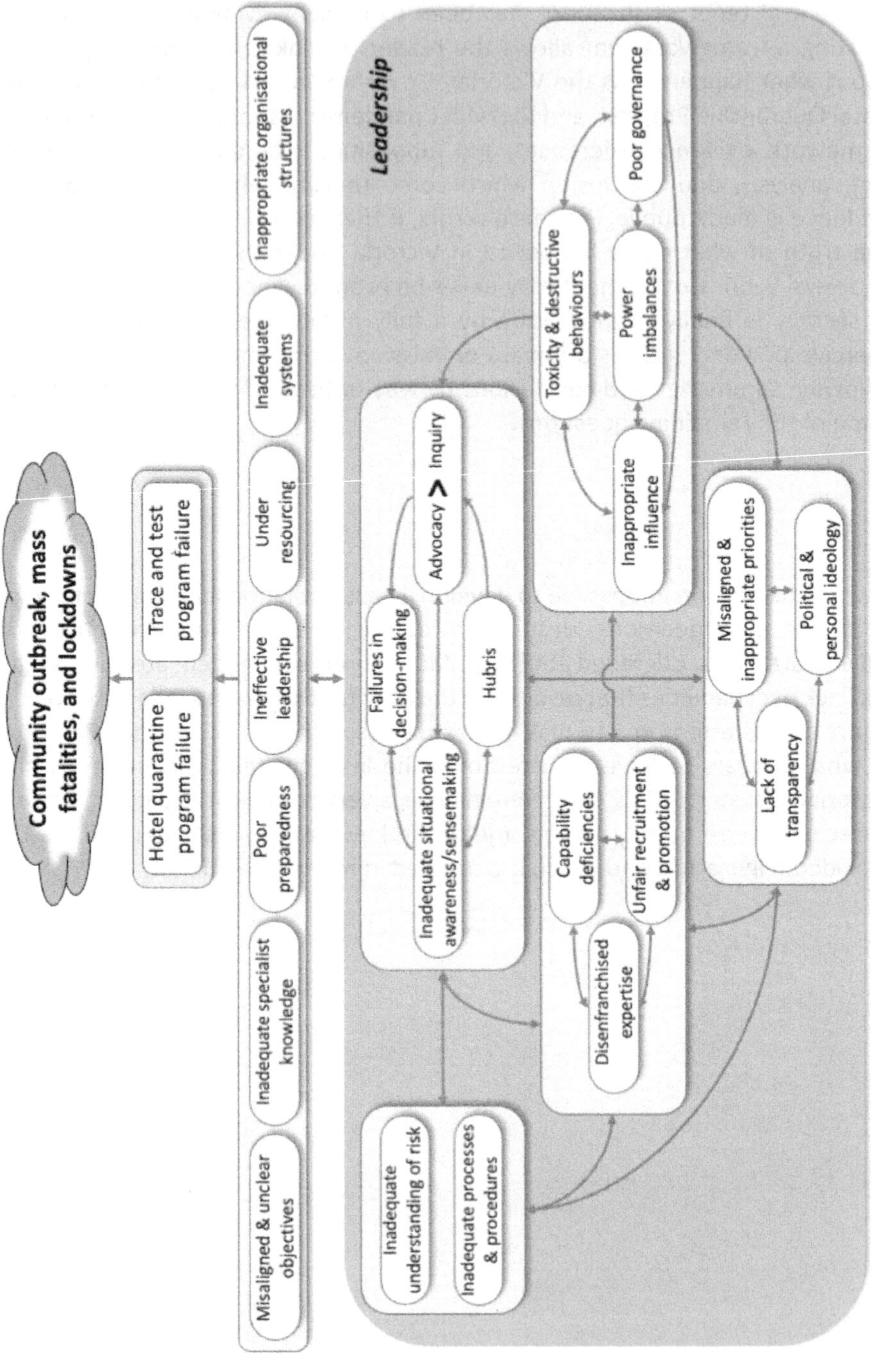

Figure 10 interrelationship map showing common themes contributing to the Victorian quarantine hotel disaster

Inevitable or avoidable program failure?

The initial set up and operation of the Victorian Hotel Quarantine program was a failure of disastrous proportions by any objective measure, and in its various resets and iterations continued to be plagued by problems and failures in its operations through 2021 and into 2022. In a similar vein, Victoria's trace and test program proved to be a disaster in the immediate aftermath of the quarantine breakdown and community transmission of COVID-19 that led to Victoria's second wave. Failing again and again in subsequent waves.

Just like the Hotel Quarantine Program, the trace and test program experienced repeated serious failures over 2020, 2021, and 2022. With hundreds of thousands of lost, abandoned, and incorrect test results, contact tracing not being undertaken, primary contact premises being misidentified and having to go into unnecessary isolation and cleaning. This culminated in one of its most embarrassing failures, when in the face of massive queues outside of test centres (with up to eight hours wait-times in some cases), over 100,000 tests had to be abandoned because they could not be analysed before the samples were degraded. Many people waited days to see if they had COVID, unnecessarily remaining in isolation just in case. Whilst others had to abandon long awaited travel interstate because they did not receive required test results. Some people received text messages days late to inform them that their tests could not be processed. Many received no information whatsoever, only realising what had happened when the media leaked news of yet another momentous failure.

Outside of the well documented failures of the initial Hotel Quarantine Program and test and trace program, there has been little in the way of detailed public disclosure about the causes of the continuing failures in both Programs over the first two plus years of the pandemic. However, it seems more than likely that those foundational factors responsible for the original failures had not been adequately addressed following the Coate Inquiry and continued to debilitate continuing efforts at managing the effects of the pandemic.

Could these various program failures have been avoided or were they inevitable given the very nature of the pandemic situation faced by Victoria. Although other jurisdictions within Australia faced similar challenges, and experienced breakouts from quarantine, they were all far more capable in managing the quarantine breaches, constraining community spread and limiting the fatality rate. At least until Australia started to more broadly open up and try to live with COVID-19. Even the New South Wales Government seemed to have learned its lessons well since the Ruby Princess cruise ship debacle at the start of the pandemic. With the benefit of hindsight and based on the experiences of others, it seems that the Hotel Quarantine Program disaster was absolutely avoidable by any competent government, assuming of course that failure was not predicated by previous years of poor decision-making and inadequate leadership.

However, for Victoria, a catastrophic failure of this nature was unavoidable. If not the Hotel Quarantine Program, then one or more different disasters would have occurred. Failure was deeply engineered into Victoria's DNA. The deep-rooted systemic problems that had developed over the previous decade had created a government that was incapable of managing a complex problem of this nature. All it need was the right sort of stressor on the system. The indicators had been growing for several years as the Victorian Government lurched from failure to failure across different programs, initiatives, service delivery, and projects. For some reason, these earlier continuing failures seem not to have been given the public prominence they warranted, a lot of media reporting continuing to contribute to building the personality cult that was becoming the government' de facto brand.

On entering the pandemic, the Victorian Government had established an abysmal scorecard for itself across multiple policy areas and projects. Was it any surprise that its response to the pandemic would not be any better?

What proximal factors were apparent?

The immediate 'causes' of the government's failure during the pandemic have been obvious (refer back to Figure 10):

<u>*Misaligned and unclear objectives*</u>: Throughout the pandemic the Victorian Government attempted to pursue a number of different objectives (political, ideological, virtue signalling, economic, societal, etc.) that were not aligned to and often conflicted with public and community health outcomes. In doing so the government had little apparent understanding of how antagonistic such objectives were to each other and accordingly failed to deliver any meaningful outcomes effectively.

In its ignorance. the government blatantly breached one of the fundamental principles of economics and public policy, the Tinbergen Rule, that government cannot pursue two or more different objectives (e.g., creating indigenous jobs *and* protecting people's health) by using the same single policy instrument (e.g., the Hotel Quarantine Program). At a minimum, one objective will not be achieved (in this case the protection of public health) and often both endeavours will fail (in this failure, it appears that little if any long term employment flowed back to indigenous Victorians). The Victorian Government did not just ignore the Tinbergen Rule once, but breached it on multiple occasions, littering the pandemic landscape with its failed policy objectives.

The Tinbergen Rule is not a new idea but has been applied in public policy across the world for decades. However, it appears to have been a complete mystery to some senior decision-makers during Victoria's pandemic response. Or was the decision made to simply ignore the 'Rule' for the sake of ideology and political expediency?

It also appears, no matter which objectives were being pursued from the 'top', that a combination of toxic cultures, poor communications, and a lack of transparency left those at the frontline confused and unclear about what actual objective they were expected to achieve. This often manifested in the de facto normalisation of deviance as workers tried to manage themselves out of the mess created from above. Such normalisation resulted in actual processes being deployed that were very different from what senior decision-makers believed to be happening. With inadequate monitoring and oversight from those 'in-charge', situational awareness was further impaired, and a common operational picture became even more degraded. With an inadequate depth of specialist knowledge within agencies involved in the Program, it was therefore unsurprising that there was very little awareness that things were going awry until the crisis suddenly became a disaster.

Inadequate specialist knowledge: it was very apparent that what should have been key skills areas before and during the pandemic, were either inadequate or completely missing, including in quarantine management, public health, infection control, disease tracking and tracing, procurement, logistics, contractor management, emergency/crisis/disaster management, and decision-making under uncertainty. In recent years there appears to have been a continuing exodus of skills and knowledge from the public sector (encouraged by poor leadership, toxic cultures, and ideology), whilst identity politics and prevailing recruitment practices (D'Abrera, 2020a) seem to have actively prevented equivalent expertise from being reinstated. Instead, there has been a steady replacement of independent public sector leadership with Labor political appointments to senior public service positions that are aligned with or subject to the Premier's ideology (Le Grand and Sakkal, 2021), and the replacement of experts with inexperienced idealogues across the public sector. It is appropriate to acknowledge that there are still a lot of good specialist expertise remaining within the Victorian Public Service. Although this is often concentrated within the middle and more junior levels, where problematic leadership and toxic cultures present often insurmountable barriers to these experts and prevent them from doing their jobs to the extent required.

Lack of preparedness: despite pandemic planning efforts going back at least two decades in Victoria, when the COVID-19 pandemic arrived, the latest revisions of these documents proved to be woefully inadequate and mismatched for the situation which they faced in early 2020. Even Victoria's specific pandemic response plan, written *after* the COVID-19 pandemic had emerged, failed to include any consideration of quarantine requirements. Despite different types of quarantine arrangements already being implemented in some other parts of the world.

Other elements of what should have been Victoria's expected 'well-oiled' emergency response, in reality proved to be superficial, cumbersome, and misplaced. This lack of preparedness was not that surprising. Experiences from earlier crises and disasters have shown just how unprepared Victoria has been in the past[275]. Time after time demonstrating that lessons were not learned or were actively unlearned. As the Delta and Omicron variants emerged and resulted in huge upswings in case numbers in 2021 and into 2022 (although with a much milder illness and with majority vaccinated populations), Victoria's lack of preparedness came to the front again with test centres, analytical laboratories, notification systems, ambulances, Triple Zero systems, and hospitals cracking under the strain. It is really scary to think about what would have happened in Victoria in 2020 if the Commonwealth had not closed down international borders and substantially limited the introduction of the COVID-19 into the country. Or if later in the pandemic, a variant more severe than Omicron had circulated. Even with two years of the pandemic to improve its capabilities, in 2022 Victoria was still 'caught with its trousers well and truly down' as Omicron spread, and the health system crumbled almost overnight.

[275] 2009 Black Saturday bushfires (Teague, 2010); Hazelwood Mine fire disaster (Teague 2014), Fiskville toxic chemical exposures (Joy, 2012; PoV, 2016).

Ineffective leadership

A combination of ideological reinforcement and 'woke' policies, along with political preferment and unmanaged conflicts of interest have resulted in the appointment of senior bureaucrats in some Victorian Government agencies that are significantly less experienced and less skilled than should otherwise have been the case. This has resulted in a dearth of effective leadership in the routine day-to-day operations of the public sector, causing the ineffective delivery (or outright failure in some cases) of many of the government's policy initiatives and major projects. The lack of capability and fragility of Victoria's leadership became even more apparent when it was faced with the uncertainty and complexity of the pandemic.

This lack of effective leadership has had long term pernicious effects on the culture and performance of many areas of the Victorian Government. Cultural toxicity and toxic management have been evident within a significant number of agencies which has resulted in continuing bullying and harassment of more junior staff. This has further exacerbated the negative effects of identity politics and increased the exodus of competent staff from the public sector. The lack of effective leadership and abysmal performance of multiple areas of government then became evident in many of the aspects of the pandemic response, well into 2022. That such leadership continued to be toxic was apparent from the various allegations of bullying, unfair blaming, and secrecy that continued long after the supposed reset of the Hotel Quarantine Program.

If further proof of the state of leadership within the Andrews government and its bureaucracy was needed, one only has to look to the performance of key individuals during the Coate Inquiry. If the collective amnesia (the Premier alone had over sixty 'memory failures' during cross examination) were not enough to be convincing, then the widespread attempts to avoid accountability and responsibility for the key decisions must surely have revealed the true nature of leadership within Victoria. That this lack of leadership was a direct contributor to the pandemic failings, in general, and the Hotel Quarantine Program in particular was exposed by the Coate Inquiry. Particularly telling on the lack of leadership is Premier Daniel Andrews' own absolute admission[276] about the Program, that *"the State.... didn't take an active role in ensuring that there was proper infection and prevention measures in place....".*

---

[276] Transcript of proceedings for Premier Daniel Andrews. Day 25, Friday 25 September 2020. Inquiry into the COVID-19 Hotel Quarantine Program P-2144. Accessed at: https://www.quarantineinquiry.vic.gov.au/hearings-transcripts.

Under-resourcing: There has been a long-term chronic under-resourcing, loss of key technical skills, and overall deterioration in capability, in many areas of the Victorian public sector over the life of the Andrews government. This has occurred despite a continuing rise in the number of public sector employees year on year, with a 21% increase in headcount from 2016 to 2021, representing over 60,000 *additional* employees of which the majority were employed well before the pandemic (VPSC, 2021). During this time period there has been a massive under resourcing of frontline health workers and a demonstrated lack of core skills and expertise in other areas of the bureaucracy, with the continuing failure to deliver on critical projects. It is reasonable to assume that a good proportion of this massive bloating of the public service has not gone to areas that have improved services to the average Victorian. Although at the same time it does not appear that any of the government's ideological vanity projects have suffered any shortage of resources.

Inappropriate structures: A common feature of many of the Victorian Government's policy and project failures (including large parts of the pandemic response) appear to be strongly influenced by inappropriate governance and management structures. This has included the way that functional areas have been organised; reporting lines established; membership of various committees, working groups, and project teams have been formulated; lines of authority established; and the interrelationships between groups, agencies, and other stakeholders have been formalised. The driving forces behind the development and continuance of these inappropriate structures appears to have a great deal to do with inadequate leadership capabilities, little deep understanding of strategic and operational contexts, ignorance of how systems of work really operate, competing personal objectives, flawed decision-making processes, and at times the fulfilment of petty rivalries.

These inappropriate structures have manifested within the bureaucracies as outdated hierarchies, unclear and confusing reporting lines, flawed systems of governance, uncertainties in accountability and responsibility, poor systems of direction and control, degraded systems of work, etc. The persistence of inappropriate structures within government has meant that any effective leadership is diluted and degraded as its effects diffuse through the organisation. Accordingly, good leaders, where they remain, have a diminishing capability to raise performance, or to discourage or counter other inadequate and toxic leadership. Decision-making capability continues to deteriorate, whilst higher performing decision-makers are discouraged from remaining within the organisation, or are actively replaced by those far less competent.

Whilst inappropriate structures do act as potent barriers to the successful management of complex change (Blackman et al, 2013), their presence can create almost unrecoverable fragility when complex change manifests in the guise of a rapidly unfolding crisis.

The senior leadership and decision-making structures that were established for the Hotel Quarantine Program did not appear to follow accepted and well-rehearsed practices as outlined in AIIMS or the Emergency Management Manual Victoria. In doing so multiple individuals were placed into key positions without either the necessary expertise and experience, whilst those with knowledge and expertise were sidelined or excluded from the key decision-making structures.

Inadequate systems: within the Victorian Government, systems of work (functions, procedures, processes, etc.) and technological systems have both proven to be unfit for the task on multiple occasions. This has included failures in:

- Political and policy development systems, which have allowed parochial ideological interests and self-serving pet projects take precedence over the public good interests.
- Effective strategy development, budgeting, resourcing, procurement, and emergency management systems have been perverted, allowing 'woke' initiatives to take precedence whilst public health and hospital systems, and preparedness have been allowed to atrophy year after year.
- Victorian Government parochialism which again refused to accept help from other states on acquiring contact management and contact tracing technology. This was combined with a bureaucratic arrogance that spent months at the start of the pandemic apparently unwilling to accept that other states had better testing and tracing regimes in place. Instead, the Victorian Government wasted millions of taxpayers' dollars on false starts and the procurement of unproven and ultimately failed technology, and persisted with inadequate and failing processes, and archaic technology that had been unfit for purpose a decade earlier.

Again, Victorian Government failure with technology is not something that was just new to the pandemic, and the government has long demonstrated its inability to effectively deliver significant IT projects. The Victorian Auditor General investigated a number of government IT projects and released a report in 2016 (Donaldson, 2016; VAGO, 2016b) which identified widespread mismanagement. IT projects were significantly delayed (some by years) or simply abandoned altogether, such as the then Department of Justice and Regulation's IT system upgrade that was abandoned after 6 years of delays, and a doubling of the cost ($60m). Other major IT projects exceeded their original budgets by many millions of dollars, whilst several projects had to be 'descoped', delivered with significantly reduced functionality to allow them to be completed. A previous report had shown that over a third of all of the state's IT projects since 2011 had significantly exceeded their budget, with just ten of these poorly delivered IT projects contributing cost overruns of $1.44 billion (Le May, 2011a; 2011b) in what was described as a *"crisis of confidence in government IT"*. The causes of these IT project disasters read like the government's conduct of the pandemic response: poor governance and management, inability to recognise the requirements that have to be delivered, poor management of contracts, failures to provide and act on advice, poor planning and implementation, and reliance on under skilled staff (Connolly, 2016).

Even when the Victorian Government established a 'state-owned enterprise' to centrally manage its IT projects, it still turned into a debacle. This enterprise, 'Cenitex', was shown by a fairly recent Victorian Auditor General's review to have problems with its relevancy to its customers and that it had failed to meet expectations. The enterprise was reliant on outdated technology, and accordingly had problems with its resilience, had suffered repeated failures with its service delivery, and was subject to poor governance and oversight from the Department of Treasury and Finance (Skatssoon, 2019).

As late as 2021, complete failure was still a hallmark of the Victorian Government's management of high cost technology projects. The Department of Justice and Community Safety had its second attempt (after the failed first attempt) to roll out a new "Victorian Infringements Enforcement Warrant" system. This latest attempt was criticised for major delays and cost overruns, inability to meet quality and functional requirements, failures in planning management, and a lack of 'situational awareness'. An independent review found that the Department was a largely *"uninformed buyer"* (sounds a like a repeat of the Hotel Quarantine security procurement approach), and had a *"misguided and poorly implemented risk strategy"* (Hendry, 2021; Talevski, 2021; VAGO, 2021i).

No real surprises there then. With such a history of failure, did anyone really expect that the Victorian Government would be capable of putting in place new technologies during the pandemic without monumental stuff-ups occurring?

The contribution of poor leadership and failed management

Effective leadership was missing in action many times during the first two years of the pandemic response. That many aspects of the pandemic response were poorly managed is absolutely evident from the findings of the Coate Inquiry, subsequent leaks of secret reports, and revelations in the media. This included significant problems in the management of: capability development; resourcing; budgeting; preparedness; planning; systems of; governance and oversight; establishment and conduct of hotel quarantine processes; COVID-19 testing; contact tracing; home isolation supervision; contractor management; front line security; PPE provision; information sharing and communications; specialist training; inter-agency liaison and coordination; intergovernmental relations; surge management; and the list goes on.

The Coate Inquiry clearly identified many examples of failed management and leadership associated directly with the Hotel Quarantine Program. These were problems that were not just unique to the Program itself, but subsequently became apparent in other areas of the pandemic response. Nor were these problems that were just unique to, or that arose because of the pandemic. These problems were just the most recent public reflections of the systemically ineffectual leadership in many areas of the Victorian Government that had been building over the life of the Andrews government.

The pandemic required leadership that strove for transparency, honesty, and skilled decision-making. Instead, leadership seemed more often than not to have been replaced by political spin, self-interest, and secret agenda. Many key decisions appear to have been made on the strength of ideology and political strategists, rather than by experts using sound scientific and economic evidence. Millions of dollars of public money were diverted to political consultants during the pandemic, to allegedly advise on spin and protecting the 'Andrews' brand' (Johnston, 2021a). This was millions of taxpayers' dollars that could have, instead, been directed to better resourcing public health and contact tracing capability, or for bolstering ambulances and hospitals well before the entirely predictable surges in demand occurred.

Effective leadership makes decisions, and then holds itself accountable for those decisions and their outcomes. Instead, in Victoria we saw the Premier, key Ministers, and multiple senior bureaucrats suffer convenient mass collective memory loss, or make repeated attempts to deny any involvement in critical decisions. When accountability could not be avoided, then there were attempts to diffuse that accountability by implicating others in decisions and actions, or just outright blaming someone else. In some cases, it appears that the truth was deliberately hidden and the media given a scapegoat to tear into, remember the 'Nebuliser Man'.

Effective leadership establishes a positive culture which promotes integrity, transparency, and personal responsibility, and within which people trust their leaders and colleagues. Instead, we have seen multiple Victorian Government agencies where highly toxic cultures have prevailed for years. Where political and bureaucratic 'leadership' in those agencies have ignored or failed to address the toxicity, and in some circumstances may have been the direct cause of that toxicity.

Whilst there are good and effective leaders remaining within the Victorian public sector, their number has diminished significantly over recent years, to the extent that their abilities are easily overwhelmed by the mediocre and the incompetent. Inadequate leadership seems to be so pervasive (as evidenced by the failure or dismal performance of many different government programs[277], not just those associated with responding to the pandemic) that there is no simple solution, such as capability development, that will address this systemic and deep-rooted problem. Regardless of what shade of politics forms government (whether Labor, Liberal, or some other mix), a complete transformation of the system of government is urgently required in Victoria. Democratic and accountable governance systems need to be reinstated, incapable Ministers need to be removed and the whole Victorian public sector needs a complete overhaul. Victoria desperately needs a public sector leadership that is fit-for-purpose. Progressive deskilling of the workforce needs to be halted and reversed, many of the current entrenched 'box tickers' need to be replaced by fresh blood from outside of the current public service and partisan political system. The practice of ideological preferment needs to be replaced by a fair meritocracy to ensure that the Victorian Public Service can return to providing expert advice without fear or favour.

The current political and bureaucratic systems are so fundamentally dysfunctional that, if the only change that occurs is the replacement of one lot of inadequate leaders by another set of inadequate leaders, then Victoria will

[277] For example, the poor performance of a number of other health and social services programs (such as the failed homelessness program), youth detention centres, the terrible performance of a majority of the largest of the State's major infrastructure construction projects, etc.).

continue to fail in the face of even minor stressors well into the foreseeable future.

The contribution of poor decision-making

The decision-making engaged in by relevant Ministers and senior bureaucrats were the key direct causes of the Hotel Quarantine Program failure. Decisions that also caused the trace and test program failure, the public health failures of the burgeoning pandemic waves, the multiple failures of the subsequent resets to hotel quarantine, and the failure to adequately anticipate and prepare for the emergence of new SARS-COV-2 variants. These were the same decisions that in 2021 and 2022 were responsible for the failure to prepare for the inevitable surges of COVID-19 cases as the State tried to return to normal. The same decisions that caused failures in testing laboratories, hospitals, the triple zero system, and ambulance service, and resulted in even more preventable premature deaths and unnecessary trauma for Victorian families.

The scarcity of good decision-making within Victoria throughout the pandemic has been evidenced by the appalling outcomes achieved. It is often said that bad outcomes can come from good decisions. However, the scale, frequency, and consistency of failures over a number of years (and not just during the pandemic) points strongly to a pattern of poor decision-making rather than simply bad luck, and points to a State bereft of effective leadership.

A lack of transparency?

The Victorian Government's decision-making processes occurring through most of the pandemic response remain largely opaque. The significant lack of transparency raises questions about why there was such a need for secrecy at the time and why the government has fought so hard since to keep these matters secret? Spending many hundreds of thousands of dollars on lawyers and the Courts to stop people from accessing information, and then refusing to provide information when directed to do so by the government's own regulators.

This is a level of secrecy that is unacceptable in the Westminster system of government and is more akin to the behaviour of totalitarian regimes and tin-pot dictatorships, than a modern democracy. This secrecy would appear to have little to do with observing the normal rules of confidentiality within governments. Especially since Daniel Andrews himself appears to be only too willing to breach confidentiality requirements when it suits him, allegedly bullying senior public servants into providing him with confidential documents on the decision-making of the previous Liberal Government and then making this information public (Johnston, 2021f; Wahlquist, 2018). Just what was the Victorian Government hiding (and continues to hide) from the public about key decisions made during the pandemic?

Systemically flawed decision-making processes

That insufficient situational awareness and flawed sensemaking would give rise to serious failures in decision-making during the pandemic response is a more than reasonable assumption. However, even if a realistic operating picture could have been achieved by senior decision-makers, would this have resulted in more effective decision-making about the pandemic response and particularly about the Hotel Quarantine Program?

The various strands of evidence indicate that the decision-making processes and capabilities were so unfit for the required task, that irrespective of the quality of situational awareness and sensemaking, similar disastrous outcomes would still have likely occurred. The inability of senior leadership to say when, how, and who made a number of key decisions is a strong indicator of a highly flawed process. What otherwise should have been key decision-making groups as part of an effective emergency and crisis response, such as the meetings at the State Control Centre, turned into a simplistic delivery of high-level summaries of decisions already made 'in secret'. Another telling indicator of a failed system.

Where we do get the occasional glimpse of what actually happened, it appears that complex and far-reaching decisions were made with the attention and analysis of purchasing stationary, rather than running a pandemic response. It is almost certain that multiple major decisions were made that were based upon false assumptions. Decisions were made with little evidence and with little attempt to identify, validate or challenge critical assumptions. Instead, it appears that these critical assumptions were blindly accepted without any further consideration.

The Coate Inquiry found that the decision-making process (if this could even be described as a 'process') breached the acceptable *"principles of the*

Westminster system of responsible government"[278], an appalling indictment of those involved.

These flawed decision-making processes were further degraded by tackling complex problems with what would have passed as barely acceptable processes even in routine day-to-day operations. There is no evidence that key participants even understood or recognised the difference between reversible and non-reversible decisions, and so treated all decisions as though they could be simply reversed if things did not work out as expected.

Dealing with such situations does not require a PhD in complexity theory. These should have been basic concepts fully understood by all managers and executives within the Victorian Public Service and by Ministers. That they appear not to have been understood at all is yet another indicator of the true capabilities of government and its bureaucracy. It is of course possible that those in positions of authority fully understood that the decision-making processes where not capable of solving the problems to which they were applied. Perhaps there was no desire to actually solve complex problems, when it was far easier to use simple processes that provided an outcome more acceptable to those in more senior positions of power. For those in authority, it may simply be that an ineffective advocacy based approach was more preferable to inquiry and problem solving. Especially when inquiry based decision-making might have come up with ideologically unpalatable options.

It is likely that a number of major bureaucratic decisions were driven by fear and the need to conform to the ideology and dictates of power, and were driven by predetermined outcomes that served vested interests, rather than the overall public good.

A low capability base?

Given the poor outcomes from apparently inadequate decision-making processes during the Hotel Quarantine Program, to what extent could inexperience and inadequate skills have contributed to the situation, compared with potential acts of wilful negligence, self-advancement, or self-protection?

The Coate Inquiry clearly demonstrated that a significant number of those appointed to senior decision-making roles were not up to the task. A

[278] Coate, 2020a, p. 20.

combination of long-term serious problems[279] all combined to a degrading of cognitive capability and complex problem-solving skills within senior levels of the public service. Even if a number of key decisions were not driven by advocacy, it is questionable as to what extent some of these senior bureaucrats could have even used inquiry mode decision-making effectively. Particularly in an environment of a declining and often ignored system of good governance.

Were decisions politically and ideologically motivated?

There have been multiple commentators that have written and spoken about the government's poor decision-making and, in particular, that on a number of occasions that the public good and public health were sacrificed for political expediency. Political decision-making seems to have driven key decisions about health resourcing; the use of hotels for quarantine; the use of private security (and Unified Security in particular); restrictions, lockdowns, and curfews; the appointment of multiple senior bureaucrats; structures; reporting lines; and governance arrangements. As more information comes to light, the credibility of the government's statements about the use of health advice in making many of these decisions, and the government's overall integrity is becoming even more tenuous.

To what extent was the Premier involved in key decisions?

Previous behaviours

When various decisions made before and during the pandemic were shown to be problematic or resulted in visible failure, Daniel Andrews was quick to distance himself from any appearance of involvement. This saw, at various times, his public denials and sixty plus memory failures during the Coate Inquiry; attempts to deflect the highly contentious curfew decision onto both Health and Victoria Police before finally admitting his involvement; denying that he made specific statements (despite media recordings to the contrary); denials about his involvement in collusion and secret deals with the firefighters union (at the time of writing an area of an ongoing corruption investigation); denial of

---

[279] The issues included toxic cultures, poor leadership, woke ideology and cancel culture, political preferment in senior appointments, a lack of ongoing capability development, and the continuing exodus of skilled specialists.

involvement in the red shirts corruption scandal and misuse of public funds, and in branch stacking corruption (the subject of Victoria's first ever joint investigation by the Ombudsman and the Independent Broad-based Anti-corruption Commission); and of course his denial of any involvement in the disastrous decision to use private security in the Hotel Quarantine Program. Questions about Daniel Andrews' integrity stretch back to the earliest days of his ministry (Gordon, 2014), and will continue to dog him long after he departs politics.

Daniel Andrews during his tenure has shown time after time his willingness to get involved in the micromanagement of different areas of government. Part of his enduring appeal through much of his time as Premier has been the carefully crafted and cultivated image of the Premier as a hands-on leader. Afterall, it was his direct intervention in the Country Fire Authority industrial dispute that saw the departure of the Chief Fire Officer, the Emergency Services Minister, the CFA Board and the CEO, and a resolution in favour of the United Firefighters Union. An intervention that has subsequently seen the Independent Broad-based Anticorruption Commission (IBAC) launch a two-year (and continuing) investigation into alleged secret deals between the union and the Premier and his government (ABC News, 2021c; Bucci, 2021b; McKenzie et al, 2021; Talbot, 2021; Tuffield and Piovesan, 2021; Willingham, 2021).

Over the same time period, IBAC conducted other corruption investigations into Victoria's Labor party and the possible involvement of the Andrews government in branch stacking and misuse of public funds (Bucci, 2021b; Durkin, 2021) including during the 2014 election campaign. Again, allegations were made, from the media and from Labor insiders about Daniel Andrews' involvement (AAP, 2021a; Clarke, 2021b), which again the Premier denied. For the first time in the State's history, the Ombudsman and IBAC conducted a joint investigation into corruption allegations in government, finding that *"widespread misuse of public resources for political purposes"* had occurred (IBAC, 2022). That there was a *"catalogue of unethical and inappropriate behaviour and concerning practices", "range from bullying to the hiring of unqualified people into publicly funded roles...rampant nepotism, forging signatures, and attempts to interfere with government grants to favour factionally aligned community organisations"*.

Labor Party corruption, or Premier Daniel Andrews possible involvement, are not core subjects of this Chapter (or of this book in general). The above summary is merely included to provide some context within which judgements about credibility and plausibility of government decision-making can be made. One of the major unresolved questions about the Victorian Government's management of the pandemic revolves around who was involved in the fatal decision to use private security as the 'main line of defence' in the quarantine hotels. A great deal of weight has been placed on Premier Daniel Andrews possible involvement and the credibility of his denials.

This book has traced a number of events, communications, and activities that argue that this decision about private security was not made at the 4.30pm SCC meeting on 27th Match 2020, that it did not occur as a result of a 'creeping assumption', or occurred as a collective process that individuals were *unaware* of participating in, as intimated by the Coate Inquiry. This public diluting of responsibility has served the interests of the potentially responsible key decision-maker(s) well, and helped them avoid accountability for what subsequently occurred.

Strong circumstantial evidence that the decision was made much earlier in the day, has been explored in previous Chapters. Who then are the most plausible candidates for this decision?

Is there evidence of the Premier's potential involvement?

There is a range of evidence, assertions, and denials that have centered around Premier Daniel Andrews' possible role in the decisions about private security in the Hotel Quarantine Program. Argument mapping provides a tool that can be used to look at the balance of evidence, and help the reader to make up their own mind about the Premier's culpability or otherwise. Argument mapping looks at the plausible relationship patterns amongst obviously related and seemingly unrelated occurrences. The tool maps out the available information as either supporting or opposing a set of contentions, and in doing so looks at supporting and opposing evidence in a cascade (Figure 11), with each subsequent information box serving as a new de facto contention in its own right.

The overall map provides a summary of support or opposition for each piece of information that is looked at. The reader can then examine the relationships across the available information and make their own judgement about the plausibility and probability of the head contention by determining whether on balance there is more or less support (solid line) or opposition (dotted line) *for each individual information box.*

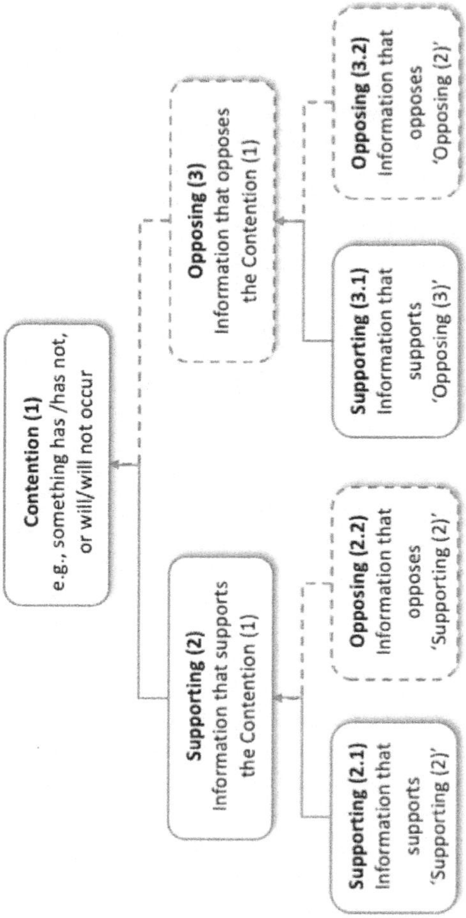

Figure 11: Basic argument map

In the first argument map (Figure 12) the 'head' contention is that Premier Daniel Andrews knew about and had a significant role in making the decision about private security.

In light of such mapping, suggestions about unidentifiable collective decision-making being responsible and the Premier's denials about involvement in, and early knowledge about the decision become much less plausible. With a weight of direct and circumstantial evidence supporting the contention that the Daniel Andrews was in some way involved in the decision.

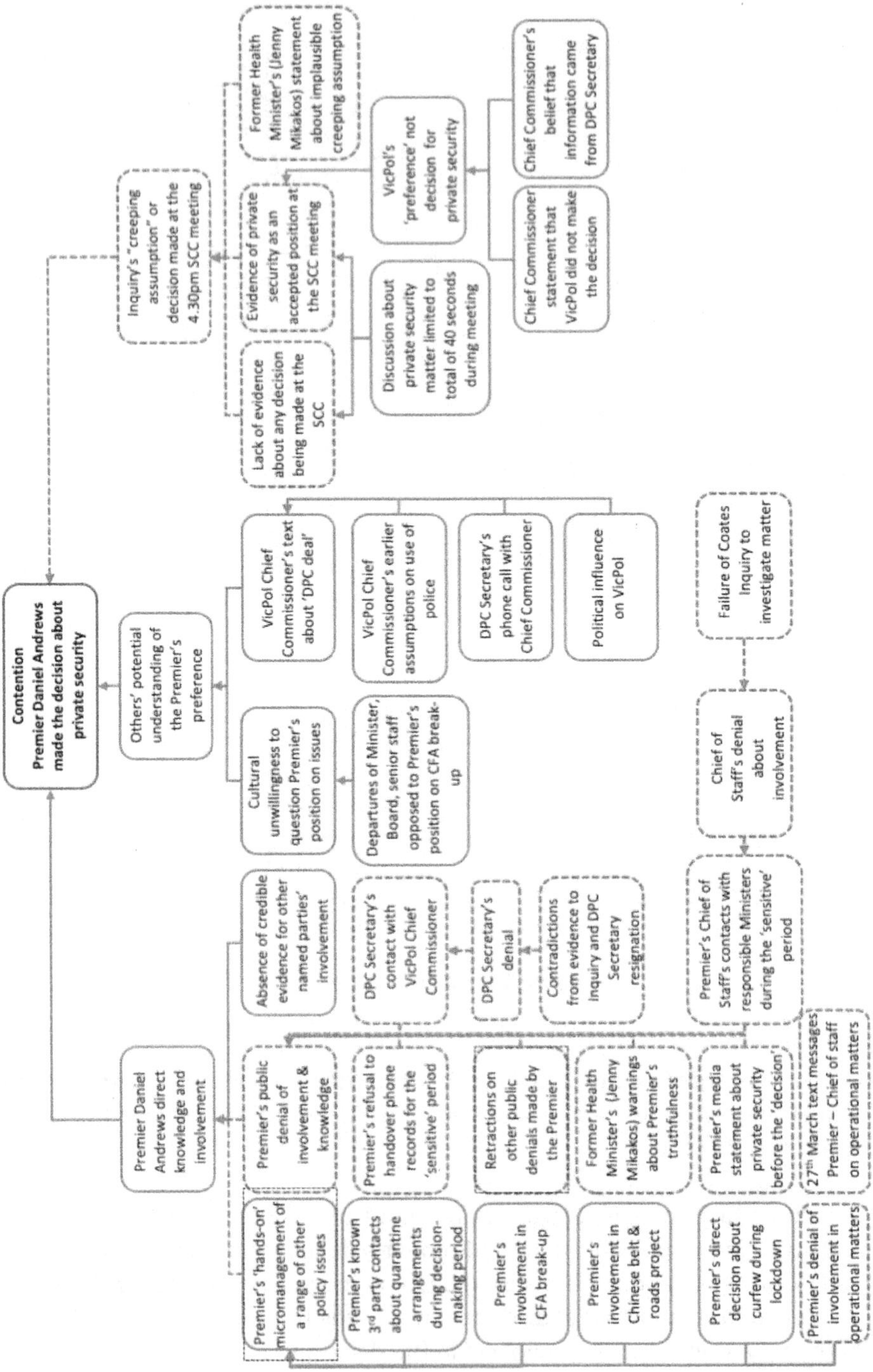

Figure 12: Argument map: Daniel Andrews – directly involved in the 'decision?

For those readers that may still believe that a group of bureaucrats unknowingly made the fateful private security decision collectively at the 4.30pm SCC meeting, and without anyone close to the Premier knowing about this decision, the argument map at Figure 13 is provided.

The influencing and contributing factors

Did poor situational awareness and sensemaking play a role in the disaster?

Various studies (summarised in Schippers and Rus, 2021) have shown that policy mistakes result generally from failures in seeking and sharing information, failures to analyse new information that conflicts with prior information and assumptions, and failures to revise and change conclusions and (ultimately) policies based on this new information. In many cases these information-related failures do not just happen as part of the crisis, they are usually chronic conditions that have affected a whole range of different decision-making in the months and even years before the crisis situation occurs. In other words, a crisis or disaster does not just suddenly happen because of some 'bad event' occurring. Before any crisis or disaster can occur, there needs to be a range of pre-conditions in place within the broad system and within institutions that allow a developing situation to run out of control.

In most crisis situations, and during the COVID-19 response in particular, it is the situational awareness and sensemaking capabilities of decision-makers under high uncertainty that plays a major role in the success of their decisions What the Coate Inquiry and a multitude of media articles have shown is that, within the Andrews government and its bureaucracy, situational awareness was consistently inadequate and that sensemaking was seriously flawed on many occasions. A number of systematic and individual leadership factors (Figure 14) could have acted as filters and manipulators of information about the real world of the pandemic response. This resulted in parts of the Victorian Government creating their own false version of the world around them, providing an aberrant and unrealistic operating picture on which critical (but ultimately doomed) decisions were made.

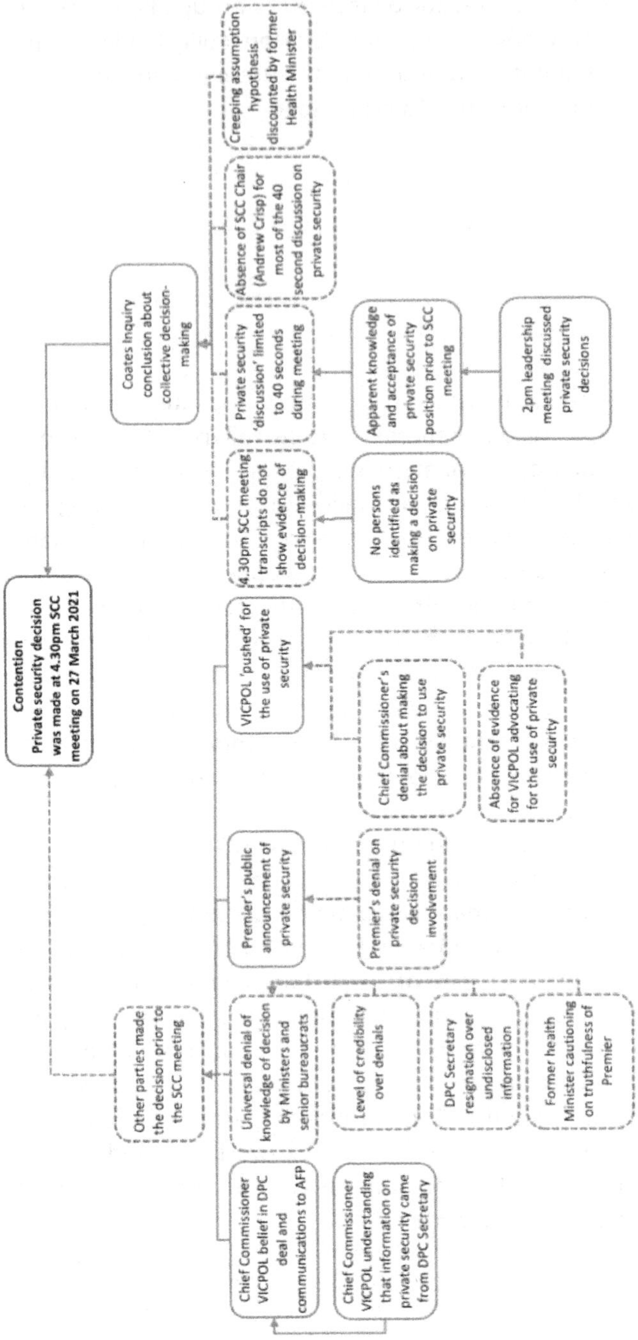

Figure 13: Argument map: SCC or faceless bureaucrats– directly involved in the 'decision?

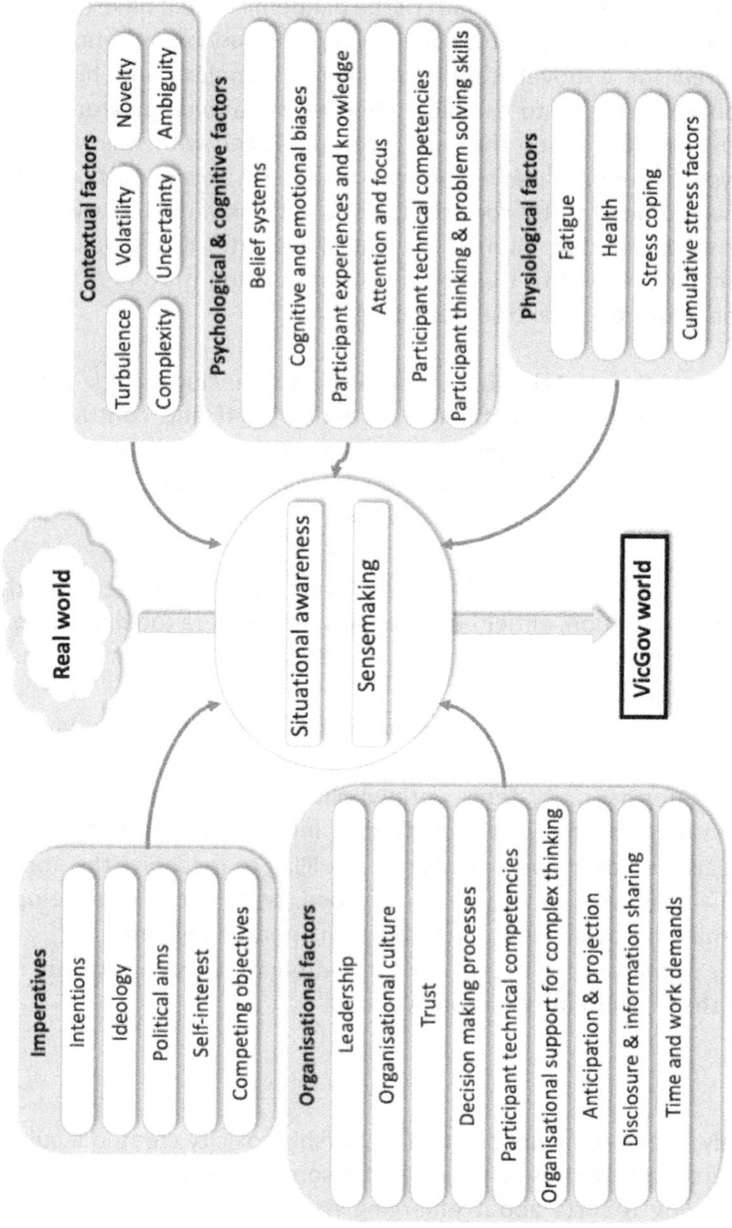

Figure 14: factors affecting situational awareness and sensemaking

Contextual issues in the early part of the pandemic would have made a material contribution to impaired situational awareness. Any organisation that is really *unprepared* for a novel, rapidly changing, complex, and highly uncertain situation will struggle to establish effective situational awareness and make sense of the information they are receiving. Faced with such a situation and being woefully unprepared would have resulted in a lot of mistakes being made which would need to be corrected, along with undertaking a whole range of activities (waste) that ultimately would have little if any value. This would naturally have added to the stress load of decision makers further impairing situational awareness and sensemaking.

Throughout the Hotel Quarantine Program, including its reset, serious problems were being identified by frontline staff and contractors, but this information in many circumstances was not being acted upon by more senior decision-makers. Depending upon the individual issue, some or all of the following are likely to have been involved.

- Reporting systems that had been set up were not gathering and collating this information, either because the systems were too difficult to use, staff were reluctant to make reports, or were actively prevented or discouraged from doing so.
- Information did not get to senior decision-makers in an understandable and useable format.
- The information systems were wholly inadequate for the intended tasks, information transfer was delayed, or information was lost.
- Decision-makers were unable or unwilling to recognise the importance of what information was being provided, or to use it to develop effective situational awareness and a common operating picture.
- The significance of the quality and content of reporting was not recognised in the midst of information overload.

Certainly, there was evidence that leadership toxicity created a culture where staff were fearful of raising issues, and in some cases were actively discouraged from making reports about emerging issues. Alongside which, the adverse effects of political and ideological imperatives, long term inadequacies in organisational leadership and culture, along with deficiencies in technical and cognitive capabilities of some key leaders all *appear* to have contributed to an inadequate understanding of what was happening during the Hotel Quarantine

Program. An understanding that was majorly divorced from the actuality of the real world.

It does seem that in the first couple of months of operation of the Hotel Quarantine Program that there was a high degree of overconfidence, even arrogance, about its 'successful' performance. This could have led senior decision-makers to unconsciously or deliberately disregard any information which did not fit this official narrative of success, whilst only paying attention to information that they believed supported this narrative.

Starting with a fundamental misunderstanding of the reality of what was happening on the ground could only lead to flawed decision-making, inappropriate and ineffective solutions, and the disaster that was Operation Soteria. What is not certain is the extent to which these problems were ultimately the result of well intentioned, but flawed approaches, or instead occurred because of more venal and self-serving interests.

To what extent did power relationships and toxicity play a role?

Whilst the situational awareness and competency of some senior bureaucrats involved in the Hotel Quarantine Program has rightly been called into question, to what extent could other factors have been even more influential? That toxic cultures were present (and remain) in many parts of the Victorian Government is absolutely certain. One only needs to look at the extent of serious bullying and harassment dealt with by regulators, recorded in published investigations, and reported in the media over many years in Victoria to realise how insidious toxicity had become in many government organisations. That such toxicity would instantly be resolved and vanish when the pandemic arrived stretches credulity too far. Instead, there are numerous pieces of evidence for continuing toxicity that were identified during the Coate Inquiry and in subsequent media reporting. Anecdotally, I have yet to speak to a previous or current Victorian public servant that does not speak privately about their experiences of widespread and embedded toxic cultures and toxic leadership.

Such toxicity will have both immediate and long-term effects on organisational performance. The more capable employees (those that can more readily find alternative employment) will be more willing to leave, resulting in a progressive deskilling of the public service. Whilst those that remain can suffer increasingly adverse physical and mental health impacts (Robinson, 2022; Ellis, 2021; Hickock, 2021; McCall, 2021; Shell, 2021; Rossheim, 2021; Bailey, 2009). As a result, organisations become increasingly dysfunctional, especially since those individuals remaining become increasingly unwilling to make decisions or take personal risks that may expose them to future retribution.

Toxic cultures are at their heart a deep reflection of the nature of senior leadership. Toxic cultures emerge and are sustained for only one of two reasons: either senior leadership behaviours and actions create and grow the toxicity, or their inaction allows toxicity to become established and perpetuate. Either way, a toxic culture is yet more evidence of failed leadership at multiple levels of an organisation.

Toxicity can often be created when there is an unfair and significant imbalance in power relationships, that is unconscionably exploited by the holder of that power in their own interests. The exploitation of such a power imbalance seems to have occurred within Victorian Labor against their own, and was at the heart of unethical behaviours and bullying uncovered by Operation Watts (IBAC, 2022). Similar power imbalances were most likely present in many of the Premier's own dealings, such as the in the way in which he dealt with those that had a different viewpoint during the CFA industrial dispute, which saw the sacking or 'resignation' of a Minister, a CEO, a Board, and a Chief Fire Officer. Or the sudden departure of the Head of WorkSafe in the aftermath of the Fiskville debacle, or the loss of the Health Minister during the Coate Inquiry. It is certainly plausible that such behaviours would have made any other Minister or senior bureaucrat exceptionally cautious about voicing any opinion or making a decision that did not align with the Premier's viewpoint on pandemic-related matters.

Did ideology drive inappropriate priorities for the pandemic response?

The pervasive lack of transparency that has mired much of the Victorian Government's pandemic response makes it exceptionally difficult to determine the extent to which the prevailing socio-political ideology derailed the government's efforts. However, we have had the occasional glimpse of the insidious nature of ideology and the resulting misplaced prioritisation of decisions, actions, and resources in many aspects of the pandemic response.

We have also seen public health concerns take a back seat to what appear to have been a mix of personal and political (and possibly 'polling' data) objectives in repeated breaches of the Tinbergen Rule. Perhaps, one of the most blatant was the decision to appoint an unqualified, inexperienced, under-resourced, and unapproved security company (Unified Security) on the apparent sole basis of their self-declared 'indigenous' ownership. Although many other similarly doubtful decisions were made: the debacle with the enforced lock down of the Flemington public housing towers; the selection of CBD hotels as quarantine facilities; the long-term underfunding of health services, and public health in particular; and the diversion of public funds to woke vanity projects with little if any direct benefit to the people of Victoria.

Such ideological misalignments may also have included the appointment of inexperienced and under skilled individuals into positions for which they were wholly unsuited, and which subsequently contributed to the disastrous pandemic response. This has also included a number of other decisions, such as the apparent support for the BLM protests compared to the subsequent heavy-handed response to other non-politically aligned demonstrations. As well as the possible role of ideology and politics on a range of decisions on mandatory restrictions, such as the imposition of the 8pm curfew for Melbourne. This latter decision, despite the Premier's early denials, was made by Daniel Andrews himself without advice or requests from Health or Police. More recent information also indicated that the imposition of the curfew had little or no effect on severity or duration of the pandemic wave.

A recent Independent Broad-based Anticorruption Commission report (IBAC 2021b) identified the use of unreasonable political pressure on the public service, quoting individual public servants:

"Bad or inconsistent decisions get made because of political pressure".

"The influence on politicians from external forces (money, industry, lobby groups) pushes an agenda that is not in the interest of Victorians at large. This transforms into influence from politicians".

Good policy decision-making, development, and implementation in government has always depended upon a degree of contestability of advice. At least one prior Premier in the last thirty years enshrined the notion of contestability by ensuring that political, ideological, experiential, and cognitive diversity drove the appointment of bureaucrats and advisors. This even included appointing former operatives from the *opposing political party* into influential senior positions.

Under Daniel Andrews' premiership it appears that that such diversity has substantially diminished, with the appointment of more and more closely aligned political appointments into what should be impartial and independent public service positions. With this removal of independent advice, along with the continuing consolidation of control into his Private Office, Daniel Andrews has further increased the power imbalance. To the extent that there appeared to be few senior people within government and the bureaucracy that are not purposefully aligned to his worldview, or where those who do think differently were just too fearful to speak out.

11
Conclusions

There is a lot of 'evidence' that has been revealed about Victoria's mismanagement of the pandemic. A mix of reliable and unreliable, substantiated and unsubstantiated, and supporting and conflicting information has been published into the public domain since March 2020. Absolute clarity has been unachievable because of what appears to be deliberate misinformation, obfuscation, cover-ups, and avoidance of the facts.

It is likely that a great deal of other evidence exists that would reveal the truth of what happened in Victoria during the first two years of the pandemic. However, this would require an investigation with coercive powers (such as a Royal Commission) to establish the facts about the Victorian Government's decisions, actions, and the advice it was provided. Something that the Coate Inquiry was not empowered to do. If the Coate Inquiry revealed anything, it was that the Victorian Government had sought to keep a range of matters secret, and in the face of multiple media reports, apparently continues to do so. The Inquiry was successful in scratching the surface and revealed some of the murky details about government's decision-making, although much remained hidden. A whole litany of bad decisions and systemic failures were eventually identified that led to the tragic breakdown in the Hotel Quarantine Program and caused hundreds of avoidable deaths and economic devastation. Impacts that will continue to be felt for years, if not decades to come.

The very nature of the Coate Inquiry looked mainly to proximate causes, and was unable (or was prevented from) to probe deeply into the 'spiders web' of interlinked causal, contributing, and influencing factors, many of which predated the pandemic by several years. The Inquiry was marked by multiple witnesses that either claimed not to have participated in key decisions or could not remember what happened. Because of this collective amnesia, definite evidence of all causal relationships has been difficult to find, requiring plausible explanations to decisions and actions to be put forward instead. Supposition and inference have had to be used where a lack of transparency has prevented direct evidence from coming to light. Therefore, many of the conclusions that can be drawn are highly dependent upon these suppositions and inferences, and hence some may be in error. However, on the balance of probabilities the conclusions appear reasonable and fair, given the circumstances.

Capability – missing in action

We now know that a whole range of systemic problems within the Victorian Government and its bureaucracy had developed over the months and years before the pandemic struck. These inherent weaknesses and vulnerabilities within the government manifested as a litany of errors and inadequate decision-making during the response to the pandemic. Although the government and its supporters have tried to lay the blame for many of the failures on the existence of an 'unprecedented' and highly infectious disease, the pandemic in Victoria was a *man-made disaster* of titanic proportions. Resulting in what has been described as the largest failing of public policy and government administration in Australia's history.

What is very clear is that the Victorian Government failed to put in place even the most basic arrangements that would be expected in the management of a public health emergency of this nature. This was not a case of a fast-moving situation overwhelming an otherwise capable system. Instead, it was yet another example of a fractured, unprepared, and poorly led government lurching from one mismanaged problem to the next, eventually being overtaken by a disaster of its own making. The government was not overwhelmed by a major disease outbreak. Its already struggling capabilities and systems were incapable of meeting the demands of fairly simple quarantine requirements and a relatively moderate number of COVID-19 cases. Lessons were repeatedly not learned, and the ailing health system continued to fail catastrophically as case numbers increased in late 2021 and 2022. COVID case levels that were entirely predictable, that should have been expected, but for which Victoria proved to be again wholly unprepared.

More tragically still this disaster was completely avoidable, there were multiple occasions where different decisions and actions could have been taken to interrupt the various causal pathways. Such interventions, such as improved preparedness, appropriate leadership capabilities, and resourcing could have been addressed years ago. However, decisions were made to pursue more narrow ideological objectives which left Victoria woefully under-prepared for a major crisis. It is certainly possible that had it not been COVID-19 that had stressed and broken Victoria's systems, then some other event would have exposed the government's underlying vulnerability and fragility.

This book has tried to avoid using counterfactuals wherever possible, and we cannot say that a different government in power or different bureaucracy would not have experienced quarantine breaches and have needed to impose harsh restrictions. However, Victoria's lack of preparedness, long term neglect, inadequate resources, lack of effective leadership, and poor decision-making raised the risk of quarantine breaches, subsequent pandemic waves, and severe lockdowns to a level where they became a certainty.

Some commentators have praised the tenacity of the Premier for enforcing repeated lockdowns, and eventually bringing each pandemic wave under control. Praise for managing a disaster that was of the government's own making. Despite the absolute responsibility of the Andrews government for turning the pandemic into a health, social, and economic disaster, and for many a personal tragedy, Daniel Andrews retained his popularity and electoral appeal until his resignation in September 2023. It has been suggested that this had more to do with adroit political manoeuvring and clever spin that has distracted Victorians, rather than displaying any real leadership during the pandemic (Brook and Hutchinson, 2021; Flower, 2021c; Johnston, 2021b; 2021c, Simpson, 2020). If we look past this smoke and mirrors, we need to remember that these draconian measures, locking down its citizens for 263 days, may not have been required had the Victoria Government been prepared, capable people had been in place to make better decisions, and the Victoria's health system had not been allowed to atrophy.

In years past I have designed and conducted a number of emergency and crisis management desktop and live exercises for both government and private sector organisations. An absolute requirement for these types of simulations is that the scenarios are believable. Many consultants develop exercises that rely on scenarios that are so unrealistic and improbable that all sense of realism and connection is lost, and the exercise fails.

If anyone was to design an exercise that represented a large scale disaster, they would probably consider *some* of the following elements to include in scenario development (depending upon the objectives of the exercise):

- Select a facility that is manifestly ill designed for a quarantine facility, such that:
    - It cannot be easily cleaned to a basic hospital standard;
    - ventilation and air conditioning flows cannot be easily isolated, and do not have suitable filtration, but instead guarantee that virus will be spread to other rooms and public areas;
    - have communal areas where infected 'guests' can easily come into contact with uninfected 'guests';
    - where facility staff (such as those actually running the hotel, maintenance, security, etc), are not trained to work in a high risk facility.

- Ensure that facility is placed in a major urban setting:
  - best of all, place it in the central business district (CBD) or city centre, where tens of thousands of people commute into and out of each day. Meaning that should a breach occur, then it can be quickly transported into multiple other metropolitan areas. Health experts, including Associate Professor Philip Russo[280] have supported the movement of quarantine outside of major population centres on the basis that it "just makes logical sense" (see Mannix and Ilanbey, 2020);
  - place the facility where there is a temptation for guests to try to temporarily leave (e.g., visit shops, cafes, etc), or allow staff to visit such retail outlets during breaks for personal reasons, or to go shopping for those in quarantine;
  - place the facility in a dense urban area (CBD) with highly restricted and very expensive car parking, thereby forcing a majority of those working in the quarantine hotels to travel by public transport.

- Establish outsourcing arrangements with an industry that has a long history of serious capability, supervision, and quality problems.

- Outsource to private providers without adequate procurement or due diligence being undertaken, thereby almost guaranteeing unsuitable service delivery.

- Allow rampant uncontrolled subcontracting, so that there is no real idea of who is doing what, and no adequate supervision.

- Make sure that contracted staff are paid as little as possible:
  - make arrangements that allow outsourced staff on the front line to be paid minimum wages, be generally poorly skilled, and do not have English as a first language;
  - use a casualised workforce, that has difficulty accessing paid sick leave, thereby almost guaranteeing that they will continue to work when they are feeling unwell with symptoms of COVID-19 infection;
  - ensure that they are in a sufficiently low socioeconomic bracket that requires them to have second and third jobs (such as taxi drivers, delivery drivers, supermarket workers, etc.), whilst making sure that these jobs provide even more opportunity for community spread.

---

[280] Associate Professor Russo, President of the Australian College for Infection Prevention and Control and Deputy Chair of the Federal Government's Infection Control Expert Group.

    - make sure that the prevailing organisational culture makes staff too fearful to complain or raise issues of concern.

- Do not provide contract staff with the necessary training:
    - make inferior NOT-fit-for-purpose online training mandatory;
    - ensure that specialist training is not provided, and wait for contractors to work for two months without necessary guidance material being made available;
    - set up a system where workers are likely to be confused about and have difficulty in accessing required personal protective equipment;
    - make sure that untrained staff work across multiple sites, thereby further increasing the chance of a breach and more rapid spread of disease.

- Do not put in place anything regarding adequate contract management and assurance, thereby ensuring that vulnerabilities in the system are not detected and corrected before serious breaches occur.

- Establish multiple objectives that conflict with each other, and in doing create confusion, a lack of cooperation, the pursuit of unnecessary activities, and the waste of resources.

- Do not establish effective incident control arrangements across the whole program.

- Allow critical decisions to be made by individuals without the requisite knowledge, experience, or skill about infectious diseases, infection control, and quarantine management. Then sideline those medical and health experts that may be able to help.

- Make sure that there is no clear leadership and put in mechanisms that instead actually hinder or prevent communications within and across different government agencies.

- Do not undertake any effective risk assessment, and instead believe that waiting to act until well after an adverse event or incident is good mitigation.

- Do not plan for the possibility of a breach, and because no risk assessment has been conducted it can be assumed that such a risk is negligible.

- Ensure that that specialist technical capability and capacity is not available by:
    - under-resourcing key areas over several years;
    - diverting funding to fringe 'popular' issues;
    - establishing toxic cultures and ineffective leadership;
    - deskilling the workforce, making more and more senior appointments and promotions not on performance and skills, but instead on the basis of identity politics, political connections, and personal relationships. Also do little to encourage skilled staff to remain, but instead work actively to facilitate their departure.

- Remove anything resembling good governance, and instead establish a fog of opaque decision-making and unaccountability.

- When the outbreak does occur, make sure that the trace and test systems are slow to respond, are under-resourced, inadequately coordinated and rely on 50 year old technology. To reinforce this, ensure that no learning about better practices from other jurisdictions can influence your own decision-making or practices.

- When someone else identifies a problem, just keep denying that anything is wrong, or better yet find a scapegoat and blame them.

- Ensure that no formal effective lessons learned capability is established, so that continued failures occur time after time.

A good crisis management exercise may seek to capture one or two of these dot points. If one was to include any more than that, the exercise participants would rightly complain that the scenario was unrealistic, that so many things going wrong could never occur in a real life situation. This, perhaps, is one of the key issues with the Hotel Quarantine Program. All of the above dot points did occur and, although many of these problems were present in Victoria for several years, they all came together during the pandemic. That leadership and senior decision-makers seemed largely unaware (or chose to ignore) many of these issues individually, makes it highly likely that they were totally incapable of imagining that even a small number of these issues could be problematic at the same time.

However, most of the issues on the above list were entirely predictable and were the subject of discussion within a small group of risk professionals shortly after the Program was announced. That these risks could be identified, but little attempt was made within government to consider these risks is yet a further indictment on those making the major decisions within Victoria during the pandemic. Perhaps the Victorian Government should have spent less time on blaming others during the pandemic (the list of those blamed is long but included: the then Health Minister, some private security providers, the Commonwealth Government, the 'nebuliser man', other international travellers, the Jewish community, the unvaccinated, interstate removalists, other state jurisdictions, (non-existent) right wing infiltrators at CFMEU protests, and on multiple occasions the people of Victoria). If Victoria's leadership had avoided thinking that everyone else was at fault, then more attention might have been given to understanding and dealing with a situation spiralling out of control.

That the Victorian Hotel Quarantine Program was a debacle is without argument. The evidence presented to, and the conclusions of the Coate Inquiry demonstrated multiple egregious failures in almost every aspect of establishing and conducting the Program. Since then, various media reports have revealed that many of the core problems had not been fixed and continued to plague the reset Program, and other acute and public health associated activities including testing and contact tracing, triple zero, ambulance, and hospital systems. This catalogue of failures continued to mount as further outbreaks from quarantine, community transmissions, and six lockdowns occurred.

With over two years of the pandemic under its belt, the Victorian Government still appeared to be surprised and unprepared as 2022 progressed. The evidence of systematic failures continued to mount in the testing system, as queues for testing extended up to eight hours wait time, holiday makers heading off interstate had to cancel their plans as the required PCR test results did not arrive in time. Until the entire system collapsed and 100,000 COVID-19 PCR test sample that had to be abandoned because they could not be processed before the samples deteriorated. It was no surprise, to many Victorians, when the contact tracing system again failed, with Victorians finding out about their exposures through friends rather than through the Health Department (Schubert and Miles 2021; Wahlquist, 2021).

With the spread of the 'milder' Omicron variant of SARS-CoV-2, and exponentially increasing number of infected Victorians, the problems within the contact tracing system became intractable and it was effectively secretly abandoned. Eventually the public were told they would have to do their own contact tracing if they tested positive and notify close contacts, as the Health Department would no longer undertake this function, nor would they continue to provide lists of exposure sites. Yet despite exposure site listing and contact tracing no longer occurring, all Victorians were still required to log in at shops, restaurants, pubs, and workplaces with the contact tracing app. This mandatory requirement remained in place for months after the data was no longer required for its intended health purpose.

This continuing use of QR codes within Victoria in 2022 was described by epidemiologists as "useless" (Kolovos and McGowan, 2022; Mills et al, 2022), criticism that as usual fell on deaf ears. This continuing requirement for using the QR code check-in system, without any apparent valid health need, combined with real concerns about government's ability to access and use the QR data for non-health purposes, started to drive increasing non-compliance with the check in requirements. Again, the government appears to have had little foresight and no consideration of the risks associated with their decision, that significantly increased the likelihood for future non-compliant behaviours should QR tracing be really needed in the future.

It is likely that COVID-19 will be with us for some time, and the emergence of new variants of concern or even an entirely different pandemic pathogen is likely at some time in the future. Whilst it is still highly uncertain if COVID-19 will remain a 'pandemic' problem for the foreseeable future, become a seasonal illness (like influenza), or just disappear (like MERS), it is certain that Australia will continue to be threatened with emerging potentially pandemic diseases for years to come. At the moment, it is doubtful if Victoria has really learned its lessons from the pandemic thus far, and if it is anywhere near prepared enough for future threats whether disease-related, due to other large-scale natural disasters, terrorism, or civil or economic unrest. What is even more worrying is the government's lack of appetite for learning those lessons with its prevailing desire for continuing secrecy.

That multiple failures of the Victorian Government contributed directly to 801 deaths is without doubt. That other lives were and will be lost in the future[281], all as a result of the Victorian Government's poor decisions and mismanagement, is an almost certainty. We may never know the full extent of harm created by the government, but it is not unreasonable to suppose it will amount to many thousands more untimely deaths even when things return to 'normal'.

---

[281] As a result of mental health issues and suicide; restricted access to health services during lockdowns resulting in undiagnosed and untreated serious health conditions, longer term psychological impacts on general health, etc.

Conclusions

The pandemic did not cause the failure of Victorian Government capabilities. This failure was the result of decisions and actions made by the Andrews government over several years before COVID-19 even emerged. Many of the government's systems were already close to failure before the pandemic arrived. Years of inadequate leadership, toxic cultures, degraded capability, misaligned objectives, the pursuit of venal ideology instead of the public good, all created a perfect storm. It was never a question of *if*, it was merely a matter of *when* an increasingly fragile system would eventually fail. All that the pandemic did was to lift part of the veil of secrecy and spin that the government had relied on for far too long.

We are still no closer to knowing who was responsible for the various key decisions that led to much of Victoria's mismanagement of the pandemic, or on what advice those decisions were made. To date, there has been a total failure to hold to account those that made decisions and created the environment which made a pandemic disaster a certainty. That many of the same unidentified individuals that got Victoria into its pandemic mess may still be in their positions (or even promoted) and will still be decision-makers for the next major disease outbreak or other major crisis is a really scary prospect.

To paraphrase and mash quotations from Oscar Wilde and Albert Einstein:

"to lose at one attempt at quarantine is unfortunate, to lose twice looks like carelessness............. To keep failing and not learn is insanity".

Note that Figure 15 includes inferences and suppositions based upon an interpretation of publicly available evidence. The coloured lines are included to make it easier to follow relational pathways. A full colour version of the map is available at:
www.executiveimpact.com.au

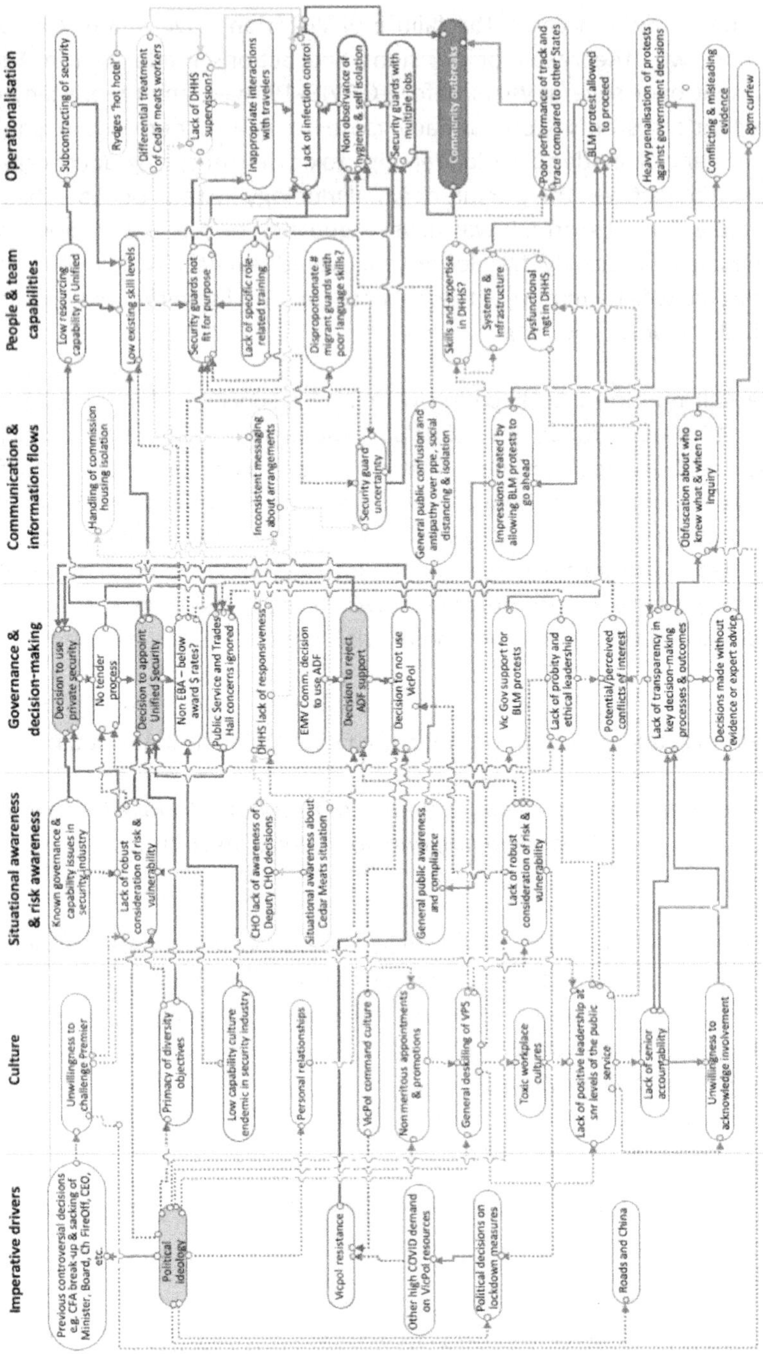

Figure 15: causal relationships in the Victorian hotel quarantine failure

Epilogue

My home growing up was on a large 'notorious' public housing project, my father worked for the railways, my mother worked as a waitress. I was the first member of my extended family to attend school after the age of 15, and the first to go to university, a feat that was unimaginable for all of my school friends. The Labor Party was our party, the Labor Prime Minister was literally all of my friends' schoolboy hero. My father was a staunch trade unionist, that is until he saw ideology triumph over representing the rank and file workers and suborned doing what was right. Over time my political views moved more to the centre, seeing both good and bad in policies across the political spectrum.

As an adult I have worked for Ministers on both the left and right of politics. As a public servant, my philosophy was to provide advice without fear or favour, serving whatever party was in power to the best of my abilities. Accordingly, when I started to research and write this book, I tried to approach it with a politically impartial perspective.

As I near the completion of this book, I can see that this exploration of the Hotel Quarantine Program disaster and second wave response has become a significant critique of the capabilities and performance of Daniel Andrews and the Victorian Government. In doing so, it has become a review of governmental failure that extends well beyond the management of the Hotel Quarantine Program.

This is not a political axe that has been ground. It is a review of a government that lost its way, many years ago, probably at the very start of the Andrews ministry. Where dogged slavery to misplaced ideologies replaced common sense, and where incompetence and poor decision-making became a defining feature of many parts of the bureaucracy. Leadership was frequently replaced by PR spin, and compliant media sound bites. Systems of governance became eroded, and accountability was replaced by blaming others: targeting the Commonwealth Government, other state governments, private business, the Victorian public in general, or individual citizens specifically. Victoria became a state where the police became increasingly seen as politically controlled rather than serving the people. A government where continuing misrepresentation pushed honest transparency out of the door.

This is a narrative of a failing government and bureaucracy, where there are too many people on the public purse that have neither the knowledge nor competencies to undertake the tasks expected of them. My mantra has always been to blame the systems, not the people. Writing this book has opened my eyes somewhat. The systems and decisions that brought Victoria to its knees are not a reflection of just the effects of the pandemic. These were decisions made by individuals, at senior levels of government and the bureaucracy, many of whom have not been identified and called to account for the disaster that they created. Nor is this a story of just multiple failures that occurred over a few months during the first year of the pandemic. These were repeated failures that were piling up, one on top of the other, years before the pandemic even started. COVID-19 just provided another lens that revealed the inadequacies of the government, inadequacies that have not been resolved and that will persist unless serious and concerted action is taken.

To fix these failures will be a long and difficult journey, a journey that will require major reform from the top, and right down to the grass roots, and will be a journey that will probably need to be taken over decades rather than just a few years. Victoria has been generationally harmed, and it will take more than a single generation to fix. Irrespective of which shade of politics is in government, the entire bureaucracy will require a stiff broom to sweep through it and remove the incompetent and the compromised. To poorly paraphrase Alfred Einstein: the definition of insanity is to think that same decision-makers that got us into this mess, will be the same decision-makers that can get us out of it.

Many lessons have not yet been identified, let alone learned, and Victoria is now arguably in a far worse position than it was heading into the 2020 start of the pandemic. Prime Minister Anthony Albanese's much promised Royal Commission or equivalent should have provided the mechanism for ensuring that circumstances around critical decisions were exposed, and that lessons could be learned. However, the Prime Minister's announcement in September 2023, that this would now be watered down to a non-judicial inquiry with 3 panel members[282], with no coercive powers, and that the states would be exempted from any inquiry into their unilateral actions. This has caused a number of commentators to allege yet another cover up and a political attack on the previous government.

We need to learn to keep the politics out of pandemics.

[282] One of whom is former Labor staffer and public supporter of the Andrews government's lockdowns.

References

9News Staff (2021). *Chief Health Officer Describe 'terrible' Consequences of Victorian Lockdowns. But all 'necessary'*. 9 News, 3 August 2021. Accessed at: https://www.9news.com.au/national/coronavirus-victoria-update-four-new-local-cases-recorded-all-in-quarantine-while-infectious/bc410eec-9069-4f4c-9c76-f191da7430a1.

3AW (2021). *The Story behind the Hotel Quarantine Security Company That's Since Folded*. 3AW Radio. Accessed at: https://www.3aw.com.au/the-story-behind-the-hotel-quarantine-security-company-thats-since-folded/.

Aaronson E. and Tavris C. (2020). *The Role of Cognitive Dissonance in the Pandemic*. The Atlantic 12 July 2020. Accessed at: https://www.theatlantic.com/ideas/archive/2020/07/role-cognitive-dissonance-pandemic/614074/.

AAP (2020). *Vic Health Secretary Quits Amid Hotel Saga*. 12 November 2020. Accessed at: https://www.theleader.com.au/story/7010589/vic-health-secretary-quits-amid-hotel-saga/.

AAP (2021a). *Daniel Andrews Named in Branch Stacking Probe*. Canberra Weekly, 8 November 2021. Accessed at: https://canberraweekly.com.au/daniel-andrews-named-in-branch-stacking-probe/.

AAP (2021b). *Victorian Government Refusal to Upgrade Contact Tracing Cost Lives*. In Daily, 15 December, 2020. Accessed at: https://indaily.com.au/news/2020/12/15/victorian-govt-refusal-to-upgrade-contact-tracing-cost-lives/.

AAP (2022). Victoria Hospitals Underfunded Before Pandemic. 1 February 2022. Accessed at: https://thenewdaily.com.au/news/state/vic/2022/02/01/victoria-hospitals-underfunded-before-pandemic/

AAP (2023). *Dan Andrews to Shirk Federal and State Comm Games Inquiries*. Canberra Daily, 3 August, 2023. Accessed at: https://canberradaily.com.au/dan-andrews-to-shirk-federal-and-state-comm-games-inquiries/.

Abbas AH. (2020). *Politicizing the Pandemic: A Schemata Analysis of COVID-19 News in Two Selected Newspapers*. International Journal for the Semiotics of Law 2020. https://doi.org/10.1007/s11196-020-09745-2.

ABC News (2020). *Melbourne's Carey Baptist Grammar School Confirms Teacher Tested Positive for Coronavirus COVID-19*. ABC News, 9 March 2020. Accessed at: https://www.abc.net.au/news

ABC (2020). *Brett Sutton has 'Enough to Get on with' During Victoria's Coronavirus Crisis Without State Controller Role, Daniel Andrews Says*. ABC News, 11 September 2020. Accessed at: https://www.abc.net.au/news/2020-09-11/brett-sutton-state-controller-daniel-andrews/12653930.

ABC News (2020a). *Coronavirus Hotel Quarantine Issues Have Been Dealt With, Victorian Premier Daniel Andrews Says*. ABC News, 9 October 2020. Accessed at: https://www.abc.net.au/news/2020-10-09/victoria-coronavirus-hotel-quarantine-premier-daniel-andrews/12743460.

ABC News (2020b). *Victoria's COVID-19 Hotel Quarantine Inquiry Has Delivered its Final Report. Here Are the Key Findings*. ABC News 21 December 2021. Accessed at: https://www.abc.net.au/news/2020-12-21/victoria-covid-19-hotel-quarantine-inquiry-final-report/13002956.

ABC News (2021a). Reports of Victorian Quarantine Staff Working at Multiples Sites. ABC News 6 March, 2021. Accessed at:
https://www.msn.com/en-au/money/other/reports-of-victorian-quarantine-staff-working-at-multiple-sites/vi-BB1eij1J.
ABC News (2021b). *Dozens of Human Rights Breaches Detailed in Victorian Ombudsman's Report*. ABC News, 4 August 2021. Accessed at:
https://www.abc.net.au/news/2021-08-04/victorian-human-rights-breaches-hotel-quarantine-lockdown/100348396.
ABC News (2021c). *Victorian Premier Daniel Andrews Knocks Back Questions on IBAC Investigation into Firefighting Saga*. ABC News, 6 October 20021. Accessed at:
https://www.abc.net.au/news/2021-10-06/ibac-premier-daniel-andrews-cfa-volunteers-pay-dispute/100517280.
ABC News (2022). *Victoria Police Office Charged with Recklessly Causing Injury in Flinders Street Station Arrest*. Accessed at:
https://www.abc.net.au/news/2022-01-21/police-officer-charged-flinders-street-arrest-filmed/100773532.
AAP (2019). *MFB Top Firefighter Pulls Pin on Vic Job*. AAP/9 News, 12 July 2019. Accessed at: https://www.9news.com.au/national/mfb-chief-quits-amid-leadership-turmoil/f0d1a9fc-ecdc-43f6-a275-ea6f835a34a2.
/2020-03-09/victoria-records-new-coronavirus-covid-19-cases/12038048.
Accountability Round Table (2015). *Strengthening the Victorian Government Integrity System - Does Victoria Have a Government Corruption Problem?* Accessed at:
https://www.accountabilityrt.org/wp-content/uploads/2015/08/Vic-Corruption-190715-submission.pdf.
Acharya K.P., Subramanya S.H., and Neupane D. (2020). *Emerging Pandemics: Lesson for One Health Approach*. Veterinary Medicine and Science 7(1) pp. 273-275.
Achenbach J. (2023). Lab-leak Fears are Putting Virologists Under Scrutiny. The Washington Post 20 January 2023. Accessed at:
https://www.washingtonpost.com/health/2023/01/18/lab-leak-theory-virologist/.
Adams M. J., Tenney Y. J., and Pew, R. W. (1995). *Situation Awareness and the Cognitive Management of Complex Systems*. Human Factors 37(1) pp. 85-104.
Adams G.B. and Balfour D.L. (2010). *Market-Based Government and the Decline of Organisational Ethics*. Administration and Society 42(6) pp.615-637.
Adini B., Goldberg A., Cohen R., Laor D., and Bar-Dayan Y. (2012). *Evidence-based Support for the All-hazards Approach to Emergency Preparedness*. Israel Journal of Health Policy Research 1 pp. 40-47.
AEIR Staff (2020). *Lockdowns Do Not Control the Coronavirus: The Evidence*. American Institute for Economic Research, 19 December 2020. Accessed at:
https://www.aier.org/article/lockdowns-do-not-control-the-coronavirus-the-evidence/.
Ahern S. and Loh E. (2020). *Leadership During the COVID-19 Pandemic: Building and Sustaining Trust in Times of Uncertainty*. BMJ Leader Published Online First: 30 September 2020.
AJMC Staff (2021). *A Timeline of COVID-19 Developments in 2020*. AJMC 2 January 2021. Accessed at:
https://www.ajmc.com/view/a-timeline-of-covid19-developments-in-2020
Alas R. and Vadi M. (2004). *The Impact of Organisational Culture on Attitudes Concerning Change in Post-soviet Organisations*. Journal for East European Management Studies 9 (1) pp. 20-39.

References

Albanese A. (2020). Quoted in: *"Labor's Most Woke Policies Mean the Culture Wars Will Live"*. Accessed at: https://www.news.com.au/national/politics/labors-most-woke-policies-mean-the-culture-wars-will-live-on/video/66620b0c727b82a29998514aaff56038.

Albeck-Ripka L. (2020). *'Nightmare' Australia Housing Lockdown Called Breach of Human Rights*. The New York Times, 17 December 2020. Accessed at: https://www.nytimes.com/2020/12/17/world/australia/melbourne-lockdown-covid-human-rights.html.

Albrechtsen J. (2021). *It's Easy as ABC to Push for Harsher Coronavirus Lockdowns*. The Australian 5 January 2021. Accessed at: https://www.theaustralian.com.au/commentary/its-easy-as-abc-to-push-for-harsher-coronavirus-lockdowns/news-story/bfd06f282b296d21cc7c8a21b514af04.

Albu O.B. and Wehmeier S. (2013). *Organizational Transparency and Sense-Making: The Case of Northern Rock*. Journal of Public Relations Research 26(2) pp. 117-133.

Alcalde Cuesta, F. Sequeiros P.G., and Rojo A.L. (2016). *Exploring the Topological Sources of Robustness Against Invasion in Biological and Technological Networks*. Scientific Reports 6 Article 20666.

Aldred M. (2022). *Inside Daniel Andrews' New 'Big Brother' Style Data Agency He Tried to Keep Secret as it Watches Every Move of Victorians from How They Spend Their Money to Personal Health Records*. Daily Mail Australia, 5 June 2022.

Alfanzo V. and Ercolano S. (2020). *The Efficacy of Lockdown Against COVID-19: A Cross-Country Panel Analysis*. Applied Health Economics and Health Policy (2020) 18 pp. 509–517.

Ali S.H. and Keil R. (2006). *Global Cities and the Spread of Infectious Disease: The Case of Severe Acute Respiratory Syndrome (SARS) in Toronto, Canada*. Urban Studies 43(3) pp. 491-509.

Allen J. (2020). *The Ethics of Leadership*. Professional Learning Hub: Thought Leadership. Griffith University, Brisbane, Australia. Accessed at: https://www.griffith.edu.au/engage/professional-learning/content-centre/the-ethics-of-leadership

Allen D.W. (2021). *Covid Lockdown Cost/Benefits: A Critical Assessment of the Literature*. International Journal of the Economics of Business 29(1) pp. 1-32.

Allington N.F.B., McCombie J.S.L. and Pike M. (2012). *Lessons not Learnt: From the Collapse of to Long-Term Capital Management to the Subprime Crisis*. CCEPP WP03-12. Cambridge Centre for Economic and Public Policy, University of Cambridge, Cambridge, UK.

Allison G.T. (1969). *Conceptual Models and the Cuban Missile Crisis*. The American Science Review. 63(3) pp. 689-728.

Allison G.T. and Zelikow P. (1999). *Essence of Decision: Explaining the Cuban Missile Crisis, Second Edition*. Longman, New York.

Almohtaseb A.A., Almahameed M.A., Sharari F.E.A., and Dabbouri E.A. (2020). *The Effect of Transformation Leadership on Government Employee Job Satisfaction During Covid-19*. Management Science Letters 11 pp.1231-1244.

Alvesson M. and Spicer A. (2016). *The Stupidity Paradox: The Power and Pitfalls of Functional Stupidity at Work*. Profile Books, London, UK.

Amaratunga D., Haigh R.P., and Hettige S. (2016). *The Role of Accountability Within Disaster Risk Governance*. 6th International Conference on Building Resilience, September 2016, Massey University and the University of Auckland, New Zealand.

ANAO (2008). *Australia's Preparedness for a Human Influenza Pandemic*. Australian National Audit Office Report No6 2007-08. Accessed at: https://www.anao.gov.au/sites/default/files/ANAO_Report_2007-2008_06.pdf.

Anderson L. (2018). *Leadership During Crisis: Navigating Complexity and Uncertainty*. Leader to Leader: Executive Forum, University of Pittsburgh.

Andrews D. (2020a). *A Stronger Quarantine Program to Protect What We've Built*. 30 November 2020. Accessed at: https://www.premier.vic.gov.au/stronger-quarantine-program-protect-what-weve-built.

Andrews D. (2020b). *Huge Expansion of our Health System to Fight Coronavirus*. Media Release by Premier of Victoria, The Hon Daniel Andrews, 1 April, 2020. Accessed at: https://www.premier.vic.gov.au/huge-expansion-our-health-system-fight-coronavirus.

Andrews D. (2020c). *Transcript of Premier's Media Conference held on 27 March, 2020*. Provided as Exhibit to the Coate Inquiry. Accessed at: https://www.quarantineinquiry.vic.gov.au/exhibits.

Andrews D. (2020d). *More Restrictions Put in Place in The Fight Against COVID-19*. Media Release, Premier of Victoria, 18 March 2020. Accessed at: https://www.premier.vic.gov.au/more-restrictions-put-place-fight-against-covid-19.

Andrews D. (2021). *Seven Day Lockdown to Keep Victorian Safe*. Media release by the Premier of Victoria, the Hon Daniel Andrews. 5 August, 2021. Accessed at: https://www.premier.vic.gov.au/seven-day-lockdown-keep-victorians-safe.

Anon. (2007). *Crisis Management – Easy to do Badly, Hard to do Right. Differing Experiences of Wal-Mart, Enron and Arthur Andersen*. Strategic Direction 23(2) pp.26-29.

Anon. (2015). *Health Service Defends Dorevitch Pathology*. The Ararat Advertiser, 4 September, 2015. Accessed at: https://www.araratadvertiser.com.au/story/3328013/provider-enjoys-service-support/.

Anon. (2019). Employee Reviews. Glassdoor. Accessed at: https://www.glassdoor.co.in/Reviews/Employee-Review-Emergency-Management-Victoria-RVW21294178.htm.

Anon (2021). *'Nonsense' Rule Requiring Residents to Display QR Code Outside Their Homes*. Sydney Morning Herald, 14 May 2021. Accessed at: https://www.smh.com.au/national/nonsense-rule-requiring-residents-to-display-qr-code-outside-their-homes-20210514-p57s5w.html.

Ansell C. and Bartenberger M. (2016). *Tackling Unruly Public Problems*. In: Governance in Turbulent Times (Editors: C. Ansell, J. Trondal, and M. Øgård). Oxford, UK: Oxford University Press Oxford, UK.

ANZSOG (2021). *Behavioural Insights Teams in Australia and Aotearoa – New Zealand*. The Australia and New Zealand School of Government. Accessed at: https://www.anzsog.edu.au/resource-library/research/behavioural-insights-teams-in-australia-and-aotearoa-new-zealand.

Appelbaum S. (2007). *Toxins in the Workplace: Affect on Organizations and Employees. Corporate Governance*. International Journal of Business in Society 7(1) pp. 17-28.

Ardebili A.A. and Padoano E. (2021). *A Literature Review of the Concepts of Resilience and Sustainability in Group Decision-making*. Sustainability 12 Article 2602.

Ariely D. (2010). *Good Decisions. Bad Outcomes*. Harvard Business Review, December 2010.

Asher N. (2021). *Coronavirus Contact Tracing Inquiry Told Victoria's DHHS had Problems with Open Disclosure*. ABC News, 16 November 2020. Accessed at: https://www.abc.net.au/news/2020-11-16/victoria-dhhs-coronavirus-contact-tracing-system-inquiry-hearing/12887410.

ASIC (2021). *Notice of Appointment as Liquidator -for Unified Security Group*. Australian Securities and Investments Commission/ Accessed at:

https://publishednotices.asic.gov.au/browsesearch-notices/notice-details/UNIFIED-SECURITY-GROUP-AUSTRALIA-PTY-LTD-138976397/651ce3df-f01e-4e57-b5fe-81451904d3cb

Aubrey D.W. (2012). *The Effect of Toxic Leadership*. Strategy Research Project. United States Army War College. Carlisle Barracks, PA.

Australian Government (2014). *Skill set details: CPPSS00044 - Provide Security Services in a Health Care Environment (Release 1)*. Accessed at: https://training.gov.au/Training/Details/CPPSS00044.

Australian Government (2019). *Unit of Competency Details: CPPSEC1004A - Apply Health Care Security Procedures (Release 1)*. Accessed at: https://training.gov.au/Training/Details/CPPSEC1004A.

Australian Government (2021). Joint Statement on the WHO-Convened COVID-19 Origins Study. Accessed at: https://www.dfat.gov.au/news/media-release/joint-statement-who-convened-covid-19-origins-study.

Aven T. (2017). *Improving Risk Characterisations in Practical Situations by Highlighting Knowledge Aspects, with Applications to Risk Matrices*. Reliability Engineering and System Safety 167 pp. 42-48.

Aven T. and Ylönen M. (2019). *The Strong Power of Standards in the Safety and Risk Fields: A Threat to Proper Developments of these Fields?* Reliability Engineering and System Safety l89 pp. 279-286.

Ayyub B.M., McGill W.L., and Kaminskiy M. (2007). *Critical Asset and Portfolio Risk Analysis: An All-Hazards Framework*. Risk Analysis 27 pp. 789-801.

Babiak P. and Hare R.D. (2007). *Snakes in Suits: When Psychopaths go to Work*. Harper Collins. New York, NY.

Babiak P., Neumann C.S., and Hare R.D. (2010). *Corporate Psychopathy: Talking the Walk*. Behavioral Sciences and the Law. 28 pp. 174-193.

Babiak P. and O'Toole M.E. 92012). *The Corporate Psychopath*. Law Enforcement Bulletin 1 November 2012. Accessed at: https://leb.fbi.gov/articles/featured-articles/the-corporate-psychopath.

Bachrach P. and Baratz M. (1963). *Decisions and Nondecisions: An Analytical Framework*. American Political Science Review 57 pp. 641–51.

Bachrach P. and Baratz M. (1970) *Power and Poverty: Theory and Practise*. Oxford University Press, New York NY.

Badie D. (2010). *Groupthink, Iraq, and the War of Terror: Explaining US Policy Shift Toward Iraq*. Foreign Policy Analysis 6 pp. 277-296.

Bagaric M. (2020). *Coronavirus: Victoria Can't Blame Bad Luck for Coronavirus Failures. The Australian 23 June 2020*. Accessed at: https://www.theaustralian.com.au/commentary/victoria-cant-blame-bad-luck-for-coronavirus-failures/news-story/dc4d8d49218156e029f0fcd7dbb15678.

Bahalla A.S. (2021). *Leadership Challenges and the COVID-19 Pandemic*. ORF Occasional Paper No. 229, February 2021, Observer Research Foundation.

Bailey L. (2009). *Toxic Cultures and Organizations: NASA and the Columbia Shuttle Disaster*. Indiana Journal of Political Science 12 pp. 69-76.

Baker D.P., Day R., and Salas E. (2006). *Teamwork as an Essential Component of High-Reliability Organizations*. Health Services Research 41 (4, Part II) pp. 1576-1598.

Baker J., Côté J., and Abernethy B. (2003). *Sport-specific Practice and Development of Expert Decision-making in Team Ball Sports*. Journal of Applied Sport Psychology 15 (12-25).

Baker R., Mills T., Fowler M., and Le Grand C. (2020). *Previously Withheld Hotel Quarantine Emails Show Sutton's Turf War with Emergency Managers*. Sydney Morning Herald, 27 November 2020. Accessed at: https://www.smh.com.au/national/victoria/previously-withheld-hotel-quarantine-emails-show-sutton-s-turf-war-with-emergency-managers-20201127-p56iom.html.

Balkin J.M. (1999) *How Mass Media Simulate Political Transparency*. Cultural Values 3 pp. 393-413.

Ball D. and Watt J. (2013). *Further Thoughts on the Utility of Risk Matrices*. Risk Analysis 33(11) pp. 22068-22078.

Ball G. (2020). *Leadership During the COVID-19 Crisis and Beyond*. Canadian Journal of Surgery 63(4) pp. E370-E371.

Barabba V. (2011). *Back to the Private Sector with Eastman Kodak*. In: The Decision Loom: A Design for Interactive Decision-Making in Organizations. Triarchy Press, Axminister UK.

Baraniuk C. (2020). *What the Diamond Princes Taught the Word About COVID-19*. The British Medical Journal 369 Article m369.

Barclay E. (2020). *The Conspiracy Theories About the Origins of the Coronavirus, Debunked*. Vox, 12 March 2020. Accessed at: https://www.vox.com/2020/3/4/21156607/how-did-the-coronavirus-get-started-china-wuhan-lab.

Baric R.S. (2008). *SARS-CoV: Lessons for Global Health*. Virus Research 133(1) pp.1-3.

Barron J. and Flower W. (2020). *Victorian Health Minister Who Resigned Over Deadly Second Wave Scandal Slams Dan Andrews and Tells Him to Release his Phone Records so People Can 'know the truth' About Hotel Quarantine*. Daily Mail Australia, 21 December 2020. Accessed at: https://www.dailymail.co.uk/news/article-9074839/Ex-Health-Minister-Jenny-Mikakos-takes-swipe-Daniel-Andrews-refused-resign.html.

Barry J.M. (2004). *The Site of Origin of the 1918 Influenza Pandemic and its Public Health Implications*. Journal of Translational Medicine 2 Article 3.

Başkan B. (2020). *Toxic Leadership in Education: A Systematic Review*. International Journal of Educational Administration, Management, and Leadership 1(2) pp.97-104.

Baxendale R. (2020a). *Coalition Motion to Lift Curfew Passes on Voices*. The Weekend Australian, September 2020. Accessed at: https://www.theaustralian.com.au/nation/coronavirus-australia-live-news-pms-covid-troops-offer-to-daniel-andrews/news-story/f33b853e037280fff0163d2725e0f8d9.

Baxendale R. (2020b). *Leaders Play Pass the Buck Over Curfew Order*. The Weekend Australian, September 2020. Accessed at: https://www.theaustralian.com.au/nation/leaders-play-pass-the-buck-over-curfew-order/news-story/769efa3dbdc38bff549c289fa90ad29f.

Baxendale R. (2020c). *Police Refusal to Punish Melbourne Protestors 'Unlawful', QC Finds*. The Australian 21 July 2020. Accessed at: https://www.theaustralian.com.au/nation/police-refusal-to-punish-melbourne-protesters-unlawful-qc-finds/news-story/63e1910a6a31f9aa794b658b01f4db61.

Baxendale R. (2020d). *Coronavirus: QR Code Won't Fit with IT Platform*. The Australian 24 December 2021. Accessed at: https://www.theaustralian.com.au/nation/politics/coronavirus-qr-code-wont-fit-with-it-platform/news-story/db8db6f1c82995333fe4362844e70e2c.

Baxendale R. and Varga R. (2020). *Coronavirus: Private Guards Decision mMade Early, says Daniel Andrews*. The Australian, 14 August 2020. Accessed at: https://www.theaustralian.com.au/nation/politics/coronavirus-defence-confirms-100-troops-were-on-standby-for-victoria/news-story/1b63799aa629caa729fd3a570e30ce0c.

References

Baxendale R. and Snowden A. (2021). *Victoria's Public Hospital System on Verge of Collapsing*. The Australian, 2 September 2021. Accessed at: https://www.theaustralian.com.au/nation/victorias-public-hospitals-buckling-may-not-cope-as-covid19-infections-soar/news-story/c73b2b2251a3d552437c592d1a76d5b3.

Bazermann M.H. and Tenbrunsel A.E. (2011). *Ethical Breakdowns*. Harvard Business Review, April 2011.

BBC (2020a). *Coronavirus Tenerife Hotel Quarantine: 'We Don't Believe it's* Safe'. BBC News, 27 February 2010. Accessed at: https://www.bbc.com/news/av/world-europe-51660762.

BBC (2020b). *Covid: Melbourne Towers Lockdown 'Breached Human Rights'*. BBC News, 17 December 2020. Accessed at: https://www.bbc.com/news/world-australia-55342990.

BBC (1998). *Special Report: 50 years of the WHO – Successes and Failures*. Accessed at: http://news.bbc.co.uk/1/hi/special_report/1998/health/47191.stm.

Beaumont P. (2021). *UK and US Criticise WHO's Covid Report and Accuse China of Withholding Data*. The Guardian, 31 March, 2021. Accessed at: https://www.theguardian.com/world/2021/mar/30/who-criticises-chinas-data-sharing-as-it-releases-covid-origins-report.

Beers L.M. (2021). *Victoria's COVID QR Code System Flaws After People Failed to Check in at Melbourne's Curry Vault*. 7 NEWS, 13 May 2021. Accessed at: https://7news.com.au/lifestyle/health-wellbeing/victorias-covid-qr-code-system-flaws-after-people-failed-to-check-in-at-melbournes-curry-vault-c-2827292.

Begg M. (2020). *Victoria Police Potentially Acted Unlawfully in Allowing Black Lives Matter Protest: Legal Advice.* Institute of Public Affairs, 21 July 2020. Accessed at: https://ipa.org.au/publications-ipa/victoria-police-potentially-acted-unlawfully-in-allowing-black-lives-matter-protest-legal-advice.

Bekker M.P.M., Greer S.L., Azzopardi-Muscat N., and McKee M. (2018). *Public Health and Politics: How Political Science Can Help Us Move Forward*. European Journal of Public Health 28(suppl 3) pp.1-2.

Belido H., Olmos L., and Román-Aso J.A. (2021). *The Influence of Government Ideology on Corruption: The Impact of the Great Recession*. Economia Politica 38 pp. 677-798.

Belizaire J. (2021). *The Proven Method for Making Irreversible Decisions*. CEO Playbook. Accessed at: https://www.ceoplaybook.co/the-proven-method-for-making-irreversible-decisions/.

Bell K.H., O'Sullivan M., Frodé K., Jones A.O., and Rebebechi C. *Inquiry into the Government's Response to the COVID-19 Pandemic*. Submission on Behalf of the Castan Centre for Human Rights Law, Faculty of Law, Monash University, Melbourne, Australia. Accessed at: https://www.parliament.vic.gov.au/images/stories/committees/paec/COVID-19_Inquiry/Submissions/68a._Castan_Centre_for_Human_Rights_Law.pdf

Bell L. and Traxler B. (2021). *Effectiveness of Masks*. ABC Science Collaborative, Final Report, June 2021. South Carolina Department of Health. and Environmental Control. Accessed at: https://scdhec.gov/sites/default/files/media/document/Evidence-For-Mask-Use-K-12-Schools.pdf

Ben-Ami S. (2020). *Why Democracies are Better at Managing Crises*. The Strategist 20 May 2020. Australian Strategic Policy Institute. Accessed at: https://www.aspistrategist.org.au/why-democracies-are-better-at-managing-crises/.

Bendavid E., Oh C, Bhattacharya J. Ioannidis J.P.A.(2021). *Assessing Mandatory Stay-at-home and Business Closure Effects on the Spread of COVID-19*. European Journal of Clinical Investigation. 51(4) Article: e13484.

Benlahcene A. and Abdullah N.S.B (2020). *Public Leadership in Times of Crisis: Lessons from the Covid-19 Pandemic in Malaysia*. The International Seminar on Regional Politics,

Administration and Development 2020, STISIPOL. Raja Haji, Riani, Indonesia, 14-15 October 2020.

Benn J., Healey A. N., and Hollnagel E. (2007). *Improving Performance Reliability in Surgical Systems*. Cognition, and Work 10(4) pp. 323–333.

Bennett C. (2020). *Where did Victoria go so Wrong with Contact Tracing and Have They Fixed it?* The Conversation 13 October 2020. Accessed at: https://theconversation.com/where-did-victoria-go-so-wrong-with-contact-tracing-and-have-they-fixed-it-147993.

Bennet C. (2020). *Transcript of Evidence,* Inquiry into the Victorian Government's COVID–19 Contact Tracing System and Testing Regime. Parliament of Victoria: Legislative Council Legal and Social Issues Committee. Accessed at: https://www.parliament.vic.gov.au/images/stories/committees/SCLSI/Inquiry_into_the_Victorian_Governments_COVID19_Contact_Tracing_System_and_Testing_Regime_/report/LCLSIC_59-05_Vic_Gov_COVID-19_contact_tracing_testing.pdf.

Bennett G., Young E., Butler I., and Coe S. (2021). *The Impact of Lockdown During the COVID-19 Outbreak on Dietary Habits in Various Population Groups: A Scoping Review*. Frontiers in Nutrition doi.org/10.3389/fnut.2021.626432.

Berg C. (2014). *Shining a Light on the Dangers of Royal Commissions*. ABC news 1 July 2014. Accessed at: https://www.abc.net.au/news/2014-07-01/berg-shining-a-light-on-the-dangers-of-royal-commissions/5562354

Bernardi C. (2020). *Andrews Uses Health Experts as a 'Human Shield' After Ignoring Health Advice*. Sky News, 29 September 2020. Accessed at: https://www.skynews.com.au/australia-news/andrews-uses-health-experts-as-a-human-shield-after-ignoring-health-advice/video/d1cd4c949d85f22270e1581efe997feb.

Bernstein J. (2006). *Crisis Manager University*. Crisis Manager – Internet Newsletter about Crisis Management. 7 January 2006. Accessed on 8 July 2017 at: https://www.bernsteincrisismanagement.com/newsletter/crisismgr060701.html.

BETA (2023). *Behavioural Economics Team*. Department of Prime Minister and Cabinet, Canberra. Accessed at: https://behaviouraleconomics.pmc.gov.au/about.

Bevege A. (2020). *How Victorian Authorities 'Knew a Housing Commission Tower was Infected with Coronavirus TWO MONTHS Before Horror Second Wave Crisis'.* Daily Mail Australia13 July 2020. Accessed at: https://www.dailymail.co.uk/news/article-8517311/Victorian-authorities-knew-housing-commission-tower-infected-TWO-MONTHS-covid-outbreak.html.

Bevington F. (2014). *Are Preparedness Funding Cuts Impacting the Capability of Local Health Departments to Respond to Global Health Security Threats?* Accessed at: https://www.naccho.org/blog/articles/are-preparedness-funding-cuts-impacting-the-capability-of-local-health-departments-to-respond-to-global-health-security-threats.

Bezos J. (2015). 2015 *Letter to Shareholders*. Amazon. Available at: https://s2.q4cdn.com/299287126/files/doc_financials/annual/2015-Letter-to-Shareholders.PDF.

Bezos J. (2016). 2016 *Letter to Shareholders*. Amazon. Available at: https://www.aboutamazon.com/news/company-news/2016-letter-to-shareholders/.

Bharosa N., Lee J., and Janssen M. (2010). *Challenges and Obstacles in Sharing and Coordinating Information During Multiagency Disaster Response: Propositions from Field Exercises*. Information Systems Frontier 12 pp. 49-65.

BINBS (2013). *Intuition, Analytical Skills Matter Most in Crisis*. BI Norwegian Business School. Reported in Science Daily, 23 December 2013.

Binskin M., Bennett A., and Macintosh A. (2020). *Report of the Royal Commission into Natural Disaster Arrangements, 20 October 2020*. Australian Government, Canberra, Australia.
Bircham J.S. and Connolly H.J. (2013). *Addicted to Performance: Society Demands More for Less*. Bircham-Global Publishing Ltd, Turanga New Zealand.
Bjørnskov C. (2021). *Did Lockdown Work? An Economist's Cross-Country Comparison*. CESifo Economic Studies Article ifab003.
Black N. and Mays N. (2013). *Public Inquiries into Health care in the UK: A Sound Basis for Policy-making*. Journal of Health Services Research and Policy 18(3) pp. 129-31.
Blanton R.E., Fein G.M., Kowalewski S.A., and Fargher L.F. (2020). *Moral Collapse and State Failure: A View from the Past*. Frontiers in Political Science 2, Article: 568704.
Blackman D., O'Flynn J., and Ugyel L. (2013). *A Diagnostic Tool for Assessing Organisational Readiness for Complex Change*. Australian and New Zealand Academy of Management Conference, Hobart, 4-6 December 2014.
Board B.J. and Fritzon K. (2005). *Disordered Personalities at Work*. Psychology, Crime & Law 11(1) pp. 17-32.
Boddy C. R. 2010a. *Corporate Psychopaths and Productivity*. Management Services, Spring pp. 26 - 30.
Boddy C. R. 2011. *Corporate Psychopaths: Organisational Destroyers*. Palgrave Macmillan, Basingstoke, UK.
Boddy C.R. (2013). *Corporate Psychopaths*. Journal of Corporate Citizenship 49 pp. 8-16.
Boddy C.R. (2016). *Psychopathy Screening for Public Leadership*. International Journal of Public Leadership, 12(4) pp. 254-274.
Boddy C. R. and Miles D., Sanyal C. and Hartog M. (2015). *Extreme Managers, Extreme Workplaces: Capitalism, Organizations and Corporate Psychopaths*. Organization 22 (4) pp. 530-551.
Boddy C., Boulter L., and Fishwick S. (2021). *How So Many Employees Ascend to Leadership*. In Debating Bad Leadership pp. 69-85 (Editor Anders Örtenblad). Palgrave Debates in Business and Management, SpringerLink.
Bogusky-Halper K. (2020). *Study: Organizations Rising to the Challenge of COVID-19 Communication, But Needs Persist*; Leaders Must Address Concerns and Demonstrate Transparency, Clarity and Openness. Business Wire, 3 April 2020. Accessed at: https://www.businesswire.com/news/home/20200403005278/en/STUDY-Organizations-Rising-to-the-Challenge-of-COVID-19-Communications-but-Needs-Persist-Leaders-Must-Address-Concerns-and-Demonstrate-Transparency-Clarity-and-Openness.
Boin A. (2013). *Leadership in Times of Crisis: A Framework for Assessment*. International Review of Public Administration 18(1) pp.79-91.
Boin A. and t'Hart, P. (2003). *Public Leadership in Times of Crisis: Mission Impossible?* Public Administration Review 63(5) pp. 544-553.
Boin A., McConnell A., and t' Hart P. (2008). *Governing After Crisis: The Politics of Investigation, Accountability and Learning*. Cambridge University Press, Cambridge, UK.
Bonardi J.P., Gallea Q., Kalanoski D., Lalive R. (2020). *Fast and Local: How Lockdown Policies Affect the Spread and Severity of COVID-19*. CEPR Covid Econ 23 pp.325–50.
Bond C. (2021). *'Secrecy and Lies': Vic Supreme Court Finding Reveals Govt 'not upfront' on QR Code Data*. Sky News, 28 December 2021. Accessed at: https://www.skynews.com.au/opinion/secrecy-and-lies-vic-supreme-court-finding-reveals-govt-not-upfront-on-qr-code-data/video/1acf03f5b2089e165a9104da55757740.
Bongiorno F. (2020). *Why Good Leaders Need to Hold the Hose: How History Might Read Morrison's Coronavirus Leadership*. The Conversation, 19 May 2020. Accessed at:

https://theconversation.com/why-good-leaders-need-to-hold-the-hose-how-history-might-read-morrisons-coronavirus-leadership-137785.

Boone S.A. and Gerba C.P. (2007). *Significance of Fomites in the Spread of Respiratory and Enteric Viral Disease*. Applied and Environmental Microbiology 73(6) pp. 1687-1696.

Bosomworth K., Own C., and Curnin S. (2017). *Addressing Challenges for Future Strategic-level Emergency Management*. Reframing, Networking, and Capacity-building. Disasters 41(2) pp. 306-323.

Boseley M. (2020a). *Melbourne Public Housing Covid Lockdown Violated Human Rights Victoria's Ombudsman Find*. The Guardian, 17 December 2020. Accessed at: https://www.theguardian.com/australia-news/2020/dec/17/melbourne-public-housing-covid-lockdown-violated-human-rights-victorias-ombudsman-finds.

Boseley M. (2020b). *Residents in Melbourne Covid-19 Tower Lockdown Say Food Supplies Have Been Inadequate*. The Guardian 6 July 2020. Accessed at: https://www.theguardian.com/world/2020/jul/06/residents-melbourne-covid-19-tower-lockdown-food-supplies-inadequate.

Bouafia M. and ZahariK.R. (2017). *Naturalistic Decision-making in Natural Disasters: An Overview*. Journal of Geography and Natural Disasters 7(1) Article 1000186.

Bouygues H.L (2019). *The Problem of Groupthink: How to Encourage More Independent Thinking*. Forbes, 20 April, 2019. Accessed at: https://www.forbes.com/sites/helenleebouygues/2019/04/20/the-problem-of-groupthink-how-to-encourage-more-independent-thinking/?sh=32bf42432aeb.

Bradley D. and Jancewicz J.A. (2016). *Teams: A Pathway to Organizational Success*. FBI Law Enforcement Bulletin, December 2016.

Bramston T. (2021). *Covid-19: Victoria Show World How to Bungle a Crisis*. The Australian, 8 June 2020. Accessed at: https://www.theaustralian.com.au/commentary/covid19-victoria-shows-world-how-to-bungle-a-crisis/news-story/41e26ede5b7ace1a8961f441e7920f53.

Bratteteig T. and Wagner I. (2012). *Disentangling Power and Decision-making in Participatory Design*. PDC '12, 12-16 August 2012, Roskilde Denmark.

Brauner J.M., Minderman S., Sharma M., Johnston D., Salvatier J., Gavenčiak T., Stephenson A.B., Leech G., Altman G., Mikulik V., Norman. A.J., Monnrad J.T., Besiroglu T., Ge H., Hartwick M.A., The Y.W., Chindelevitch L., Gal Y., and Kulveit J. (2021). *Inferring the Effectiveness of Government Interventions Against COVID-19*. Science 371 Article 6531.

Briley D.A., Morris M.W., and Simonson I. (2000). *Reasons as Carriers of Culture: Dynamic Versus Dispositional Models of Cultural Influence on Decision Making*. Journal of Consumer Research 27 pp. 157-178.

Brisbois M.C., Morris M., and de Loë R. (2019). *Augmenting the IAD Framework to Reveal Power in Collaborative Governance – An Illustrative Application to Resource Industry Dominated Processes*. World Development 120 pp.159-168.

Broadfoot M. (2021). *Masks Protect Schoolkids from COVID Despite what Antiscience Politicians Claim*. Scientific American 16 September 2021. Accessed at: https://www.scientificamerican.com/article/masks-protect-schoolkids-from-covid-despite-what-antiscience-politicians-claim/.

Brook S. and Hutchinson S. (2021). *Spring Street's Spin Machine Red-faced After Confidential Notes Takes Wrong Track*. The Age, 17 June 2021. Accessed at: https://www.theage.com.au/national/spring-street-s-spin-machine-red-faced-after-confidential-notes-takes-wrong-track-20210616-p581m6.html.

Brooks S.K., Webster R.K., Snith L.E., Woodand L., Wessely S., Greenberg N., and Ruben G.J. (2020). *The Psychological Impact of Quarantine and How to Reduce it: Rapid Review of the Evidence.* The Lancet 395 pp. 912-920.

Brooks J.C., Pinto M., Gill A., Hills K.E., Murthy S., Podgornik M.N., Hernandez L.F., Rose D.A., Angulo F.J., and Rzeszotarski P. (2016). *Incident Management Systems and Building Emergency Management Capacity during the 2014–2016 Ebola Epidemic — Liberia, Sierra Leone, and Guinea.* Morbidity and Mortality Weekly Reports (MMWR), Supplements 65(3) pp. 28-34.

Brooks N. and Fritzon K. (2016). *Psychopathic Personality Characteristics Amongst High Functioning Populations*. Crime Psychology Review 2(1) pp. 22-44.

Brower T. (2020). *5 Predictions about How Coronavirus Will Change the Future of Work*. Forbes, April 6. Accessed at: https://www.forbes.com/sites/tracybrower/2020/04/06/how-the-post-covid-future-will-be-different-5-positive-predictions-about-the-future-of-work-to-help-your-mood-and-your-sanity/?sh=4fe5ac073e22

Brown L.D. (2010). *The Political Face of Public Health*. Public Health Reviews 32(1) pp. 155-173.

Browne E. (2020). *Fauci Was 'Untruthful' to Congress About Wuhan Lab Research, New Documents Appear to Show.* Newsweek 9 September 2021. Accessed at: https://www.newsweek.com/fauci-untruthful-congress-wuhan-lab-research-documents-show-gain-function-1627351.

Bucci N. (2021a). *Agency Staff Allowed to Work Across Multiple Aged Care Homes During COVID Lockdown*. The Guardian, 5 June 2021. Accessed at: https://www.theguardian.com/australia-news/2021/jun/05/agency-staff-allowed-to-work-across-multiple-aged-care-homes-during-covid-lockdown.

Bucci N. (2021b). *Daniel Andrews Won't Stand Down Over Reports IBAC is Investigating his Role in Firies Dispute*. The Guardian, 6 October 2021. Accessed at: https://www.theguardian.com/australia-news/2021/oct/06/daniel-andrews-wont-stand-down-over-reports-ibac-is-investigating-his-role-in-firies-dispute.

Bucci N. (2021). *Patronage and Branch Stacking: Five Things We Learned from Adem Somyurek's IBAC Evidence This Week.* The Guardian, 13 November 2021. Accessed at: https://www.theguardian.com/australia-news/2021/nov/13/patronage-and-branch-stacking-five-things-we-learned-from-adem-somyureks-ibac-evidence-this-week.

Bullens L. (2013). *Having Second Thoughts: Consequences of Decision Reversibility*. Thesis, University of Amsterdam, Netherlands.

Bullens L., van Harrevald F., Förster J.; and Higgins T.E. (2014). *How Decision Reversibility Affects Motivation*. Journal of Experimental Psychology: General 143 pp. 835-849.

Buchan B. (2020). *Exception or the Rule? When Corruption Becomes Commonplace*. ABC Religion and Ethics, 1 December 2020. Accessed at: https://www.abc.net.au/religion/machiavellian-moment-when-corruption-becomes-commonplace/12838170.

Bundy J., Pfarrer M.D., Short C.E., and Coombs T. (2017). *Crises and Crisis Management: Integration, Interpretation, and Research Development*. Journal of Management 43(6) pp. 1661-1692.

Burgess M. (2021). Life in the World's Most Locked Down City. Bloomberg, Coronavirus Daily, 15 September 2021. Accessed at: https://www.bloomberg.com/news/newsletters/2021-09-15/life-in-the-world-s-most-locked-down-city.

Burgo J. (2015). *The Narcissist You Know. Defending Yourself Against Extreme Narcissists in an All-about-me Age*. Pan Macmillan Australia, Sydney, Australia.
Burke C.S., Wilson K.A. and Salas E. (2007). *The Use of a Team-based Strategy for Organizational Transformation:*
Guidance for Moving Toward a High Reliability Organization. Theoretical Issues in Ergonomics Science 6(6) pp. 509-530.
Burns W.A. (2017). *A Descriptive Literature Review of Harmful Leadership Styles: Definitions, Commonalities, Measurements, Negative Impacts, and Ways to Improve These Harmful Leadership Styles*. Creighton Journal of Interdisciplinary Leadership. 3(1) pp. 33-52.
Burton T. (2020). *Health Department Split Ends Victoria's Mega-agency Experiment*. Financial Review, 3 December 2020. Accessed at:
https://www.afr.com/policy/health-and-education/dhhs-split-ends-victoria-s-mega-agency-experiment-20201202-p56k25.
Burton T. (2021a). *Health Department Split Ends Victoria's mega Agency Experiment*. Australian Financial Review, 3 December 2020. Accessed at:
https://www.afr.com/policy/health-and-education/dhhs-split-ends-victoria-s-mega-agency-experiment-20201202-p56k25.
Burton T. (2021b). *Why Royal Commissions Don't Always Solve the Problem*. Financial Review, 5 March 2021. Accessed at: https://www.afr.com/policy/health-and-education/why-royal-commissions-don-t-always-solve-the-problem-20210305-p57810.
Busby E. (2022). *Evidence on Effectiveness of Face Masks in Schools 'inconclusive', New Study Finds*. Independent, 6 January 2022. Accessed at:
https://www.independent.co.uk/news/uk/nadhim-zahawi-evidence-england-government-mps-b1988082.html.
Bush R.M. (2004). *Influenza as a Model System for Studying the Cross-species Transfer and Evolution of the SARS Coronavirus*. Philosophical Transactions of the Royal Society London 359 pp. 1067-1073.
Butler B. (2020). *Essential Service? Call for Crown Casinos and Pokie Venues to be Shut During Coronavirus Outbreak*. The Guardian, 19 March 2020. Accessed at:
https://www.theguardian.com/world/2020/mar/19/crown-casinos-and-pokie-venues-should-be-shut-during-coronavirus-outbreak-say-critics.
Butt A.I. (2019). *Why Did Bush Go to War in Iraq?* Aljazeera, 20 March 2019. Accessed at:
https://www.aljazeera.com/opinions/2019/3/20/why-did-bush-go-to-war-in-iraq.
Butterworth P., Schurer S., Trinh T-A., Toscano E.V., and Wooden M. (2022). *Effect of Lockdown on Mental Health in Australia: Evidence from a Natural Experiment Analysing a Longitudinal Probability Sample Survey*. The Lancet Public Health 7 Article e427-36.
Buying for Victoria (2018). *Security Services Contract*. Accessed at:
https://www.buyingfor.vic.gov.au/security-services.
CAIB (2003). *Report Volume 1, August 2003*, Columbia Accident Investigation Board, Washington, DC.
Calbert J. and Arbuthnott G. (2021). *China, the WHO and the Power Grab that Fuelled a Pandemic*. The Australian, 17 August 2021. Accessed at:
https://www.theaustralian.com.au/life/china-the-who-and-the-power-grab-that-fuelled-a-pandemic/news-story/6b09d435842244632749e7a53aafcb83.
Calisher C., Carroll D., Colwell R., Corley R.B., Daszak P., Drosten C., Enjuanes L., Farrar J., Field H., Golding J., Gorbalenya A., Haagmans B.M., Hughes J.M., Karesh W.B., Keusch G.T., Lam S.K., Lubroth J., Mackenzie J.S., Madoff L., Mazet J., Palese P., Perlman S., Poon L., Roizman B., Saif L., Subbarrao K., and Turner M. (2020). *Statement in Support of the*

Scientists, Public Health Professionals, and Medical Professionals of China Combatting COVID-19. The Lancet 395 (10226) E42-E43.
Calloway E. and Ledford H. (2021). *How Bad is Omicron? What Scientists Know so Far.* Nature, 2 December 2021.
Cameron E. (2021). *Beware the Promises of Easy Answers When it Comes to COVID.* Sydney Morning Herald, 15 October 2021. Accessed at:
https://www.smh.com.au/national/beware-the-promise-of-easy-answers-when-it-comes-to-covid-20211014-p58zud.html.
Camm T.W. (2014). *The Dark Side of Leadership: Dealing with a Narcissistic Boss*. SME Annual Meeting, 23-26 February 2014, Salt Lake City, UT. Preprint 14-090.
Campbell C. (2021). *Health Experts Call for national Approach to COVID-19 Outbreaks, Lockdown and Quarantine*. ABC News 31 July 2021. Accessed at:
https://www.abc.net.au/news/2021-07-31/experts-call-for-national-approach-to-covid-19-lockdowns/100338080.
Campbell M. (2020). *The Carnival Cruise Ship That Spread Coronavirus Around the World.* Bloomberg Businessweek 15 September 2020. Accessed at:
https://www.bloomberg.com/news/features/2020-09-15/carnival-s-ruby-princess-cruise-ship-spread-coronavirus-around-the-world.
Carey A and Towell N. (2018). *'Promises were Made': Firefighter's Union Boss Claims Secret Deal with Daniel Andrews*. The Age, 18 April 2018. Accessed at:
https://www.theage.com.au/politics/victoria/promises-were-made-firefighters-union-boss-claims-secret-deal-with-daniel-andrews-20180418-p4zae9.html.
Caristia S., Ferranti M., Skrami E., Raffeti E., Pierannunzio D., Carle F., Saracci R., Badaloni C., Barone-Adesi F., Ancona C., and AIE Working Group on the Evaluation of the Effectiveness of Lockdowns. *Effect of National and Local Lockdowns on the Control of COVID-19 Pandemic: A Rapid Review*. Epidemiologia e Prevenzione 44(5-6 Suppl 2) pp. 60-68.
Carlson J.M. and Doyle J. (2000). *Highly Optimised Tolerance: Robustness and Design in Complex Systems*. Physics Review Letters 84(11) pp. 2529-32.
Carlström E.D. and Ekman I. (2012). *Organisational Culture and Change: Implementing Person-centred Care*. Journal of Health Organization and Management 26(2), pp. 175-191.
Carlton E, (1984). *Ideologies as Belief Systems*. International Journal of Sociology and Social Policy. 4(2) pp. 17-29.
Carmine S., Andriopoulos C., Gotsi M., Härtel C.E.J., Krzeminska A., Mafico N., Pradies C., Raza H., Raza-Ullah T., Schrage S., Sharma G., Slawinski N., Stadtler L., Tunarosa A., Winther-Hansen C., and Keller J, (2021). *A Paradox Approach to Organizational Tensions During the Pandemic Crisis.* Journal of Management Inquiry 30(2) pp. 138-153.
Carney S. (2020). How Did the Second Wave Happen? It's not Rocket Science Folks. The Sydney Morning Herald, 2 August 2020. Accessed at:
https://www.smh.com.au/national/how-did-the-second-wave-happen-it-s-not-rocket-science-folks-20200731-p55hab.html.
Carr C. *Daniel Andrews' Victoria: Scenes from a Failed State.* Quadrant Online, 12 September,2020. Accessed at:
https://quadrant.org.au/opinion/qed/2020/09/daniel-andrews-victoria-scenes-from-a-failed-state/.
Carrillo J.A., Mendoza E.G., Nuguer V., and Roldán-Peña J. (2019). *Tight Money-Tight Credit: Coordination Failure in the Conduct of Monetary and Financial Policies.* IMES Discussion Paper Series, Discussion Paper No. 2019-E-8. Institute for Monetary and Economic Studies, Bank of Japan, Tokyo, Japan.

Carrillo-Castrillo J.A., Rubio-Romero J.C. and Onieva L. (2013). *Causation of Severe and Fatal Accidents in the Manufacturing Sector.* International Journal of Occupational Safety and Ergonomics (JOSE) 19(3) pp. 423–434.

Carswell A. (2013). *Kevin Rudd – Hero or Psychopath?* The Daily Telegraph 10 August 2013. Accessed at: https://www.dailytelegraph.com.au/news/nsw/kevin-rudd--hero-or-psychopath/news-story/49e8551dd478f1eb28f5a33653b3ca62.

Castro J.L. (2017*). The World Health Organization Made a Big Mistake on TB. It Must Fix it.* STAT, 13 March 2017. Accessed at: https://www.statnews.com/2017/03/13/tuberculosis-who-antibiotic-resistance/.

Cater N. (2021a). *Daniel Andrews' Contempt for Citizenry Might Explain Loss of Trust*. The Australian, 27 September 2021. Accessed at: https://www.theaustralian.com.au/commentary/andrews-contempt-for-citizenry-might-explain-loss-of-trust/news-story/ca80042d8347f7646756c2471559baf5.

Cater N. (2021). *Victoria: A Fractured Democracy*. Menzies Research Centre. 10 March 2021. Accessed at: https://www.menziesrc.org/news-feed/victoria-a-fractured-democracy.

Cazzola M., Ora J., Bianco A., Rogliani P., and Matera M.G. (2021). *Guidance on Nebulization During the Current COVID-19 Pandemic*. Respiratory Medicine 176 Article 106236.

CDC (2022). *SARS-CoV-2 Variant Classification and Definitions*. Centers for Disease Control and Prevention. Updated 26 April 2022. Accessed at: https://www.cdc.gov/coronavirus/2019-ncov/variants/variant-classifications.html.

CDC (2019). *Public Health Emergency Preparedness and Response Capabilities: National Standards for State, Local, Tribal, and Territorial Public Health*. Centers for Disease Control and Preparedness, Center for Preparedness and Response.

***CDC** (2003a). Centers for Disease Control and Prevention Update: Outbreak of Severe Acute Respiratory Syndrome—Worldwide,* MMWR Morbidity and Mortality Weekly Report 52 pp. 241–6, 248.

CDC (2003b). *Use of Quarantine to Prevent Transmission of Severe Acute Respiratory Syndrome --- Taiwan, 2003*. MMWR Weekly 52(29) pp.680-683, 25 July 2003, Centers for Disease Control.

CERC (2019). *Psychology of a Crisis. Crisis and Emergency Risk Communication*. Centers for Disease Control and Prevention.

Certo S. T., Lester R. H., Dalton C. M., and Dalton D. R. (2006). *Top Management Teams, Strategy and Financial Performance: A Meta-analytic Examination*. Journal of Management studies 43(4) pp. 813-839.

Chadborne T. (2018). *Behavioural and Social Sciences in Public Health: The First Strategy of its Kind*. UK Health Security Agency. Accessed at: https://ukhsa.blog.gov.uk/2018/10/03/behavioural-and-social-sciences-in-public-health-the-first-strategy-of-its-kind/.

Charters C. (2021). *Oliver Dowden Aims to End the Grip of "Cultural Elite' and 'Woke' Bias*. The Times, 17 May 2021. Accessed at: https://www.thetimes.co.uk/article/oliver-dowden-end-grip-cultural-elite-woke-bias-tgq3zr632.

Cheesbrough J.S., Green J., Gallimore C.I., Wright P.A. and Brown D.W.G. (2000). *Widespread Environmental Contamination with Norwalk-like Viruses (NLV) Detected in a Prolonged Hotel Outbreak of Gastroenteritis*. Epidemiology and Infection 125 pp. 93-98.

Chellaney B. (2022). *The Great Covid Cover Up*. The Strategist. Australian Strategic Policy Institute, 17 January 2022. Accessed at: https://www.aspistrategist.org.au/the-great-covid-cover-up/.

Chen J., Wang R., Wang M., Wei G-W. (2020a). *Mutations Strengthened SARS-CoV-2 Infectivity*. Journal of Molecular Biology 432 pp. 5212-5226.

Chen N, Zhou M, Dong X, Qu J., Gong F., Han Y., Qiu Y., Wang J., Liu Y., Wei Y., Xia J., Yu T., Zhang X. and Zhang L. (2020b). *Epidemiological and Clinical Characteristics of 99 Cases of 2019 Novel Coronavirus Pneumonia in Wuhan, China: A Descriptive Study*. Lancet 395(10223) pp.507–513.

Chen N-H., Wang P-C., Hsieh M-J., Huang C-C., Kao K-C., Chen Y-H., and Tsai Y-H. (2007). *Impact of Severe Acute Respiratory Syndrome Care on the General Health Status f healthcare Workers in Taiwan*. Infection Control and Hospital Epidemiology 28(1) pp. 75-79.

Cheng A., Friedman D., Russo P., and Sim M. (2021). *Review of the Management of Variants of Concern of COVID-19 in Hotel Quarantine Settings*. Department of Health Victoria. Accessed at: https://www.google.com/url?sa=t&rct=j&q=&esrc=s&source=web&cd=&cad=rja&uact=8&ved=2ahUKEwijncTKqqzxAhWSSH0KHfCQDK8QFjAAegQIChAD&url=https%3A%2F%2Fwww.vic.gov.au%2Fsites%2Fdefault%2Ffiles%2F2021-03%2FCheng-Review-Report-final.docx&usg=AOvVaw0c17yK-YrYp1RTZwRTUYq4.

Cheriyedath S. (2021). *What are the Natural Origins of SARS-CoV-2?* Life Sciences Medical News 29 January 2021.

Chevreau F.R., Wybo J.L., and Cauchois D. (2006). *Organizing Learning Processes on Risks by Using the Bowtie Representation*. Journal of Hazardous Materials. 130 (3) pp. 276–283.

Chia J. (2009). *Inquiring into Inquiries: The Review of the Royal Commissions Act [2009]*. ALRCRefJl 42; (2009) 94 Australian Law Reform Commission Reform Journal 49 pp. 49-50.

Chokshi D.A. and Stine N.W. (2013). *Reconsidering the Politics of Public Health*. JAMA 310(10) pp. 1025-1026.

CHP (2019). *Guidelines on Infection Control and Prevention in the Hotel Industry*. Centre for Health Protection, Hong Kong. Accessed at: https://www.chp.gov.hk/files/pdf/105_guideline_on_infection_controland_prevention_in_hotel_industry.pdf.

Chung F. (2020). *Coronavirus Victoria: Brett Sutton Says He Did Not Recommend Melbourne Curfew*. News.com.au, 9 September 2020. Accessed at: https://www.news.com.au/lifestyle/health/health-problems/coronavirus-victoria-brett-sutton-says-he-did-not-recommend-curfew/news-story/43e246ebaf7e5a63286084209d0f0291.

Civil Service (2012). *Civil Service Competency Framework, 2012-2017*. Civil Service Human Resources. Accessed at: https://assets.publishing.service.gov.uk/government/uploads/system/uploads/attachment_data/file/436073/cscf_fulla4potrait_2013-2017_v2d.pdf.

Clarke J. (2005). *Working with Monsters: How to Identify and Protect Yourself from the Workplace Psychopath*. Random House Australia, Sydney, Australia.

Clarke M. and Rooney K. (2021). *Source of Latest Victorian COVID Case Confirmed as QR Fail Hampers Contact Tracing*. Herald Sun, 13 May 2021. Accessed at: https://www.heraldsun.com.au/coronavirus/source-of-latest-victorian-covid-case-confirmed-as-qr-fail-hampers-contact-tracing/news-story/9aab1dcf957f3ef5e89909db772b0e8e.

Clarke M., Ryan M., Travers B., Sum E., and Irving K. (2021). Three New COVID Cases, Alarm Over 'Stranger-to- Stranger' Infections. Herald Sun 1 June 2021. Accessed at: https://www.heraldsun.com.au/coronavirus/james-merlino-hints-at-factors-that-may-determine-end-of-victorian-lockdown/news-story/7530251c173e0bf6c4e07a500651a9e1.

Clarke T. (2021a). *Victorian Liberal Frontbencher: Andrews Government Rapidly Becoming 'Great Keepers of State Secrets'*. Sky News, 2 November 2021. Accessed at: https://www.skynews.com.au/australia-news/politics/victorian-liberal-frontbencher-andrews-government-rapidly-becoming-great-keepers-of-state-secrets/news-story/22b9123fe13cc9ed1af34d5af3d2bf5e.

Clarke T. (2021b). *Adem Somyurek Points to Daniel Andrews as a Labor Party Branch Stacking Operative in Late 1990s*. Sky News, 8 November 2021. Accessed at: https://www.skynews.com.au/australia-news/politics/adem-somyurek-points-to-daniel-andrews-as-a-labor-party-branch-stacking-operative-in-late-1990s/news-story/620b5366389b009af413baac1be914c5.

Clarke T. and Zaczek Z. (2022). *Ex Labor MP Michael Danby Backs Claims Kimberley Kitching was Bullied Within ALP*. Sky News, 16 March 2022. Accessed at: https://www.skynews.com.au/australia-news/politics/ex-labor-mp-michael-danby-backs-claims-kimberley-kitching-was-bullied-within-alp/news-story/25aa443aaba651258a425bc36b32f246.

Clemens J. and Ippolito B. (2017). *Uncompensated Care and the Collapse of Hospital Payment Regulation: An Illustration of the Tinbergen Rule*. National Bureau of Economic Research, Working Paper 23758. Accessed at: https://www.nber.org/papers/w23758

Cliff A. and Smallman-Raynor M. (2013). *Oxford Textbook of Infectious Disease Control: A Geographical Analysis from Medieval Quarantine to Global Eradication*. Oxford University Press, April 2013.

Cluff C. (2019a). *Corrections Victoria's Toxic Culture Near Ballarat: Staff Speak Out*. The Courier, 24 June 2019. Accessed at: https://www.thecourier.com.au/story/6233021/the-boys-club-sexism-homophobia-and-abuse-rife-in-this-workplace/.

Cluff C. (2019). *On Notice: Department of Justice Investigated by WorkSafe Victoria*. The Courier, 26 June 2019. Accessed at: https://www.thecourier.com.au/story/6240754/on-notice-department-of-justice-investigated-by-worksafe-victoria/.

Clun R. (2020). *Preventing Victoria's Second Wave Would Have Saved Lives in Aged Care: Colbeck*. The Sydney Morning Herald, 27 October 2020.Accessed at: https://www.smh.com.au/politics/federal/preventing-victoria-s-second-wave-would-have-saved-lives-in-aged-care-colbeck-20201027-p5692m.html.

CNBC (2020). *This Hotel is Infamous as Ground Zero for a SARS 'super spreader' Event in the 2003 Outbreak- Here's What Happened*. CNBC, 16 February, 2020. Accessed at: https://www.cnbc.com/2020/02/14/hong-kong-hotel-hosted-super-spreader-in-the-2003-sars-outbreak.html.

COAG (2009). *National Action Plan for Human Influenza Pandemic, April 2009*. Working Group on Australian Influenza Pandemic Prevention and Preparedness, Council of Australian Governments. Accessed at: https://apo.org.au/sites/default/files/resource-files/2009-05/apo-nid2995.pdf.

Coate J. (2020a). *COVID 19 Hotel Quarantine Inquiry Final Report and Recommendations, Volume 1*. December 2020. Parliamentary Paper No 191 (2018-2020), Melbourne Australia.

Coate J. (2020b). *COVID 19 Hotel Quarantine Inquiry Interim Report and Recommendations.* November 2020. Parliamentary Paper No 169 (2018-2020), Melbourne, Australia.

Cockburn G. (2021). *Experts Warn of Economic Hit from Victorian Lockdown.* News.com.au, 2 June 2021. Accessed at:

https://www.news.com.au/finance/economy/australian-economy/experts-warn-of-economic-hit-from-victorian-lockdown/news-story/ca47d44734b153c0f26cc9be27fbacc2.
Coë C. (2020). *Dan Andrews' Secret Text Messages on the Disastrous Hotel Quarantine Program that Sparked Victoria's Second Wave of Deadly Coronavirus are FINALLY Made Public - Here's What He Said*. Daily Mail Australia, 30 November 2020. Accessed at: https://www.dailymail.co.uk/news/article-8992233/Dan-Andrews-secret-text-messages-disastrous-hotel-quarantine-program-FINALLY-public.html.
Colen B.D. (2015). *An Indictment of the Ebola Response*. The Harvard Gazette, 22 November, 2015. Accessed at:
https://news.harvard.edu/gazette/story/2015/11/an-indictment-of-ebola-response/.
Cohen J. (2020). *Scientists 'Strongly Condemn' Rumors and Conspiracy Theories About Origin of Coronavirus Outbreak.* Science 19 February 2020. Accessed at:
https://www.sciencemag.org/news/2020/02/scientists-strongly-condemn-rumors-and-conspiracy-theories-about-origin-coronavirus.
Cohen J. (2021). *Fights Over Confidentiality Pledge and Conflicts of Interest Tore Apart COVID-19 Origin Probe*. Science, 18 October 2021. Accessed at:
https://www.science.org/content/article/fights-over-confidentiality-pledge-and-conflicts-interest-tore-apart-covid-19-origin-probe.
Collins P. (2019). *Avoiding Ethical Failure: Understanding How we Elude Integrity is the First Step Toward Doing the Right Thing*. IBAC Insights, 27 June 2019. Independent Broad-based Anti-corruption Commission. Accessed at: https://www.ibac.vic.gov.au/publications-and-resources/ibac-insights/issue-20/avoiding-ethical-failure-understanding-how-we-elude-integrity-is-the-first-step-toward-doing-the-right-thing.
Collins T., Akslerod S., Bloomfield A., Gankredlidze A., Jakab Z., and Placella E. (2020). *Rethinking the COVID-19 Pandemic: Back to Public Health*. Annals of Global Health 86(1): 133 pp.1-7.
Commins P. (2021). *Victorian Covid-19 Lockdown: Stay-at-home Order a $1.3bn Hit to National Economy*. The Australian Business Review, 20 June 2021. Accessed at:
https://www.theaustralian.com.au/business/economics/victorian-covid19-lockdown-stayathome-order-a-13bn-hit-to-national-economy/news-story/cd18ee1683c7b513cc1191608e2487e3.
Condon B.J. and Shina T. (2008). *The Successes and Failures of Global Health Organizations: The World Health Organization, UNAIDS, Médicins sans Frontières and PEPFAR.* In: Global Lessons from the AIDS Pandemic pp. 265-299. Springer Berlin, Heidelberg.
Connolly B. (2016). *Audit Reveals Sad State of Victorian Government IT Projects*. CIO, 9 March 2016. Accessed at:
https://www.cio.com/article/208013/audit-reveals-sad-state-of-victorian-government-it-projects.html
Coorey P. (2022). *Bully Allegations Rock Labor*. Financial Review, 16 March 2022. Accessed at:
https://www.afr.com/politics/federal/bullying-allegations-rock-labor-20220316-p5a50n.
Coorey P. and Durkin P. (2020a). *PM Questions Quality of Contact Tracing in Victoria*. Australian Financial Review 16 July 2020. Accessed at:
https://www.afr.com/politics/federal/nsw-a-better-example-of-how-to-contain-an-outbreak-pm-20200716-p55chu.
Coorey P. and Durkin P. (2020b). *Victoria's Outbreak 'Could have been Avoided': Hunt*. Australian Financial Review 8 September 2020. Accessed at:
https://www.afr.com/politics/federal/victoria-s-outbreak-could-have-been-avoided-hunt-20200908-p55tec.

Coorey P. *All Side to Blame as Victoria's Lockdown Drags on*. Financial Review, 31 May 2021. Accessed at: https://www.afr.com/politics/federal/victorian-blame-game-disguises-the-fact-that-all-sides-are-to-blame-20210528-p57w4h.

Consultancy.com.au (2020). *Victoria's Hotel Quarantine Program Spent over a Million on Consultants*. Accessed at: https://www.consultancy.com.au/news/2647/victorias-hotel-quarantine-program-spent-millions-on-consultants.

Cordero G. and Blais A. (2017). *Is a Corrupt Government Totally Unacceptable?* West European Politics 20(4) pp. 645-662.

COSO (2017). *Enterprise Risk Management—Integrating with Strategy and Performance*. Committee of Sponsoring Organisations of the Treadway Commission.

Cousins S. (2020). *Experts Criticise Australia's Aged Care Failings Over COVID-19*. Lancet 396 (10259) pp. 1322-1323.

COVID SurgCollaborative (2021). *Effect of COVID-19 Pandemic Lockdowns on Planned Cancer Surgery for 15 Tumour Types in 61 Countries: An International, Prospective, Cohort Study*. The Lancet Oncology 22(11) pp. 1507-1517.

Cowan N. (2010). *The Magical Mystery Four: How is Working Memory Capacity Limited, and Why?* Current Directions in Psychological Science 19(1) pp. 51-57.

Cowe D., Harris R., and Hatch P. (2020). *Hotels to be Quarantine Wards in Mammoth Industry Response to Virus*. The Sydney Morning Herald, 22 March 2020. Accessed at: https://www.smh.com.au/politics/federal/hotels-to-be-quarantine-wards-in-mammoth-industry-response-to-virus-20200322-p54cqj.html.

Cowper A. (2020). *The Public Health of Politics and the Politics of Public Health*. The British Medical Journal Opinion 29 May 2020. Accessed at: https://blogs.bmj.com/bmj/2020/05/29/andy-cowper-the-public-health-of-politics-and-the-politics-of-public-health/.

Cozzolino A. (2012) *Humanitarian Logistics and Supply Chain Management*. In: Humanitarian Logistics pp 5–16 Springer, Champ, Switzerland.

Cramm S. *How Sudden Failures Happen Gradually*. Crisis Management, Harvard Business Review 9 April 2009.

Crampton E. (2019). *Central Banking: Hitting Two Policy Birds with One Stone Risks Missing Them Both*. Stuff: Business. Accessed at: https://www.stuff.co.nz/business/opinion-analysis/118025004/central-banking-hitting-two-policy-birds-with-one-stone-risks-missing-them-both.

Craven G. (2015). *The Trouble with All Our Royal Commissions*. The Australian, 26 August 2015. Accessed at: https://www.theaustralian.com.au/commentary/opinion/the-trouble-with-all-our-royal-commissions/news-story/ca40f3b76660b7d1baee8a9e44da32a8.

Credlin P. (2020a). *Coronavirus, Peta Credlin: Too Much We're Not Being Told About Victoria's Hotel Quarantine Fiasco*. The Australian 14 October 2020. Accessed at: https://www.theaustralian.com.au/commentary/coronavirus-too-much-were-not-being-told-about-victorias-hotel-quarantine-fiasco/news-story/a187d9dd5f56a24cc0368d01e43920b9.

Credlin P. (2020b). *Coronavirus, Peta Credlin: Hotel Quarantine Inquiry Can't Dodge Life-and-death Question.* The Australian 20 October 2020. Accessed at: https://www.theaustralian.com.au/commentary/coronavirus-quarantine-inquiry-cant-dodge-lifeanddeath-questions-this-time/news-story/14abb46538048e0cd08a75451c6b4cd2.

Credlin P. (2020c). *Coronavirus: Victoria's Hotel Quarantine Inquiry Must Reopen Hearings*. 31 October. Accessed at: https://www.theaustralian.com.au/inquirer/coronavirus-victorias-hotel-quarantine-inquiry-must-reopen-hearings/news-story/704970dcd6446f0af62bca8bd13f7840.

Credlin P. (2020d). *Andrews Government's Hotel Quarantine Story 'Gets Murkier'*. Sky News 14 October 2020. Accessed at: https://www.skynews.com.au/australia-news/andrews-governments-hotel-quarantine-story-gets-murkier/video/0fc85a06dacbd2f32cf1851b49ec734f.

Credlin P. (2021). *'Lack of Transparency' the 'Most Concerning Thing About Victoria's Hotel Quarantine System'*. Sky News 5 May 2021. Accessed at: https://www.youtube.com/watch?v=wJ8GPMy9peA.

Credlin P. (2022). *Report Reveals 'Damning Truth' About Victorian Hospital System*. Sky News, 1 February 2022. Accessed at https://www.youtube.com/watch?v=WV9k9sfnFuo.

Crichton M.T., Lauche K., and Flin R. (2008). *Learning from Experience: Incident Management Team Leader Training*. In: Naturalistic Decision Making and Macrocognition, Chapter 6 pp. 103-120, (Editors; J.M. Schragen, L.G. Militello, Ormerod T., and R. Lipshitz), CRC Press.

Crisp A. (2020). Witness Statement. COVID-19 Hotel Quarantine Inquiry. Accessed at: https://www.quarantineinquiry.vic.gov.au/sites/default/files/2020-09/Exhibit%20HQI0144b_P%20First%20witness%20statement%20of%20Commissioner%20Andrew%20Crisp.pdf.

CSMEC (2004). *Molecular Evolution of the SARS Coronavirus During the Course of the SARS Epidemic in China*. The Chinese SARS Molecular Epidemiology Consortium. Science 303 (5664) pp. 1666-1669.

Cumin S., Brooks B., and Owen C. (2020). *A Case Study of Disaster Decision-making in the Presence of Anomalies and Absence of Recognition*. Journal of Contingencies and Crisis Management 28(2) pp. 110-121.

Cunha D. (2020). *A Condensed History of Quarantine's Success and Failure*. Atlas Obscura. Accessed at: https://www.atlasobscura.com/articles/a-condensed-history-of-quarantines-success-and-failur.

Cunningham M. (2021). *Source of Melbourne's Highly Infectious Delta Outbreak Set to Remain Mystery*. The Sydney Morning Herald, 14 June 2021. Accessed at: https://www.smh.com.au/national/source-of-melbourne-s-highly-infectious-delta-outbreak-set-to-remain-mystery-20210614-p580st.html.

Cunningham M., Mills T., and Dow A. (2020). *Health Officials Shut Sutton Out of Top Pandemic Response*. The Sydney Morning Herald. 10 September 2020. Accessed at: https://www.smh.com.au/national/health-officials-shut-sutton-out-of-top-pandemic-response-20200910-p55u91.html.

Cunningham M. and Mannix L. (2021). *Man at Centre of Holiday Inn Cluster Calls for Inquiry as Experts Query Nebuliser Theory*. The Age, 17 February 2021. Accessed at: https://www.theage.com.au/national/victoria/killed-my-trust-nebuliser-patient-at-centre-of-holiday-inn-cluster-calls-for-probe-20210217-p5738k.html.

Cunningham M. and Sakkal P. (2021). *Cracks Emerged in Digital Contact Tracing System Days Before Five-day Lockdown*. The Age, 7 March 2021. Accessed at: https://www.theage.com.au/national/victoria/cracks-emerged-in-digital-contact-tracing-system-days-before-five-day-lockdown-20210306-p578dl.html.

D'Abrera B. (2020a). *Coronavirus: Identity Politics Focus Diverts Attention from the Real Issues*. The Australian, 13 August 2020. Accessed at https://www.theaustralian.com.au/commentary/coronavirus-identity-politics-focus-diverts-attention-from-real-issues/news-story/708b372a51b63897a9cb01e6c53789cd.

D'Abrera B. (2020b). *Checked Out: When Activism Quarantines Common Sense*. Institute of Public Affairs, 13 August 2020.

Dahm D. (2016). *New pathology Pain: Warning for GP Practices: There is a Price for Certainty!* Practice Management 4 February 2016. Accessed at: https://thebusinessofhealthcare.com.au/2016/02/04/new-pathology-pain-warning-for-gp-practices-there-is-a-price-for-certainty/.

Dailey S.F. and Kaplan D. (2014). *Shelter-in-place and Mental Health: An Analogue Study of Well-being and Distress*. Journal of Emergency Management 12(2) pp. 121-131.

Dainton C. and Hay A. (2021). *Quantifying the Relationship Between Lockdowns, Mobility, and Effective Reproduction Number (Rt) During the COVID-19 Pandemic in the Greater Toronto Area*. BMC Public Health 21 Article Number 1658.

Daly N. and Clure E. (2022). *Labor MP Kaushaliya Vaghela Alleges Victorian Premier's Office Turned a Blind Eye to Systemic Bullying*. ABC News, 24 February 2022. Accessed at: https://www.abc.net.au/news/2022-02-24/labor-mp-kaushaliya-vaghela-says-premier-office-ignored-bullying/100854794.

Daly P. and Walsh J.S. (2010). *Drucker's Theory of the Business and Organisations: Challenging Business Assumptions*. Management Decision 48(4) pp. 500-511.

Daszak P. (2020). *Ignore the Conspiracy Theories: Scientists Know Covid-19 Wasn't Created in a Lab*. The Guardian, 9 June 2020. Accessed at: https://www.theguardian.com/commentisfree/2020/jun/09/conspiracies-covid-19-lab-false-pandemic.

Davey M. (2021). *Victorian Quarantine Manager Stood Down Over Allegations of Covid Infection Control Breach*. The Guardian, 5 May 2021. Accessed at: https://www.theguardian.com/australia-news/2021/may/05/victorian-quarantine-manager-stood-down-over-allegations-of-covid-infection-control-breach.

Davey M. and Rachwani M. (2021). *Decision on Lockdown Extension Looms Amid Warning Positive Case Travelled to NSW*. The Guardian, 2 June 2021.

Day T. (2004). *Predicting Quarantine Failure Rates*. Journal of Emerging Infectious Diseases 10(3) pp. 487-8.

Dayaratna K. and Vanderplas A. (2020). *Are Lockdowns Necessary? What Data form 10 Countries Show*. The Heritage Foundation 29 July 2020. Accessed at: https://www.heritage.org/public-health/commentary/are-lockdowns-necessary-what-data-10-countries-show.

Dean L. (2021). *'You May Not Know': Warning About $5,060 QR Code Fine*. Yahoo Finance, 17 May 2021. Accessed at: https://au.finance.yahoo.com/news/warning-about-5060-qr-code-fine-021903463.html.

Debnam G. (1975). *Nondecisions and Power: The Two Faces of Bachrach and Baratz*. The American Political Science Review 69(3) pp. 889-899.

DeFazio P.A. (2019). *Final Committee Report: Boeing 737 Max*. The House Committee on Transportation and Infrastructure. Washington, DC. Accessed at: https://transportation.house.gov/imo/media/doc/2020.09.15%20FINAL%20737%20MAX%20Report%20for%20Public%20Release.pdf.

Dekker S.W.A. (2009). *Just Culture: Who Gets to Draw the Line?* Cognition, Technology and Work 11 (3) pp. 177–185.

Dekker S.W.A. (2014). *Deferring to Expertise versus the Prima Donna Syndrome: A Manager's Dilemma*. Cognition, Technology and Work 16 pp. 541-548.

Dekker S.W.A. (2015a). *The Danger of Losing Situational Awareness*. Cognition, Technology and Work 17 pp. 159-161.
Dekker S. (2015b). *Safety Differently: Human Factors for a New Era*. CRC Press, London, New York.
Devine M. (2023). *New Emails Show Dr. Anthony Fauci Commissioned Scientific Paper in Feb. 2020 to Disprove Wuhan lab Leak Theory*. Accessed at: https://nypost.com/2023/03/05/new-emails-show-fauci-commissioned-paper-to-disprove-wuhan-lab-leak-theory/.
Dexter R. and Fowler M. (2021). *Infection Control Manager Stood Down Amid Damning Hotel Quarantine Reports*. The Age 5 May 2021. Accessed at: https://www.theage.com.au/national/victoria/infection-control-manager-stood-down-amid-damning-hotel-quarantine-reports-20210505-p57oyk.html
DHA (2011). *Review of Australia's Health Sector Response to Pandemic (H1N1) 2009*. Department of Health and Ageing, Report, September 2011. Accessed at: https://www1.health.gov.au/internet/publications/publishing.nsf/Content/review-2011-l/$File/lessons%20identified-oct11.pdf.
DHHS (2020). *COVID-19 Pandemic Plan for the Victorian Health Sector*. Department of Health and Human Services, Victoria, 10 March 2020. Accessed at: https://www2.health.vic.gov.au/about/publications/researchandreports/covid-19-pandemic-plan-for-vic.
Diamante D. (2020). *It Was Only a Matter of Time... How Government Can Avoid the Next Hotel Quarantine Bungle*. Mia Consulting, 12 August 2020. Accessed at: https://miaconsulting.com.au/blog/government-procurement-capabilities-quarantine-bungle/
Diederich A. and Trueblood J.S. (2018). *A Dynamic Dual Process Model of Risky Decision Making*. Psychological Review 125(2) pp. 270-292.
Dietrich C. (2010). *Decision Making: Factors that Influence Decision Making, Heuristics Used, and Decision Outcomes*. Inquiries Journal 2(2) pp. 1-3.
Dilanian K. (2021). *U.S. Intel Report Identified 3 Wuhan Lab Researchers Who Fell Ill in November 2019*. NBC News 25 May 2021.
Dirani K.M., Abadi M., Alizadeh A., Barhate B., Garza R.C., Gunasekara N., Ibrahim G. and Majzun Z. (2020). *Leadership Competencies and the Essential Role of Human Resource Development in Times of Crisis: A Response to Covid-19 Pandemic*. Human Resource Development International 23(4) pp. 380-94.
Dixit J. (2019). *How JFK Inspired the Term 'Groupthink'*. You Brain at Work, NeuroLeadership Institute. Accessed at: https://neuroleadership.com/your-brain-at-work/jfk-inspired-term-groupthink/.
Dobbs J.M. and Do J.J. (2018). *The Impact of Perceived Toxic Leadership on Cynicism in Officer Candidates*. Armed Forces and Society 45(1) pp. 3-26.
DOE (2022). *Evidence Summary: Coronavirus (COVID-19) and the Use of Face Coverings in Education Settings*. Department of Education, UK Government, January 2022. Accessed at: https://assets.publishing.service.gov.uk/government/uploads/system/uploads/attachment_data/file/1055639/Evidence_summary_-_face_coverings.pdf.
DoH (2014). Victorian Health Management Plan for Pandemic Influenza. Department of Health, Victoria, October 2014.
DoH (2019). *Australian Health Management Plan for Pandemic Influenza, August 2019*. Department of Health, Accessed at: https://www1.health.gov.au/internet/main/publishing.nsf/Content/519F9392797E2DDCCA257D47001B9948/$Fi le/w-AHMPPI-2019.PDF.

DoH (2020). *Health Emergency Preparedness and Response.* Department of Health, Australian Government, Canberra. Accessed at: https://www1.health.gov.au/internet/main/publishing.nsf/Content/health-pubhlth-strateg-bio-index.htm.

DOHA (2007). *National Pandemic Influenza Exercise. Exercise Cumpston 06 Report.* Office of Health Protection, Department of Health and Ageing, Australian Government. Accessed at: https://apo.org.au/sites/default/files/resource-files/2007-06/apo-nid972.pdf.

Doherty B. (2020). *Coronavirus: Three Cases in NSW and One in Victoria as Infection Reaches Australia.* The Guardian 25 January 2020. Accessed at: https://www.theguardian.com/science/2020/jan/25/coronavirus-five-people-in-nsw-being-tested-for-deadly-disease.

Doloi H., Crawford R.H., Langston C., and Pheng L.S. (2015). *A Social Network Based Framework for Assessing Risks and Vulnerability in Built Environment.* 5th Internal Conference on Building Resilience Conference Paper. Newcastle, July 2015.

Donahue D.A., Cunnion O., and Sochats K. (2012). *The All Needs Approach to Emergency Management.* Homeland Security Affairs 8 Article 1.

Donaldson D. (2015). *Victoria's WorkSafe Management Sacked Over Contamination.* The Mandarin, 3 March 2015. Accessed at: https://www.themandarin.com.au/24689-worksafe-management-sacked-contamination/.

Donaldson D. (2016). *A 'Bad Track Record in ICT Projects': Learn from Victoria's Mistakes.* The Mandarin. 15 March 2016. Accessed at: https://www.themandarin.com.au/61749-auditor-blasts-ict-project-budget-blowouts/.

Dorani S. (2018). *The Groupthink Model the Impact of Groupthink on Decision Making Case Study: The Afghanistan and Iraq Wars.* Political Reflection Magazine 20. Accessed at: https://cesran.org/the-groupthink-model-the-impact-of-groupthink-on-decision-making-case-study-the-afghanistan-and-iraq-wars.html.

Douglas P.K., Douglass D.B., Harrigan D.C., and Douglas K.M. (2009). *Preparing for Pandemic Influenza and its Aftermath: Mental Health Issues Considered.* International Journal of Emergency Mental Health 11(3) pp. 137-144.

Dow A. (2022a). *More Deaths Linked to Triple-zero Crisis as Long Delays Continue.* The Age, 3 May 2022. Accessed at: https://www.theage.com.au/national/victoria/more-deaths-linked-to-triple-zero-crisis-as-long-delays-continue-20220502-p5aho1.html.

Dow A. (2022). *Surf Lifesavers and Students Fill Paramedic Shifts, as Omicron Spreads.* The Sydney Morning Herald, 9 January 2021. Accessed at: https://www.smh.com.au/national/surf-lifesavers-and-students-fill-paramedic-shifts-as-omicron-spreads-20220108-p59mrq.html.

Dow A., Cunningham M., and Fowler M. (2021). *Victoria 'can't be trusted' with Hotel Quarantine, Disease Expert Says.* The Age, 16 February 2021. Accessed at: https://www.theage.com.au/national/victoria/victoria-can-t-be-trusted-with-hotel-quarantine-disease-expert-says-20210216-p572yx.html.

Dow A. and Eddie R. (2022). *More Than 1000 Victorians Could Have Been Harmed by Triple-zero Delays.* The Age, 16 August 2022. Accessed at: https://www.theage.com.au/national/victoria/more-than-1000-victorians-could-have-been-harmed-by-triple-zero-delays-20220808-p5b80p.html.

Dow A., McKenzie N., and Tozer J. (2022). *Twelve Victorians Die, Including Four Children, After Waiting for Triple-Zero to Pick Up.* The Age, 6 March 2022. Accessed at: https://www.theage.com.au/national/victoria/twelve-victorians-die-including-four-children-after-waiting-for-triple-zero-to-pick-up-20220303-p5a1dn.html.

Dowell E. and Jackson M. (2020). *"Woke-Washing" Your Company Won't Cut it"*. Harvard Business Review 27 July 2020.
DPC (2019). *Behavioural Insights*. Department of Premier and Cabinet. Accessed at: https://www.vic.gov.au/behavioural-insights.
Drews K. (2013). *A Brief History of Quarantine*. The Virginia Tech Undergraduate Historical Review 2.
Drummond D. (2020). *Daniel Andrews' VicPol: Unfit for Purpose*. Quadrant Online, 21 October 2020. Accessed at:
https://quadrant.org.au/opinion/sicktoria/2020/10/victoria-police-unfit-for-purpose/.fight the fines
DTMR (2011). *Submissions for the State of Queensland*. 11 March 2011. Department of Transport and Main Roads (DTMR) and Translink Transit Authority. Brisbane, Queensland, Australia.
Drummond J., Shephard D., and Trnka D. (2021). *Behavioural Insight and Regulatory Governance*: Opportunities and Challenges". OECD Regulatory Policy Working Papers, No. 16, OECD Publishing, Paris.
Drupsteen L. and Guldenmund F.W. (2014). *What is Learning? A Review of the Safety Literature on Learning*
from Accidents. Journal of Contingencies and Crisis Management 22(2) pp. 81-96.
DuBrin A. J. (2013). *Handbook of Research on Crisis Leadership in Organizations*, Edward Elgar Publishing, Cheltenham, UK.
Duckett S., Cuddihy M., and Newnham H. (2016). *Targeting Zero: Supporting the Victorian Hospital System to Eliminate Avoidable Harm and Strengthen Quality of Care. Report of the Review of Hospital Safety and Quality Assurance in Victoria*. Victorian Government, Melbourne Australia. Accessed at:
https://www.dhhs.vic.gov.au/sites/default/files/documents/201610/Hospital%20Safety%20and%20Quality%20Assurance%20in%20Victoria.pdf.
Duckett S. (2020). *What NSW Could Learn from Victoria About Fighting COVID-19*. Grattan Institute, 9 September 2020. Accessed at:
https://grattan.edu.au/news/what-nsw-could-learn-from-victoria-about-fighting-covid-19/.
Dueñas V. (2017). *Bay of Pigs: A Case Study in Strategic Leadership and Failed Assumptions*. The Bridge, 2 May 2017. Accessed at:
https://thestrategybridge.org/the-bridge/2017/5/2/bay-of-pigs-a-case-study-in-strategic-leadership-and-failed-assumptions.
Duijm N.J. (2015). *Recommendations on the Use and Design of Risk Matrices*. Safety Science 76 pp. 21–31.
Dunleavy J. (2021). Daszak and Scientists Stand by Lancet Letter Condemning Wuhan Lab Conspiracy Theories. Washington Examiner, 7 July 2021. Accessed at:
https://news.yahoo.com/daszak-scientists-stand-lancet-letter-192900005.html.
Dunning D., Johnson K., Ehrlinger J., and Kruger J. (2003). *Why People Fail to Recognize Their Own Incompetence*. Current Directions in Psychological Science 12(3) pp. 83-87.
Dunning D., Griffin D.W., Milojkovic J.D., and Ross L. (1990). *The Overconfidence Effect in Social Prediction*. Journal of Personality and Social Psychology 58(4) pp. 568-81.
Dunstan J. (2021). *How Victoria's Year from Hell Battling Coronavirus has Changed the State*. ABC News, 24 January 2021. Accessed at:
https://www.abc.net.au/news/2021-01-24/what-victoria-learnt-from-a-year-living-with-coronavirus/13079916.

Durkin P. (2021). *Andrews Braces for IBAC Double Trouble*. Australian Financial Review, 11 October 2021. Accessed at: https://www.afr.com/politics/andrews-braces-for-ibac-double-trouble-20211008-p58yib.

Durkin P. (2022). *Daniels Confirms He has 90 Staff, but that's Just the Start*. Australian Financial Review 11 April, 2022. Accessed at: https://www.afr.com/politics/daniel-andrews-confirms-he-has-90-staff-but-that-s-just-the-start-20220811-p5b920.

Durkin P. (2023). *PwC Scandal Casts Secrecy Over Commonwealth Games Inquiry*. Australian Financial Review 28 August 2023. Accessed at: https://www.afr.com/politics/federal/pwc-scandal-casts-shadow-over-commonwealth-games-inquiry-20230828-p5e006.

Durkin P., Wootton H, and Burton T. (2020). *Daniel Andrews Texts Reveal Hotel Quarantine Plans*. Financial Review 27 November 2020. Accessed at: https://www.afr.com/policy/economy/daniel-andrews-texts-reveal-hotel-quarantine-plans-20201127-p56ihn.

Durso F. T., and Gronlund, S. D. (1999). *Situation Awareness*. In: Handbook of Applied Cognition pp. 284-314, (Editors: F.T. Durso, R. Nickerson, R. Schvaneveldt, S. Dumais, S. Lindsay, M. Chi). Wiley, New York, NY.

Duso A. (2017). *Ideological Cognitive Dissonance*. In: Personality and Challenges of Democratic Government., pp 9-65. Palgrave Macmillan, New York, NY.

Dutton K. (2012). *The Wisdom of Psychopaths: What Saints, Spies, and Serial Killers Can Teach Us About Success.* FSG/ Scientific American.

Dyrenfurth N. (2021). *Private Gain, Public Pain: Taking Stock of Privatisation, Outsourcing and Contracting Public Sector Work.* John Curtin Research Centre Policy Report No.7, November 2021. Accessed at: https://static1.squarespace.com/static/587e1296579fb39e3199b6e9/t/618b0a1138dd2e57d9c393f7/1636502044937/Public+Pain%2C+Private+Gain.pdf.

Dyson T. (2020). *A Revolution in Military Learning? Cross-functional Teams and Knowledge Transformation by Lessons-learned Processes.* European Security 29(4) pp. 483-505.

Eagle C. (2020). *Exhibit HQ1010150b_RP Witness Statement of Mr Christopher Eagle*. COVID-19 Hotel Quarantine Inquiry. Accessed at: https://www.quarantineinquiry.vic.gov.au/exhibits.

Easton S. (2017). *How High Pressure Health and Human Services Workplaces Turn Toxic*. The Mandarin 21 July 2017. Accessed at: https://www.themandarin.com.au/81646-managers-must-keep-on-top-of-culture-or-high-pressure-health-workplaces-can-go-toxic/.

Eburn M. and Dovers S. (2015). *Learning Lessons from Disasters: Alternatives to Royal Commissions and Other Quasi-Judicial Inquiries*. Australian Journal of Public Administration 74(4) pp. 495-508.

ECDC (2019). *The Use of Evidence in Decision-making During Public Health Emergencies.* Technical Report. On an Expert Workshop, 5-6 December 2018. European Centre for Disease Prevention and Control, Stockholm, Sweden.

ECDC (2017). *Public Health Emergency Preparedness: Core Competencies for EU Member States*. European Centre for Disease Prevention and Control, Stockholm. Accessed at: https://www.ecdc.europa.eu/sites/default/files/documents/public-health-emergency-preparedness-core-competencies-eu-member-states.pdf.

Eckfeldt B. (2017). *Not All Bad Outcomes Are the Result of Bad Decisions, Here's Why*. Inc. Strategy. Accessed at: https://www.inc.com/bruce-eckfeldt/the-simple-4-box-model-that-skilled-entrepreneurs-use-to-analyze-important-decisions.html.

Eddie R. (2022). *Victorian Labor MP Treated as a 'nuisance' After Bullying Complaint*. The Age, 12 February 2022. Accessed at:

https://www.theage.com.au/politics/victoria/labor-mp-treated-as-a-nuisance-after-complaint-20220212-p59vwu.html.

Eddie R. (2023). *'Tremendous Progress' on Games One Day, Lawyers Called in the Next*. The Age, 4 October 2023. Accessed at: https://www.theage.com.au/politics/victoria/tremendous-progress-on-games-one-day-lawyers-called-in-the-next-20231004-p5e9lp.html

Eddie R., Hall B., Lucas C., and Percel N. (2020). *'You Couldn't Eat it': Food for Tower Residents Left in Corridors as Deliveries Delayed*. The Age, 6 July 2020. Accessed at: https://www.theage.com.au/national/victoria/you-couldn-t-eat-it-food-for-tower-residents-left-in-corridors-as-deliveries-delayed-20200706-p559h6.html.

Eddy B. (2019). *4 Reasons Why We Elect Narcissists and Sociopaths*. Psychology Today 6 May 2019. Accessed at:

Editorial (2020). *Outbreak Exposes Failures in Leadership and Systems*. The Australian 1 August 2020. Accessed at: https://www.theaustralian.com.au/commentary/editorials/outbreak-exposes-failures-in-leadership-and-systems/news-story/11e5f3dbe9e64db2f34c3def38f00b24.

Editorial (2021a). *A Litany of Haphazard, Sloppy Practices. The Australian 5 May 2021*. Accessed at: https://www.theaustralian.com.au/commentary/editorials/victorias-treacherous-hotel-quarantine-failure-exposed/news-story/d3a97eb7696eaed88567891574338daf.

Editorial (2021b). *Big Brother Still Calling the Shots*. The Australian, 6 July 2021. Accessed at: https://www.theaustralian.com.au/commentary/editorials/big-brother-still-calling-the-shots/news-story/a7661a2ee597c103d014fe0336606a82.

Editorial Board (2020). *Opinion: A New Report Adds to the Evidence of a Coronavirus Coverup in China*. The Washington Post, 6 December 2020. Accessed at: https://www.washingtonpost.com/opinions/global-opinions/a-new-report-adds-to-the-evidence-of-a-coronavirus-coverup-in-china/2020/12/06/81d880f2-366e-11eb-8d38-6aea1adb3839_story.html.

Editorial Board (2021). *Anthony Fauci, Rand Paul and Wuhan*. WSJ Opinion, 25 July 2021. Access at: https://www.wsj.com/articles/anthony-fauci-rand-paul-wuhan-lab-leak-11627240720.

Editorial Team (2021). *Brett Sutton Signed Off on "Frankly Dangerous" Decision to Replace St Basil's Staff, Say Doctors at Inquest*. Hellocare, 18 November. Accessed at: https://hellocare.com.au/brett-sutton-signed-off-on-frankly-dangerous-decision-to-replace-st-basils-staff-say-doctors-at-inquest/.

Edwards J. (2015a). *Former Victorian Auditor-General Sexually Harassed Colleague, Parliamentary Committee Finds*. ABC News, 10 November 2015. Accessed at: https://www.abc.net.au/news/2015-11-10/former-vic-auditor-general-john-doyle-harassment-report/6927568.

Edwards J. (2015). *WorkSafe Victoria Defends Decision Not to Prosecute CFA over Fiskville Handling*. ABC News 20 November 2015. Accessed at: https://www.abc.net.au/news/2015-11-20/worksafe-defends-no-prosecution-cfa-fiskville-handling/6960460.

Ehrlinger J., Johnson K., Banner M., Dunning D., and Kruger J. (2008). *Why the Unskilled are Unaware: Further Explorations of (Absent) Self-insight Among the Incompetent*. Organizational Behaviour and Human Decision Processes 105(1) pp. 98-121.

Elbanna S. (2017). Decision Making. In the SAGE Encyclopedia of Political Behaviour, (Editor F.M. Moghaddam). Sage Publishing, Thousand Oaks, CA.

Elder J. (2017). *Are Politicians Natural-born Psychopaths? Well, You Could Say That*. The New Daily, 17 June 2017. Accessed at: https://thenewdaily.com.au/life/wellbeing/2017/06/17/are-politicians-psychopaths/.

Ellis C.D. (2021). *Dangers of Toxic Work Culture and How to Fix it*. CEO Magazine, 29 September 2021. Accessed at: https://www.theceomagazine.com/opinion/toxic-work-culture/.

Elllis R. (2022). *Did Pandemic Lockdowns Do Little to Prevent COVID Deaths*. WebMD, 7 February 2022. Accessed at: https://www.webmd.com/lung/news/20220204/lockdowns-covid-deaths-study.

Elwyn G., Laitner S., Coulter A., Walker E., Watson P., and Thomson R. (2010). *Implementing Shared Decision Making in the NHS*. British Medical Journal 341 pp. 971-975.

Emblemsvåg J. and Kjølstad L.E. (2006*). Qualitative Risk Analysis: Some Problems and Remedies*. Management Decision 44(3) pp. 395-408.

Emmanuel Z and Moore S. (2020). *Economics, not Politics, Helps Explain Why Coronavirus and Other Diseases Started in China*. The Washington Post 1 May 2020. Accessed at: https://www.washingtonpost.com/politics/2020/05/01/economics-not-politics-helps-explain-why-coronavirus-other-diseases-started-china/.

EMV (2020). *State Emergency Plan (SEMP)*. Emergency Management Victoria: Accessed at: https://www.emv.vic.gov.au/responsibilities/semp/roles-and-responsibilities/response.

EMV (2017). *State Health Emergency Response Plan, Edition 4*. Emergency Management Victoria, Melbourne.

Endsley M. R. (1995). *Toward a Theory of Situation Awareness in Dynamic Systems*. Human Factors 37(1) pp. 32-64.

Endsley M. R. (2015). *Situation Awareness Misconceptions and Misunderstandings*. Journal of Cognitive Engineering and Decision Making 9(1) pp. 4-32.

Endsley M. R. (2000). *Theoretical Underpinnings of Situation Awareness: A Critical Review*. In: Situation Awareness Analysis and Measurement pp. 3-3. (Editors: M.R. Endsley, D.J. and Garland, D. J.), LEA, Mahwah, NJ.

Erikson R. S., and Tedin K.L. (2003). *American Public Opinion* (6th edition). Longman Press New York, NY.

Erikson T. (2018). *Surrounded by Psychopaths*. Penguin Books London UK.

Errett N.A., Sauer L.M., and Rutkow L. (2020) *An Integrative Review of the Limited Evidence on International Travel Bans as an Emerging Infectious Disease Disaster Control Measure*. Journal of Emergency Management 1 pp. 7–14.

Evans J.S. (2008*). Dual-processing Accounts of Reasoning, Judgment, and Social Cognition*. Annual Review of Psychology 59 pp. 255-278.

Evans J.S.B. and Stanovich K.E. (2013). *Dual-process Theories of Higher Cognition Advancing the Debate*. Perspectives on Psychological Science 8 (3), pp. 223- 241.

Fahlbruch B. and Schöbel M. (2011). *SOL – Safety Through Organizational Learning: A Method for Event Analysis*. Safety Science 49(1) pp. 27–31.

Fairbanks J. Plowman K.D., and Rawlins B.L. (2007). *Transparency in Government Communication*. Journal of Public Affairs 7 pp. 23-37.

Fair Work (2021). *COVID-19 Hotel Quarantine Security Report*. Fair Work Ombudsman. Accessed at: https://www.fairwork.gov.au/sites/default/files/2021-10/covid-19-hotel-quarantine-security-report.pdf/

Faruqi O. (2020). *Exclusive: Brett Sutton's Leaked Call*. 7am Podcast. Accessed at: https://7ampodcast.com.au/episodes/exclusive-brett-suttons-leaked-call.

Fast N.J. *How to Stop the Blame Game*. Harvard Business Review 13 May 2020. Accessed at:

https://hbr.org/2010/05/how-to-stop-the-blame-game.

FAU (2019). *Open Letter: FAU's Physics Department Stands Behind Gerd Schröder-Turk.* Friedrich-Alexander Universat. Accessed at: https://www.physics.nat.fau.eu/files/2019/10/2019_10_20_schroeder_turk.pdf.

Fedderson T. (2020). *What Strong Crisis Leadership Looks Like During the Pandemic.* Editorial based on insights from T. Fedderson. Kellog Insight. Kellog School of Management at Northwestern University, Evanston, Il.

Feldwisch-Drentrup H. (2020). How WHO Became China's Coronavirus Accomplice. Foreign Policy, 2 April 2020. Accessed at: https://foreignpolicy.com/2020/04/02/china-coronavirus-who-health-soft-power/.

Fennimore A., and Sementelli A. (2016). *Public Entrepreneurship and Sub-clinical Psychopaths: A Conceptual Framework and Implications.* International Journal of Public Sector Management 29(6) pp. 612-634.

Ferguson J. (2016). *Labor Link to Key Victoria Police Appointment.* The Australian, 30 May 2016. Accessed at: https://www.theaustralian.com.au/nation/politics/labor-link-to-key-victoria-police-appointment/news-story/89c8d9b22a73a70b1ca7f4914489e31d.

Ferguson J. (2020). *Coronavirus: Hypocrisy Unfettered in March of Stupidity.* The Australian, 22 October 2021. Accessed at: https://www.theaustralian.com.au/commentary/coronavirus-black-lives-matter-protest/news-story/32a8b87460e32647047b4cc570f2d39f.

Ferguson J. (2021). *Who Andrews Spoke to on Hotel D-Day.* The Australian, 11 September 2021. Accessed at: https://www.theaustralian.com.au/nation/politics/who-andrews-spoke-to-on-quarantine-dday/news-story/c2945ae577857886f7723f0db7eb5156.

Ferguson S. and Freri M. (2023). *Commonwealth Games Vice-president Challenges Daniel Andrews's Version of Games Decision.* ABC News, 19 July, 2023. Accessed at: https://www.abc.net.au/news/2023-07-19/commonwealth-games-vp-challenges-victorian-decision-730/102622720.

Fernstrom A. and Goldblatt M. (2013). *Aerobiology and Its Role in the Transmission of Infectious Diseases.* Journal of Pathogens 2013 Article number 493960.

Ferri B. (2020). *'Where's the Consistency?' Dan Andrews is Slammed for Cracking Down on Anti-lockdown Protesters after Allowing Black Lives Matter Rallies to go Ahead Despite Risk They Posed to Spread of COVID-19.* Daily Mail (Australia). 5 September 2020. Accessed at: https://www.dailymail.co.uk/news/article-8700551/Dan-Andrews-slammed-cracking-anti-lockdown-allowing-Black-Lives-Matter-rallies.html.

Feuerherd P. (2019). *How the Bay of Pigs Invasion Changed JFK.* JSTOR Daily: Politics and History, 11 April 2019. Accessed at: https://daily.jstor.org/how-the-bay-of-pigs-invasion-changed-jfk/.

Field E. (2019). *Latrobe Regional Hospital Facing Health Department Investigation into Claims of Bullying, Intimidation.* ABC News 30 April 2019. Accessed at: https://www.abc.net.au/news/2019-04-30/workplace-culture-review-at-latrobe-regional-hospital/11052676.

Figueredo A.J., Gladden P.R., Sisco M.M., Patch E.A., and Jones D.N. (2015). *The Unholy Trinity: The Dark Triad, Sexual Coercion, and Brunswik-Symmetry.* Evolutionary Psychology 13(2) [pp.435-454.

Fink J. (2021). *Timeline of What Dr. Fauci Has Said About the Wuhan Lab and COVID's Origins.* Newsweek, 25 May 2021.Accessed at:

https://www.newsweek.com/timeline-what-dr-fauci-has-said-about-wuhan-lab-covids-origins-1594698.

Finn J. and McKenna J. (2010). *Coping with Academy-to-First-Team Transitions in Elite English Male Team Sports: The Coaches' Perspective*. International Journal of Sports Science & Coaching 5(2) pp. 257-279.

Finnane M. (2000). *The Road to Mundingburra: Police Unions and Politics in Australia*. School of Humanities, Griffith University. Brisbane, Australia. Accessed at: https://research-repository.griffith.edu.au/bitstream/handle/10072/368694/finnane00.pdf?sequence=1.

Fitzsimmons C. (2021). *COVID-19 is Spreading Faster in Victoria than NSW*. Sydney Morning Herald, 12 September 2021. Accessed at: https://www.smh.com.au/national/why-covid-19-is-spreading-faster-in-victoria-than-nsw-20210909-p58qce.html.

Flower W. (2021a). *Low for Victorian Police After Dousing an Elderly Woman as She Lay Injured on the Road During Melbourne's Wild Anti-lockdown Protest*. Daily Mail Australia, 20 September 2021. Accessed at: https://www.dailymail.co.uk/news/article-10007539/Victoria-Police-fire-amid-claims-blatant-brutality-targeting-news-photographers.html.

Flower W. (2021b). *A 'Dog's Breakfast' QR System, Shutting the WRONG Woolies... and then Blaming YOU: The Full, Shocking Story of How a Single Covid Infection has Condemned Victoria to a Fourth Lengthy Lockdown.* Daily Mai Australia, 2 June 2021. Accessed at: https://www.dailymail.co.uk/news/article-9642633/How-Victorias-QR-code-abomination-DOOMED-state-fourth-lockdown.html.

Flower W. (2021c). *Fact From Dan's Fiction: Premier Andrews Says he was Forced to Impose the Latest Soul-Destroying Statewide Lockdown - but Political Spin Can't Hide the Fact Another Quarantine Fail Happened on HIS Watch*. Daily Mail Australia. 15 February 2021. Accessed at: https://www.dailymail.co.uk/news/article-9260295/Daniel-Andrews-continues-feed-trapped-Victorians-political-spin.html.

Flower W. (2021d). *He Appeared on Victorian TV Screens for 120 days Straight, and Then Just Disappeared. Surprising New Theory Reveals Why Daniel Andrews Has Been Out of Action for So Long - and Why it May Have Backfired*. Daily Mail Australia, 9 June 2021. Accessed at: https://www.dailymail.co.uk/news/article-9662441/Victorians-demanding-know-happened-injured-leader.html.

Fontanesi L., Marchetti D., Mazza C., Di Giandomenico S., Roma P., and Verrochio M.C. (2020). *The Effect of the COVID-19 Lockdown on Parents: A Call to Adopt Urgent Measures*. Psychological Trauma: Theory, Research, Practice, and Policy 12(S1) pp. S79-S81.

Ford R.C. and Richardson W.D. (2013). *Ethical Decision Making: A Review of the Empirical Literature*. In: Chapter 2, Citation Classics from the Journal 19 of Business Ethics, Advances in Business Ethics Research 2, pp. 19-41 (Editors: A.C. Michalos and D.C. Poff).

Forni D., Cagliani R., Clerici M., and Sironi M. (2017). *Molecular Evolution of Human Coronavirus Genomes*. Trends in Microbiology 25(1) pp. 35-48.

Forster B.B., Patlas M.N., and Lexa F.J. (2020). *Crisis Leadership During and Following COVID-19*. Canadian Association of Radiologists' Journal 71(4) pp. 421-422.

Forsyth W.M., Grix D.C., and Gibson C.A. (1993). *Diagnosis of Highly Pathogenic Avian Influenza in Chickens: Bendigo 1992*. Australian Veterinary Journal 70(3) pp. 118-119.

Foster G. (2020a). *Early Estimates of the Impact of COVID-19 Disruptions on Jobs, Wages, and Lifetime Earnings of Schoolchildren in Australia*. Australian Journal of Labour Economics 23(2) pp. 129-151.

Foster G. (2020b). *Inquiry into the Victorian Government's Response to the COVID-19 Pandemic.* Transcript page 1. Public Accounts and Estimate Committee, 12 August 2020). Accessed at:
https://www.parliament.vic.gov.au/images/stories/committees/paec/COVID-19_Inquiry/Transcripts_Round_2/Foster_12_August_verified_transcript.pdf.

Foster G (2021). *What are the Hidden Costs of COVID-19 Lockdowns?* Business Think, 10 June 2021. UNSW Business School. Accessed at:
https://www.businessthink.unsw.edu.au/articles/covid-19-lockdowns-cost.

Fowler M. (2020). *Bureaucrat Denied Andrews' Request for Infected Travellers to Quarantine Away From CBD.* The Age, 19 September 2020. Accessed at:
https://www.theage.com.au/national/victoria/bureaucrat-denied-andrews-request-for-infected-travellers-to-quarantine-away-from-cbd-20200919-p55x8j.html.

Fowler M. (2021). *Hotel Quarantine Costs $1.6m a Day but no Money for it in State Budget.* The Age 21 May 2021. Accessed at:
https://www.theage.com.au/politics/victoria/hotel-quarantine-costs-1-6m-a-day-but-no-money-for-it-in-state-budget-20210521-p57tzg.html.

Fowler M., Ilanbey S., and Sakkal P. (2021). *Hotel Quarantine Manager Fired After 51 Incident Reports in FIrst Four Weeks.* The Sydney Morning Herald, 6 May 2021. Accessed at:
https://www.smh.com.au/national/victoria/hotel-quarantine-manager-fired-after-51-incident-reports-in-first-four-weeks-20210505-p57p6g.html.

Fraher A.I. and Grint K. (2016). *Agonistic Governance: The Antinomies of Decision-making in US Navy SEALs.* 14(4) 395-414.

Franken E. and Plimmer G. (2019). *Mediocre and Harmful Public Sector Leadership.* International Journal of Public Leadership 15(4) pp. 274-286.

Fraser D.W, Tsai T.R., Orenstein W., Parkin W.E., Beecham H.J., Sharrar R.G., Harris J., Mallison G.F., Martin S.M., McDade J.E., Shepard C.C., Brachman P.S., and the Field Investigation Team (1977). Legionnaires' Disease: Description of an Epidemic. Journal of Medicine 297(22) pp. 1189-1198.

Fraser M.R. and Blumenstock J. (2021). Lessons Relearned? H1N1, COVID-19, and Vaccination Planning. Journal of Public Health Management and Planning 27(1) pp. S106-S110.

Frey D. (1981). *Reversible and Irreversible Decisions: Preference for Consonant Information as a Function of Attractiveness of Decision Alternatives.* Personality and Social Psychology Bulletin 7(4) pp. 621-626.

Frieden T., Koplan J., and Satcher D., and Besser R. (2020). *We Ran the CDC. No President Ever Politicized its Science the Way Trump Has.* The Washington Post. July 14, 2020.
https://www.washingtonpost.com/outlook/2020/07/14/cdc-directors-trump-politics.

Fritz M., Gries T., and Redlin M. (2023). *The Effectiveness of Vaccination, Testing, and Lockdown Strategies Against COVID-19.* International Journal of Health Economics and Management 23 pp. 585–607

Funabashi Y. and Kitazawa K. (2012). *Fuskushima in Review: A Complex Disaster, a Disastrous Response.* Bulletin of the Atomic Scientists 68(2). Accessed on 3 April 2017 at:
http://thebulletin.org/2012/march/fukushima-review-complex-disaster-disastrous-response.

Fung C., Tsui B., and Hon A.H.Y. (2020). *Crisis Management: A Case Study of Disease Outbreak in the Metropark Hotel Group.* Asia Pacific Journal of Tourism Research 25(10) pp. 1062-10709.

Furnham A., Richards S.C., and Paulhus D.L. (2013). *The Dark Triad of Personality: A 10 year Review.* Social and Personality Psychology Compass 7(3) pp.199-216.

Fuss G.K., Weizman Y., and Tan A.M. (2022). *COVID-19 Pandemic: How Effective Are Preventive Control Measures and Is a Complete Lockdown Justified? A Comparison of Countries and States*. COVID 2022 2(1) pp. 18-46.

Garstang J, Debelle G, Anand I, Armstrong J., Botcher E., Chaplin H., Hallett N., Morgans C., Price M., Tan E.E.H., Tudor E., Taylor J. (2020). *Effect of COVID-19 Lockdown on Child Protection Medical Assessments: A Retrospective Observational Study in Birmingham, UK*. British Medical Journal Open 10 Article e042867.

Gal D. and Rucker D.D. (2010). *When in Doubt, Shout! Paradoxical Influences of Doubt on Proselytizing*. Psychological Science 21(11) pp. 1701-1707.

Galloway A. (2021). *'Breach of Trust': Police Using QR Check-in Data to Solve Crimes*. The Sydney Morning Herald, 6 September 2021. Accessed at: https://www.smh.com.au/politics/federal/breach-of-trust-police-using-qr-check-in-data-to-solve-crimes-20210903-p58om8.html.

Gans J. (2016). *The Disruption Dilemma*. MIT Press, Cambridge MA.

Garrett N., Tapley A., Andriesen J., Seocharan I., Fisher L.H., Bunts L., Espy N., Wallis C., Randhawa A.K., Goga A., Bekker L-G., Gray G.E., and Corey L. (2021). *High Rate of Asymptomatic Carriage Associated with Variant Strain Omicron*. MedRxiv, doi: https://doi.org/10.1101/2021.12.20.21268130.

Garvin D.A. and Roberto M.A. (2001). *What You Don't Know About Making Decisions*. Harvard Business Review, September 2001, Article R0109G.

Gentlin D. (2020). *Why Ethical Leadership Needs to be Practiced before a Crisis*. The Ethics Centre. Accessed at: https://ethics.org.au/ethical-leadership-in-a-crisis/.

Geraets N. and Dow A. (2022). *Code Red Chaos: Victorian Ambulance Staff Resort to Paper and Pen After IT Failure*. Accessed at: https://www.theage.com.au/politics/victoria/code-red-chaos-victorian-ambulance-staff-resort-to-paper-and-pen-after-it-failure-20220527-p5aoza.html.

Ghaemi N. (2011). *A First Rate Madness. Uncovering the Links Between Leadership and Mental Illness*. Penguin Books. London, UK.

Gibb A. G., Lingard H., Behm M., and Cooke T. (2014). *Construction Accident Causality: Learning from Different Countries and Differing Consequences*. Construction Management and Economics 32(5) pp. 446 - 459.

Gibson B., Miles D., and Burns A. (2020). *Advocates Say Cost-cutting by Private Pathology Providers Jeopardising Regional Health Care*. ABC News, #0 May 2020. Accessed at: https://www.abc.net.au/news/2020-05-30/pathology-cost-cutting-in-country-victoria/12296186?nw=0.

Gibson C.A. (2020). *Monograph: Perspectives in Resilience*. In: Monographs in Risk and Resilience, Australian Risk Policy Institute. Canberra, Australia. Accessed at: https://static1.squarespace.com/static/5cc7b079e666697c8ea24697/t/5f67fd97eb716a35bc4a3248/1600650686305/monographs+in+risk+and+resilience+volume+1+2020+pub3.pdf

Gibson C.A. and Gibson K.I.J. (2023). *A Critical Incident Field Guide: Integrating Risk, Business Continuity, Emergency, and Crisis Management. Volume 1: Concepts, Second Edition*. Executive Impact Press, Melbourne, Australia.

Gibson C.A. and Pupulidy I. (2015a). *Margin of Manoeuvre: A Safe Space for Emergency and Disaster Responders*. Planet@Risk 3(2) pp. 201-208.

Gibson C.A. and Pupulidy I. (2015b). *Using Your Brain: Improving Safety and Performance on the Fireground*. Asia Pacific Fire July 2015 pp. 96-98.

Gidley S. (2018). 'They Day' Victorian Government Backs Gender-Neutral Pronouns. SBS News 2 August 2018. Accessed at:

https://www.sbs.com.au/news/they-day-victorian-government-backs-gender-neutral-pronouns/3285a29d-a2a2-45e7-ad48-086342f45416.

Gigerenzer G. and Gaissmaier W. (2015. *Decision Making: Nonrational Theories*. In: International Encyclopedia of the Social & Beviousral Sciences, 2nd Edition, Volume 5, pp. 911-916.

Gilbert L. and Lilly A. (2020). *Independent Review of COVID-19 outbreaks at St Basil's Home for the Aged in Fawkner, Victoria; Heritage Care Epping Gardens in Epping, Victoria.* 30 November 2020. Accessed at: https://www.health.gov.au/sites/default/files/documents/2020/12/coronavirus-covid-19-independent-review-of-covid-19-outbreaks-at-st-basil-s-and-epping-gardens-aged-care-facilities.pdf.

Gilchrist A.L., Cowan N., and Naveh-Benjamin M. (2008). *Working Memory Capacity for Spoken Sentences Decreases with Adult Ageing: Recall of Fewer but Not Smaller Chunks in Older Adults*. Memory 16(7) pp. 773-87.

Gillespie D. (2017). *Taming Toxic People: The Science of Identifying & Dealing with Psychopaths at Work & at Home*. Pan Macmillan Australia, Sydney Australia.

Gilovich T., Griffin D., and Kahneman D. (2002). *Heuristics and Biases: The Psychology of Intuitive Judgment*. Cambridge University Press, Cambridge, UK.

Gjøsæter T., Radianti J., Vhen W. (2019). *Understanding Situational Disabilities and Situational Awareness in Disasters*. In: Universal Design of ICT in Emergency Management Proceedings of the 16th ISCRAM Conference, WiPe Paper (Editors: Z. Franco, J.J. González and J.H. Canós), May 2019, València, Spain.

Glare K. (2022). *Vic Police no Longer Independent of Govt*. Sky News, 27 January 2022. Accessed at: https://www.youtube.com/watch?v=S5FzQlbJsbY.

Glasgow W. (2020). *Wuhan Lab Door Slammed on Covid Inquiry by China*. The Australian, 13 August 2021. Accessed at: https://www.theaustralian.com.au/world/head-of-who-team-investigating-origins-of-covid19-calls-fo-closer-look-at-china-lab/news-story/7d07fa106afca54faa7387bf792a036a.

Glenn J., Chaumont C., and Dintrans P.V. (2021). *Public Health Leadership in the Times of COVID-19: A Comparative Case Study of Three Countries*. International Journal of Public Leadership 17(1) pp. 81-94.

Glick J.A. and Barbara J.A. (2013). *Moving from Situational Awareness to Decisions During Disaster Response: Transition to Decision Making*. Journal of Emergency Management 11(6) pp. 423-32.

Godde C. (2022). *Rebel MP Accuses Vic Premier of Bullying*. 7 News, 9 March 2022. Accessed at: https://7news.com.au/politics/rebel-mp-accuses-vic-premier-of-bullying-c-5988486.

Godlock G.C., Miltner R.S., and Sullivan D.T. (2017). *Deference to Expertise: Making Care Safer*. Creative Nursing 23(1) pp. 7-12.

Goerlandt F. and Reniers G. (2016). *On the Assessment of Uncertainty in Risk Diagrams*. Safety Science 84 pp. 67-77.

Goldberg D.S. (2012). *Against the Very Idea of the Politicization of Public Health*. American Journal of Public Health 102(1) pp. 44-49.

Goldhammer J.G. (2008). *Wildland Fires: Creeping and Sudden Disasters – Part 1*. Crisis Response Journal 3(4) pp. 51-52.

Goldin M. (2021). *Why is the So-called 'Health Advice' Kept Secret from Us?* The Australian, 29 October 2021. Accessed at: https://www.theaustralian.com.au/inquirer/why-is-the-socalled-health-advice-kept-secret-from-us/news-story/252543a472242a7c26809ed0585446c2.

Goldstein P., Yeyati E.L., and Sartori L. (2021). *Lockdown Fatigue: The Declining Effectiveness of Lockdowns*. VoxEU CEPR, 20 March 2021. Accessed at: https://voxeu.org/article/declining-effectiveness-lockdowns.

Golightly D., Wilson J. R., Lowe E., and Sharples S. (2010). *The Role of Situation Awareness for Understanding Signalling and Control in Rail Operations*. Theoretical Issues in Ergonomics Science, 11(1-2) pp. 84-98.

Goode C. (2020). *Cedar Meats Cleared in Vic COVID-19 Probe*. The West Australia, 25 December 2020. Accessed at: https://thewest.com.au/news/health/cedar-meats-cleared-in-vic-covid-19-probe-ng-s-2042117.

Goodwin G.F., Blacksmith N., and Coats M.R. (2018). *The Science of Teams in the Military: Contributions from Over 60 Years of Research*. American Psychologist 73(4) pp. 322-333

Gordon J. (2014). *Daniel Andrews Under Pressure Over Tape Denials*. The Age, 28 July 2014. Accessed at: https://www.theage.com.au/national/victoria/daniel-andrews-under-pressure-over-tape-denials-20140728-zxsjv.html.

Gorman J. and Zimmer C. (2021). *Scientist Opens Up About His Early Email to Fauci on Virus Origins*. The New York Times 14 June 2021. Accessed at: https://www.nytimes.com/2021/06/14/science/covid-lab-leak-fauci-kristian-andersen.html

Gorman L. and Stoney C. (2015). *Missed Opportunities: Public Health Disaster Management in Canada*. Journal of Public Management & Social Policy 22(2) Article 6.

Gostin O.L. (2018). *Language, Science, and Politics: The Politicization of Public Health*. JAMA 319(6) pp. 541-542.

Gottliebsen R. (2019). *Victoria's Virtue Signalling on Gas Ignores Common Sense*. Accessed at: https://www.theaustralian.com.au/business/mining-energy/victorias-virtue-signalling-on-gas-ignores-common-sense/news-story/49398491953b33099a05308279edd968.

Gottliebsen R. (2020a). *Questions Over Cover-ups at Victoria's Department Health and Human Services*. The Australian Business Review, 12 November 2020. Accessed at: https://www.theaustralian.com.au/business/economics/questions-over-coverups-at-victorias-department-health-and-human-services/news-story/a6fb0cf980ce4e686f96b290b21d7b9d.

Gottliebsen R. (2020b). *Pressure on WorkSafe Victoria to Turn Blind Eye on Hotel Quarantine*. The Australian Business Review, 17 November 2020. Accessed at: https://www.theaustralian.com.au/business/pressure-on-worksafe-victoria-to-turn-blind-eye-on-hotel-quarantine/news-story/d6a1209b6c4a81e266f22d37e736b509.

Government of South Australia (2020), *Independent Review of South Australia's 2019-20 Bushfire Season*.

Goyal N. and Howlett M. (2018). *Lessons learned and Not Learned: Bibliometric Analysis of Policy Learning*. In: Learning in Public Policy, Chapter 2 pp. 27-49 (Editors: C.A. Dunlop, C.M. Radaelli, P. Trein). International Series in Public Policy, International Public Policy Association.

Goyette K. (2020). *How Ethics Play a Role in Your Strategic Response to Crisis*. Chief Executive, 23 September 2020. Accessed at: https://chiefexecutive.net/how-ethics-play-a-role-in-your-strategic-response-to-crises/.

Graham R.L. and Baric R.S. (2020). *SARS-CoV-2: Combating Coronavirus Emergence*. Immunity 52(5) pp. 734-736.

Graham R.N.J. and Woodhead T. (2020). *Leadership for Continuous Improvement in Healthcare During the Time of COVID-19*. Clinical Radiology 76(1) pp.67-72.

Gray R. (1998). *Organisational Culture and the Psychological Contract: A Review of the Literature*. Practitioner Papers. Accessed at:

http://rodericgray.com/orgcultureandpsycontract.pdf
Grayson L. (2020). *Exhibit HQI0001_P Witness Statement of Prof. Lindsay Grayson, 19 [75].* Accessed at: https://www.quarantineinquiry.vic.gov.au/exhibits.
Green B.C. (2005). *Building Sport Programs to Optimize Athlete Recruitment, Retention, and Transition: Toward a Normative Theory of Sport Development.* Journal of Sport Management 19 pp. 233-253.
Greyling T.; Rossouw S.; and Adhikari T. (2020). *A Tale of Three Countries: How did Covid-19 Lockdown Impact Happiness?* GLO Discussion Paper No. 584. Global Labor Organization (GLO), Essen.
Grimes P. (2020). *Good Intentions are not Enough: Building the Infrastructure to Support Ethical Leadership.* Independent Broad-based Anti-corruption Commission. Accessed at: https://www.ibac.vic.gov.au/publications-and-resources/ibac-insights/issue-15/good-intentions-are-not-enough-building-the-infrastructure-to-support-ethical-leadership.
Grimmelikhuijsen S., Jilke S., Olsen A.L., and Tummers L. (2017). *Behavioral Public Administration: Combining Insights from Public Administration and Psychology.* Public Administration Review 77(1) pp. 45-56.
Grout L., Katar A., Ouakrim A.A., Summer J.A., Kvalsvig A., Baker M.G., Blakely T., and Wilson N. (2021). *Estimating the Failure Risk of Hotel-based Quarantine for Preventing COVID-10 Outbreaks in Australia and New Zealand.* MedRxiv, https://doi.org/10.1101/2021.02.17.21251946.
Grupe D.W. and Nitschke J.B. (2013). *Uncertainty and Anticipation in Anxiety.* Nature Reviews in Neuroscience 14(7) pp. 488-501.
Gubler D.J., Vasilakis N., and Musso D. (2017). *History and Emergence of Zika Virus.* The Journal of Infectious Diseases 216(Suppl 10) pp. 2860-S867.
Gudmundsson A. and Southey G. (2011) *Leadership and the Rise of the Corporate Psychopath: What can Business Schools do about the 'Snakes Inside'?* e-Journal of Social and Behavioural Research in Business 2(2), pp. 18-27.
Guerrieri V. (2020). *'Unclean! Unclean!:' The Questionable History of Quarantines.* Popular Mechanics 6 March 2020. Accessed at: https://www.popularmechanics.com/science/health/a31260166/quarantine-history-coronavirus/
HACSU (2019). *Submission to the Royal Commission into Victoria's Mental Health System.* Health and Community Services Union. Accessed at: https://hacsu.asn.au/file/56953/21453.
Hadida A., Travainen W., and Rose J. (2014). *Organizational Improvisation: A Consolidating Review and Framework.* International Journal of Management Reviews 17(4) pp.437-459.
Hafner R. J., White M. P., and Handley S. J. (2012*). Spoilt for Choice: The Role of Counterfactual Thinking in the Excess Choice and Reversibility Paradoxes.* Journal of Experimental Social Psychology 48 pp. 28–36.
Hahnel U.J.J., Mumenthaler C., Spampatti T., Brosch T. (2020). *Ideology as Filter: Motivated Information Processing and Decision-Making in the Energy Domain.* Sustainability 12(20) Article 8429.
Halal W.E. (2015). *Business Strategy for the Technology Revolution: Competing at the Edge of Creative Destruction.* Journal of the Knowledge Economy 6(1) pp. 31-47.
Hald E.J., Gillespie A., and Reader T.W. (2020). *Causal and Corrective Organisational Culture: A Systematic Review of Case Studies of Institutional Failure.* Journal of Business Ethics https://doi.org/10.1007/s10551-020-04620-3.
Hales H. (2022a). *Chaos as Ambulance Victoria Declares Code Red for Melbourne Services.* The West Australian 11 January 2022. Accessed at:

https://thewest.com.au/news/chaos-as-ambulance-victoria-declares-code-red-for-melbourne-services-c-5258685.

Hales H. (2022b). *Victorian MP Kaushaliya Vaghela Launches New Bullying Claims Against Premier Daniel Andrews and Colleagues*. News.com.au, 9 March 2022. Accessed at: https://www.news.com.au/national/victoria/politics/victorian-mp-kaushaliya-vaghela-launches-new-bullying-claims-again-premier-daniel-andrews-and-colleagues/news-story/d5099170bf233f22af0a9fad7e1337a3.

Hall B. and Eddie R. (2020*). Department Apologies for Delays in Getting Food to Tower Residents*. The Age, 7 July 2020. Accessed at: https://www.theage.com.au/politics/victoria/department-apologises-for-delays-in-getting-food-to-tower-residents-20200707-p559ok.html.

Hallsworth M., Egan M. Rutter J., and McCrae J. (2018). *Behavioural Government: Using Behavioural Science to Improve How Governments Make Decisions.* Behavioural Insights Team. UK Government and NESTA.

Halpern D. *Inside the Nudge Unit: How Small Changes Can Make a Big Difference*. WH Allen, London, UK.

Halpern D. (2016). *Behavioural Insights and Healthier Lives: VicHealth's Inaugural Leading Thinking Residency*. VicHealth. https://www.vichealth.vic.gov.au/-/media/ResourceCentre/PublicationsandResources/General/2016-Behavioural-Insights-and-Healthier-Lives.pdf

Halse D. (2011). *The Thin Blue Bottom Line: How Victoria's Police Re-Defined Public Pay Battles*. The Conversation 7 November 2011. Accessed at: https://theconversation.com/the-thin-blue-bottom-line-how-victorias-police-re-defined-public-pay-battles-4167.

Halverson P.K., Yeager V.A., Menachemi N., Fraser M.R., and Freeman L.T. (2021). *Public Health Officials and COVID-19: Leadership, Politics, and the Pandemic.* Journal of Public Health Management and Practice 50(1 Supp) pp 11-13.

Hams P.D. and Spain S.M. (2015). *Beyond the Bright Side: Dark Personality at Work*. Applied Psychology 64(1) pp. 15-24.

Hanger I. (2014). *Report of the Royal Commission into the Home Installation Program*. Commonwealth of Australia, Canberra.

Hannan E. and Johnston D. (2021a). *What Caused the State's Third Lockdown*. The Australian 6 July 2021. Accessed at: https://www.theaustralian.com.au/nation/hotel-quarantine-corridor-swab-ignited-outbreak-lockdown/news-story/00e845db02f968be24f2c71c9006776a.

Hannan E. and Johnston D. (2021b). *Vic Official Stood Down Over Breaches*. 4 May 2021. Accessed at: https://www.theaustralian.com.au/nation/hotel-quarantine-top-official-matiu-bush-caught-breaching-covid19-protocols/news-story/3cf2767dcb9b3046f35bcc587720fc44.

Hannan E. and Johnston D. (2021c). *Ex-hotel Quarantine Boss Matiu Bush Hired Gym Buddies for $101k-a-Year Roles.*

Hannan E. and Johnston D. (2021d). Victorian Hotel Boss Matiu Bush Resigns. The Australian, 12 June 2021. Accessed at: https://www.theaustralian.com.au/nation/victorian-hotel-quarantine-boss-matiu-bush-resigns/news-story/09e967b09f1a4537d369f66d057453c8.

Hansard (2023). House of Representatives, Monday 4 September 2025. Commonwealth of Australia. Accessed at:

https://parlinfo.aph.gov.au/parlInfo/download/chamber/hansardr/27162/toc_pdf/House%20of%20Representatives_2023_09_04.pdf;fileType=application%2Fpdf#search=%22chamber/hansardr/27162/0167%22

Hansen M.T. (2013). How John F. Kennedy Changed Decision Making for Us All. Harvard Business Review, 22 November 2013. Accessed at: https://hbr.org/2013/11/how-john-f-kennedy-changed-decision-making

Harcourt V., Massaro A., Courtney A., and Goessler M. (2021). *COVID-19 Outbreaks: WorkCover Investigates Residential Aged Care Providers*. Russel Kennedy Lawyers, 25 October 2021. Accessed at: https://www.russellkennedy.com.au/insights-events/insights/covid-19-outbreaks-workcover-investigates-residential-aged-care-providers.

Harris A. (2021). *Failure of Political Leadership and Imagination is Holding Back the COVID-19 Recovery*. Wellcome, 19 May 2021. Accessed at: https://wellcome.org/news/failure-political-leadership-and-imagination-holding-back-covid-19-recovery.

Harris A. and Jones M. (2018). *The Dark Side of Leadership and Management*. School of Leadership and Management 38(5) pp. 475-477.

Harris R. (2020). *Offer of ADF Support: Morrison's Letters to Daniel Andrews Revealed*. The Sydney Morning Herald, 23 September 2020. Accessed at: https://www.smh.com.au/politics/federal/offer-of-adf-support-morrison-s-letters-to-daniel-andrews-revealed-20200923-p55yld.html.

Harrison D. (2017). *Investigation Finds 'Insufficient Evidence' To Prosecute Falls Festival Organisers Over 2016 Stampede*. The Music, 6 November 2017. Accessed at: https://themusic.com.au/news/investigation-finds-insufficient-evidence-to-prosecute-falls-festival-organisers-over-2016-stampede/0fPCxcTHxsk/06-11-17/.

Hart P.S., Chinn S., and Soroka S. (2020). *Politicization and Polarization in COVID-19 News Coverage*. Science Communication 42(5) pp. 679-697.

Härtel C.E.J. (2008). *How to Build a Healthy Emotional Culture and Avoid a Toxic Culture*. In: Research Companion to Emotion in Organization, pp.1260-1291. (Editors: C.L. Cooper and N.M. Ashkanasy). Edwin Elgar Publishing, Cheltenham, UK.

Harvey A., Koloff S., and Wiggins N. (2021). *How Australia's COVID Vaccine Rollout has Fallen Short and Left us 'in a Precarious Position'*. ABC News, 24 May 2021. Accessed at: https://www.abc.net.au/news/2021-05-24/australia-covid-vaccine-rollout-what-went-wrong/100151396.

Harvey P., and Martinko M.J. (2008) *An Empirical Examination of the Role of Attributions in Psychological Entitlement and its Outcomes*. Journal of Organisational Behavior 30(4) pp. 459–476

Haslam A.A., Steffens N.K., Reicher S.D., and Bentley S.V. (2021). *Identity Leadership in a Crisis: A 5R Framework for Learning from Responses to COVID-19*. Social Issues and Policy review 15(1) pp. 35-83.

Haseltine W.A. (2022). *Omicron Less Virulent but Still Dangerous*. Forbes, 11 January 2022. Accessed at: https://www.forbes.com/sites/williamhaseltine/2022/01/11/omicron-less-virulent-but-still-dangerous/?sh=2d4f75b92ea6.

Haug N., Geyrhofer L., Londei A., Dervic E., Desvars-Larrive A., Loreto V., Pinoir B., Thurner S., and Klimek P. (2020). *Ranking the Effectiveness of Worldwide COVID-19 Government Interventions*. Nature Human Interventions 4 pp. 1303-1312.

Hausken K., Bier V., Zhuang J. (2009*). Defending Against Terrorism, Natural Disaster, and All Hazards*. In: Game Theoretic Risk Analysis of Security Threats, pp. 65-97, (Editors: V.M. Bier and M.N. Azaiez). International Series in Operations Research and Management Science vol 128., Springer, Boston, MA.

HBP (2020). *COVID-19 Heightens the Leadership Gap*. Special Report, Harvard Business Publishing.

Head E. and van Elsand S.L. (2021). *Omicron Largely Evades Immunity from Past Infection or Two Vaccine Doses*. Imperial College London, 17 December 2021. Accessed at: https://www.imperial.ac.uk/news/232698/omicron-largely-evades-immunity-from-past/.

Health Department (2021). *Behavioural Insights and Interventions*. Accessed at: https://www.health.gov.au/health-topics/medicare-compliance/how-we-ensure-compliance/behavioural-insights-and-interventions.

HealthVic (2020). *Leading Thinkers Initiative Residency 1: Behavioural Insights and Healthier Lives*. Accessed at: https://www.vichealth.vic.gov.au/programs-and-projects/leading-thinkers-initiative-residency-1.

Heinrich H.W. (1931). *Industrial Accident Prevention*. McGraw-Hill, New York.

Hendry J. *'Significant Failures' Marred Victoria's Fines IT System Upgrade: Auditor*. IT News, 5 May 2021. Accessed at: https://www.itnews.com.au/news/significant-failures-marred-victorias-fines-it-system-upgrade-auditor-564174.

Henriques-Gomes L. (2020). *Experts Say Aged Care Royal Commission's Covid Review Does Not Address Wider Problems*. The Guardian, 2 October 2020. Accessed at: https://www.theguardian.com/australia-news/2020/oct/02/experts-say-aged-care-royal-commissions-covid-review-does-not-address-wider-problems.

Heller V.L. and Darling J.R. (2011). *Toyota in Crisis: Denial and Mismanagement*. Journal of Business Strategy 32(5) pp. 4-13.

Henderson P.G. (2018). *Anatomy of a National Security Fiasco: The George W. Bush Administration, Iraq, and Groupthink*. Humanitas 31-2(1) pp. 46+.

Henderson G. (2021). *Media Watch Dog: Covid Central Victoria and Dan's Run of 'Bad Luck'*. The Australian, 19 February 2021.

Heneghan S. and Mahtani K.R. (2020). *Leadership in COVID-19: The Dangers of Groupthink in Crisis Leadership.* The Centre for Evidence-Based Medicine, 26 May 2020. Accessed at: https://www.cebm.net/covid-19/leadership-in-covid-19-the-dangers-of-groupthink-in-crisis-leadership/

Heneghan C. (2022). *Masks in Schools: How Convincing is the Evidence?* The Spectator, 8 January 2022. Accessed at: https://www.spectator.co.uk/article/masks-in-schools-how-convincing-is-the-government-s-evidence-

Herby J., Jonung L., and Hanke S.H. (2022*). A Literature Review and Meta-analysis of the Effects of Lockdowns on COVID-19 Mortality*. Studies in Applied Economics 200 pp. 1-61.

Hess K.M. and Hess O.C. (2012). *Management and Supervision in Law Enforcement (6th edition)*. Derlmar Cengage Learning, Clifton Park, NY.

Hewett J. (2020). *Inside Victoria's Coronavirus Meltdown*. Financial Review 10 July 2020. Accessed at: https://www.afr.com/policy/health-and-education/inside-victoria-s-coronavirus-meltdown-20200709-p55amo

Hickey S. and Nedim U. (2020). *Victorian Government Wants COVID-19 powers to be Permanently Expanded.* Sydney Criminal Lawyers, 22 May 2020. Accessed at: https://www.sydneycriminallawyers.com.au/blog/victorian-government-wants-covid-19-powers-to-be-permanently-expanded/.

Hickock H. (2021). *Why Toxic Workplace Cultures Follow You Home.* BBC, 5 April 2021. Accessed at:

https://www.bbc.com/worklife/article/20210330-why-toxic-workplace-cultures-follow-you-home.

Hiekkataipale M-M. and Lämsä A-M. (2017). *(A)moral Agents in Organisations? The Significance of Ethical Organisation Culture for Middle Managers' Exercise of Moral Agency in Ethical Problems*. Journal of Business Ethics, DOI 10.1007/s10551-017-3511-9.

Hilbert M. (2012). *Toward a Synthesis of Cognitive Biases: How Noisy Information Processing Can Bias Human Decision Making*. Psychological Bulletin 138(2) pp. 211-237.

Hiles A. (2014). *The Anatomy of Crisis: How Crises Develop*. Accessed on 7 July 2017 at: https://www.linkedin.com/pulse/20141110135620-1967426-the-anatomy-of-crisis-how-crises-develop.

Hill C. (2016). *5 Signs that a Politician is a Narcissistic Psychopath*. Market Watch 30 January 2016. Accessed at: https://www.marketwatch.com/story/5-signs-that-a-politician-is-a-narcissistic-psychopath-2016-01-29.

Hill J. (2019). *Tackling Victoria Police's Culture of Misogyny*. The Saturday Paper, 6 September 2019. Accessed at:
https://www.thesaturdaypaper.com.au/news/law-crime/2019/08/31/tackling-victoria-polices-culture-misogyny/15671736008684#hrd.

Hodge J.G., Gostin L.O., and Vernick J.S. (2007). *The Pandemic and All-Hazards Preparedness Act: Improving*
Public Health Emergence Response. JAMA 297(15) pp. 1708–1711.

Hodge N. (2019). *Learning From Corporate Collapse*. Risk Management, 1 February 2019. Accessed at:
http://www.rmmagazine.com/2019/02/01/learning-from-corporate-collapse/.

Hodgins M., MacCurtain S., and Mannix-McNamara P. (2014). *Workplace Bullying and Incivility: A Systematic Review of Interventions*. International Journal of Workplace Health Management *7* pp. 54-72.

Hogan-Doran (2019). *Lessons for Government from Recent Royal Commissions and Public Inquiries*. Paper Presented to the Law Society of New South Wales, Government Solicitors' Conference, 30 September 2019.

Hollingsworth T.D., Ferguson N.M., and Anderson R.M. (2007). *Frequent Travelers and Rate of Spread of Epidemics*. Emerging Infectious Diseases 13(9) pp. 1288-1294.

Hollyer J.R. and Wantchekon L. (2014). *Corruption and Ideology in Autocracies*. Journal of Law, Economic and Organization 31(3) pp. 499-533.

Holmes C.E. (2011). *Queensland Floods Commission of Inquiry – Interim Report*.

Holmes C.E. (2012). *Queensland Floods Commission of Inquiry – Final Report*.

Holmes E.C. and Rambaut A. (2004). Viral Evolution and the Emergence of SARS Coronavirus. Philosophical Transactions of the Royal Society London B. 359 pp, 1059-1065.

Holmes E.C., Goldstein S.A., Rasmussen A.L. Robertson D.L., Crits-Christoph A., Wertheim J.O., Anthony S.J., Barclay W.S., Boni M.F, Doherty P.C., Farrar J., Geoghegan J.L, Jiang X., Leibowitz J.L., Neil S.J.D., Skern T., Weiss S.R., Worobey M., Andersen K.G., Garry R.F., Rambaut A. (2021). *The Origins of SARS-CoV-2: A Critical Review*. Preprint, accessed at: https://zenodo.org/record/5075888#.YRs13y0Rond.

HK Government (2003). *Preventing Severe Acute Respiratory Syndrome (SARS) Guidelines for Hotels*. Accessed at:
https://www.info.gov.hk/info/sars/en/GuidelinesForHotels.htm.

Honigsbaum M. (2020). *Revisiting the 1957 and 1968 Influenza Pandemics*. The Lancet 295 pp. 1824-1826.

Hope Z. (2020). *'Dangerous Virtue Signalling': Police Union Fury at Public Drunkenness Laws Putting 'The Cart Before the Horse'*. The Age, 28 November 2020. Accessed at:

https://www.theage.com.au/national/victoria/dangerous-virtue-signalling-police-union-fury-at-public-drunkenness-laws-putting-the-cart-before-the-horse-20201128-p56iro.html.

Hooper P.T., Lunt R.A., Gould A.R., Hyatt A.D., Russell G.M., Kattenbelt J.A., Black S.D., Reddacliff L.A., Kirkland P.D., Davis R.J., Durham P.J.K., Bishop A.L., and Waddington J. (1990). *Epidemic of Blindness in Kangaroos – Evidence of a Viral Aetiology*. Australian Veterinary Journal 77 (8) pp. 529-536.

Hopkins A. (2006). *Studying Organisational Cultures and their Effects on Safety*. Working Paper 44. National Research Centre for OHS Regulation, Australian National University, Canberra, Australia.

Houston C. (2021a). *Licence Renewed for Security Firm at Centre of Hotel Quarantine Fiasco*. The Age, 12 January 2021. Accessed at:
https://www.theage.com.au/national/victoria/licence-renewed-for-security-firm-at-centre-of-hotel-quarantine-fiasco-20210112-p56ti4.html.

Houston C. (2021b). *Group to Mount Legal Challenge to Force Prosecution of Premier Over Hotel Quarantine Disaster*. The Age, 11 December 2021. Accessed at:
https://www.theage.com.au/national/victoria/group-to-mount-legal-challenge-to-force-prosecution-of-premier-over-hotel-quarantine-disaster-20211209-p59gcl.html.

Houston C. and Preiss B. (2018). *Police Frustration Grows Amid Claims of Red Shirts Probe Interference*. The Age, 25 October 2018. Accessed at:
https://www.theage.com.au/politics/victoria/police-frustration-grows-amid-claims-of-red-shirts-probe-interference-20181024-p50bpi.html.

Howlett M. (2017). *The Criteria for Effective Policy Design: Character and Context in Policy Instrument Choices*. ICPPIII Conference, 28-30 June 2017. LKY School of Public Policy, National University of Singapore.

Hovden J., Størseth F., and Tinmannsvik R.K. (2011). *Multilevel Learning from Accidents—Case Studies in Transport*. Safety Science 49(1) pp. 98–105.

Howlett M., How Y.P., del Rio P. (2015). *The Parameters of Policy Portfolios: Verticality and Horizontality in Design Spaces and their Consequences for Policy Mix Formulation*. Environment and Planning C: Government and Policy 47 pp. 1-13.

Hu B., Guo H., Zhou P., and Shi Z-L. (2021). *Characteristics of SAR-COV-2 and COVID 19*. Nature Reviews: Microbiology 19pp. 141-154.

Huanca W.T. (2020). The Failure of Leadership in the Face of COVID-19. Heconomist, Switzerland, 21 April 2020. Accessed at:
https://heconomist.ch/2020/04/21/the-failure-of-leadership-in-the-face-of-covid-19/.

Huang Y. (2004). *The SARS Epidemic and its Aftermath in China: A Political Perspective*. In Learning from SARS: Preparing for the Next Disease Outbreak: Workshop Summary, (Editors: S. Knobler, A. Mahmoud, S. Lemon, A. Mack, L. Sivitz, K. Oberholtzer). Institute of Medicine (US) Forum on Microbial Threats. National Academies Press (US).

Huang Y. (2020). *How the Origins of COVID-19 Became Politicized*. Think Global Health. 14 August 2020.
https://www.thinkglobalhealth.org/article/how-origins-covid-19-became-politicized.

Hubbard D.W. (2009). *The Failure of Risk Management: Why it's Broken and How to Fix it*. John Wiley and Sons, Hoboken, NJ.

Hubbard D. and Evans D. (2010). *Problems with Scoring Methods and Ordinal Scales in Risk Assessment*. IBM Journal of Research and Development 54(3) Paper 2.

Hughes I. (2019). *Unpicking Donald Trump's Psychopathology Helps Explain the Toxic Reality Facing America*. Euronews 14 August 2019. Accessed at:
https://www.euronews.com/2019/08/14/unpicking-donald-trump-s-psychopathology-helps-explain-the-toxic-reality-facing-america-vi.

Huitson J. (2022). *Victorian Premier's Toxic Culture of 'Retribution' Exposed by Whistleblower in Peta Credlin Documentary 'The Cult of Daniel Andrews'*. Sky News, 15 November 2022. Accessed at: https://www.skynews.com.au/australia-news/politics/victorian-premiers-toxic-culture-of-retribution-exposed-by-whistleblower-in-peta-credlin-documentary-the-cult-of-daniel-andrews/news-story/2ee49d7928f76766035a3814b0874613.

Human Rights Watch (2021). *Covid-19 Triggers Wave of Free Speech Abuse*. 11 February 2021. Accessed at: https://www.hrw.org/news/2021/02/11/covid-19-triggers-wave-free-speech-abuse.

Human Rights Watch (2020). *Australia: Harsh Police Response During COVID-19: Victoria's Parliament Shouldn't Broaden Police Powers*. 24 September 2020. Accessed at: https://www.hrw.org/news/2020/09/24/australia-harsh-police-response-during-covid-19.

Huang Y. (2016). *How to Reform the Ailing World Health Organization*. Council on Foreign Relations. Accessed at: https://www.cfr.org/expert-brief/how-reform-ailing-world-health-organization.

Hung K.K.C., Mark C.K.M., Yeung M.P.S., Chan E.Y.Y, and Graham C.A. (2018). *The Role of the Hotel Industry in the Response to Emerging Epidemics: A Case Study of SARS in 2003 and H1N1 Swine Flu in 2009 in Hong Kong*. Globalisation and Health 14 Article number: 117.

Hunt G. (2020). *First Confirmed Case of Novel Coronavirus in Australia*. Federal Minister for Health, Media Release, 25 January 2020). Accessed at: https://www.health.gov.au/ministers/the-hon-greg-hunt-mp/media/first-confirmed-case-of-novel-coronavirus-in-australia.

Huremović D. (2019). *Mental Health of Quarantine and Isolation*. In: Psychiatry of Pandemics: A mental Health Response to Infection Outbreak (Editor D. Huremović), Springer Nature, Switzerland.

Hung K.C., Mark C.K.M., Yeung M.P.S., Chan E.Y.Y., and Graham C.A. (2018). *The Role of the Hotel Industry in the Response to Emerging Epidemics: A Case Study of SARS in 2003 and H1N1 Swine Flu in 2009 in Hong Kong*. Globalisation and Health 14 Article 117.

Hunt G. and Murphy B. (2020). *First Confirmed Case of a Novel Coronavirus in Australia*. Parliament of Australia. Accessed at: https://parlinfo.aph.gov.au/parlInfo/download/media/pressrel/7158085/upload_binary/7158085.pdf;fileType=application%2Fpdf#search=%22media/pressrel/7158085%22.

Hutala M., Kangas M., Lämsä A-M., and Feldt T. (2013). *Ethical Managers in Ethical Organisations? The Leadership-culture Connection Among Finnish Managers*. Leadership and Organisational Development Journal 34(3) pp. 250-270.

Hutchinson S. (2017). *Opposition Takes Aim at Victoria Police Chief Over 'Independence'*. The Australian 3 June 2017. Accessed at: https://www.theaustralian.com.au/nation/politics/opposition-takes-aim-at-victoria-police-chief-over-independence/news-story/ac332d6ea390148bfd18bfe661b45b74.

IBAC (2017). *Corruption Risks Associated with the Public Health Sector*. Independent Broad-based Anti-Corruption Commission, 25 October 2017. Accessed at: https://www.ibac.vic.gov.au/publications-and-resources/article/corruption-risks-associated-with-the-public-health-sector.

IBAC (2019). *Managing Corruption Risks Associated with Conflicts of Interest in the Victorian Public Sector*. Independent Broad-based Anti-corruption Commission, October 2019. Accessed at: https://www.ibac.vic.gov.au/docs/default-source/research-documents/managing-corruption-risks-associated-with-conflicts-of-interest-in-the-victorian-public-sector.pdf?sfvrsn=fdda4f90_2/.

IBAC (2020). *Unauthorised Access and Disclosure of Information Held by the Victorian Public Sector an Analysis of Corruption Risks and Prevention Opportunities*. Independent Broad-based Anti-corruption Commission, February 2020. Accessed at: https://www.ibac.vic.gov.au/docs/default-source/research-documents/unauthorised-access-and-disclosure-of-information-held-by-the-victorian-public-sector.pdf?sfvrsn=d76fc48_6.

IBAC (2021a). *Special Report on Corrections: IBAC Operations Rous, Capabarra, Nsidia, and Molara*. Independent Broad-based Anti-corruption Commission, Melbourne Australia, June 2021. Accessed at: https://www.ibac.vic.gov.au/docs/default-source/special-reports/special-report-on-corrections---june-2021.pdf?sfvrsn=ee450c8c_2.

IBAC (2021b). *Corruption and Integrity: Perceptions of Victorian Public Sector Employees*. Independent Broad-based Anti-corruption Commission, June 2021. Accessed at: https://www.ibac.vic.gov.au/docs/default-source/research-documents/research-report---perception-of-corruption---state-government---june-2021.pdf?sfvrsn=600ba74b_2.

IBAC (2022). *Operation Watts. Investigation into Allegations of Misuse of Electorate Office and Ministerial Office Staff and Resources for Branch Stacking and Other Party-related Activities*. Independent Board-based Anti-corruption Commission Victoria, and Victorian Ombudsman. Accessed at: https://www.ibac.vic.gov.au/publications-and-resources/article/operation-watts-special-report-july-2022

Ilanby S. (2022). *Labor MP Crosses Floor to Back Fresh Investigation into Red Shirts Scandal*. The Age, 9 February 2022. Accessed at: https://www.theage.com.au/politics/victoria/labor-mp-crosses-floor-to-back-fresh-investigation-into-red-shirts-scandal-20220209-p59v17.html.

Ilanby S. and Baker R. (2020). *Top Bureaucrats Warned a Year Ago Victoria's Key Public Health Team was Starved of Money and Staff.* The Age, 29 July 2020. Accessed at: https://www.theage.com.au/politics/victoria/top-bureaucrats-warned-a-year-ago-victoria-s-key-public-health-team-was-starved-of-money-and-staff-20200729-p55ggh.html.

IMLC (2020). *Ombudsman's Public Housing Report Scathing of Human Rights Violations, Validating Resident Concerns*. Inner Melbourne Community Legal, 17 December 2020. https://imcl.org.au/news/media-releases-1/response-victorian-ombudsman-investigation-public-housing-hard-lockdown.

Ireton E. (2018). *How Public is a Public Inquiry*. Public Law, April 2018, pp. 277-298.

Jacobsson A., Sales J., and Mushtaq F. (2009). *A Sequential Method to Identify Underlying Causes from*
Industrial Accidents Reported to the MARS Database. Journal of Loss Prevention in the Process Industries. 22 (2) pp. 197–203.

Jackson S. and Ross D. (2021). *Coronavirus Quarantine Security Operator Dumped*. The Australian, 20 March 2021. Accessed at: https://www.theaustralian.com.au/nation/politics/coronavirus-quarantine-security-operator-dumped/news-story/0e75e35c4a12125abe0a857a6acaf525.

Jain A.K., Thompson J.M., Chaudry J., McKenzie S., and Schwartz R.W. (2008). *High-performance Teams for Current and Future Physician Leaders: An Introduction*. Journal of Surgical Education 65(2) pp.145-50.

James E. and Wooten L.P. (2005). *Leadership as (un)Usual: How to Display Competence in Times of Crisis*. Organizational Dynamics 34(2) pp. 141-152.

James K. (2021). *Quarantine Hotels: A History of Controversy and Occasional Comfort*. The Conversation, 14 May 2021. Accessed at:

https://theconversation.com/quarantine-hotels-a-history-of-controversy-and-occasional-comfort-160132.
Jamieson H. (2020). *Are You at Risk of Woke-washing Your Workplace*. Training and Industry. Accessed at: https://trainingindustry.com/blog/diversity-equity-and-inclusion/are-you-at-risk-of-woke-washing-your-workplace/.
JDD (2017). *Leadership*. Executive Series ADDP 00.6. Joint Doctrine Directorate, Department of Defence, Canberra, Australia.
Jenkins S. (2020a). *Major Victorian Government Department Split in Two, New Secretary Appointed*. The Mandarin, 30 November 2020. Accessed at:
https://www.themandarin.com.au/146089-major-victorian-government-department-split-in-two-new-secretary-appointed/.
Jenkins S. (2020b). *Vic Public Servants Requested Police Support for Hotel Quarantine Days into Scheme, Emails Show*. The Mandarin 14 July 2020. Accessed at:
https://www.themandarin.com.au/136118-vic-public-servants-requested-police-support-for-hotel-quarantine-days-into-scheme-emails-show/.
Jerrard J. (2012). *Advice of John Jerrard QC Concerning the Examination of Material Provided to the Crime and Misconduct Commission Pursuant to Recommendation 16.1 of the Queensland Floods Commission of Inquiry's Final Report. Crime and Corruption Commission Queensland*. Accessed on 12 December 2017, at:
https://www.ccc.qld.gov.au/publications/advice-johnjerrard-qc-concerning-examination-material-provided-crime-and-misconduct.
Jhangiani R. and Tarry H. (2014). *Group Decision Making*. In: Principles of Social Psychology, 1st International Edition. BC Campus OpenEd, Victoria, BC, Canada.
Johal S.S. (2009). *Psychosocial Impacts of Quarantine During Disease Outbreaks and Interventions That May Help to Relieve Strain*. The New Zealand Medical Journal 122(1296) pp. 53-58.
Johnson C.E. (2019). *Shaping Ethical Contexts*. In: Meeting the Ethical Challenge of Leadership, 7th Edition, part 4. Sage Publishing, Thousand Oaks, CA.
Johnson B. and Turner-Cohen A. (2021). *Whistleblower Claims Victoria's Hotel Quarantine System is Still Flawed*. 7 News, 7 March, 2021. Accessed at:
https://7news.com.au/lifestyle/health-wellbeing/whistleblower-claims-victorias-hotel-quarantine-system-is-still-flawed-c-2301339.
Johnson D.D.P., Blumstein D.T., Fowler J., and Haselton M.G. (2013). *The Evolution of Error: Error Management, Cognitive Constraints, and Adaptive Decision-making Biases*. Trends in Ecology and Evolution 28(8) pp. 474-481.
Johnston D. (2023a). *Witnesses Grilled About Daniel Andrews: IBAC Probe*. The Australian 3 August 2023. Accessed at:
https://www.theaustralian.com.au/nation/politics/witnesses-grilled-about-daniel-andrews-ibac-probe/news-story/093a025af9ee5ef33b80986e52c64248.
Johnson D. (2023b). *Daniel Andrew 'Fireys Probe' by IBAC in the Offing*. The Australian 28 September 2023. Accessed at:
https://www.theaustralian.com.au/nation/politics/daniel-andrews-fireys-probe-by-ibac-in-the-offing/news-story/0d51d30daa759781b348b4673370ed72.
Johnston D. (2022a). *Labor 'has Betrayed IBAC Witnesses*. The Australian, 6 June 2022. Accessed at:
https://www.theaustralian.com.au/nation/labor-has-betrayed-ibac-witnesses/news-story/d8e38adb6b13c238c3d6caae6e7978df,
Johnston D. (2022b). *'Significant number of witnesses' in Secret Union Probe*. The Australian, 1 June 2022. Accessed at:

https://www.theaustralian.com.au/nation/significant-number-of-witnesses-in-secret-union-probe/news-story/536ecd295089776abbe097778f45b0d1.
Johnston D. (2022c). *Watchdog: Daniel Andrews' Pandemic Documents Must be Released.* The Australian 31 May 2022. Accessed at:
https://www.theaustralian.com.au/nation/watchdog-daniel-andrews-pandemic-documents-must-be-released/news-story/2648f699df493386e9d69468ad3646e8.
Johnston D. (2022d). *Independent Broad-based Anti-corruption Commission's Infuriated After Labor MP Harriet Shing Ignored Concerns*. The Australian, 11 August 2022. Accessed at:
https://www.theaustralian.com.au/nation/independent-broadbased-anticorruption-commissions-infuriated-after-labor-mp-harriet-shing-ignored-concerns/news-story/538d76f04ec377d6e1e4a6b201336a2b.
Johnston D. (2021a). *Taxpayer-funded Strategist Advises Ministers on Premier Daniel Andrews' Brand*. The Australian, 8 February 2022. Accessed at:
https://www.theaustralian.com.au/nation/taxpayerfunded-strategist-advises-ministers-on-premier-daniel-andrews-brand/news-story/8c590f0d675439f587fa084610c1da1e.
Johnston D. (2021b). *The Secret Virus Surveys by Daniel Andrews' Spin Doctor John Armitage.* The Australian, 13 July 2021. Accessed at:
https://www.theaustralian.com.au/nation/the-secret-virus-surveys-by-daniel-andrews-spin-doctor-john-armitage/news-story/688fd26fc89f113353cfabf6027dd488.
Johnston D. (2021c). *Daniel Andrews' Spin Doctor Writes the Playbook*. The Australian, 13 July 2021. Accessed at:
https://www.theaustralian.com.au/nation/politics/daniel-andrews-spin-doctor-writes-the-playbook/news-story/9b889dd5287a8cdbf1b1a392598e9f22.
Johnston D. (2021d). *Victorian Budget 2021: Project Cost Blowouts Dig a $3.8bn Hole*. The Australian, 20 May 2021. Accessed at:
https://www.theaustralian.com.au/nation/politics/victorian-budget-2021-project-cost-blowouts-dig-a-38bn-hole/news-story/03018c5eafacedb4faa1ebe11635cae4.
Johnston D. (2021e). *Hubris Rules: Labor's Great Moral and Ethical Failure on Daniel Andrews' Watch*. The Australian, 15 October 2021.
Johnston D. (2021f). *Dan Andrews' Order: Hand Over Secret Liberal Files*. The Australian, 23 August 2021. Accessed at:
https://www.theaustralian.com.au/nation/politics/dan-andrews-order-hand-over-secret-liberal-files/news-story/eb034a2f425e263fb694f610e1a09c34.
Johnston D. and Varga R. (2021). *Victorian Labor Minister Lisa Neville Feels Heat of IBAC Watchdog*. The Australian 8 October 2021. Accessed at:
https://www.theaustralian.com.au/nation/politics/victorian-labor-minister-lisa-neville-feels-heat-of-ibac-watchdog/news-story/d0956fcdd550fe07059d4ac8115b774c.
Johnson J.G. and Busemeyr J.R. (2010). *Decision Making Under Risk and Uncertainty.* Interdisciplinary Reviews: Cognitive Science 1(5) pp. 736-749.
Jofee A.R. (2021). COVID-19: Rethinking the Groupthink. Frontiers in Public Health https://doi.org/10.3389/fpubh.2021.625778.
Joint Committee on Human Rights (2021). *The Government Response to Covid-19: Freedom of Assembly and the Right to Protest*. House of Commons, House of Lords Joint Committee on Human Rights. Thirteenth Report of Session 2019-2021. Accessed at:
https://committees.parliament.uk/publications/5153/documents/50935/default/.
Jones J.B., Hyatt, A.D., Hine, P.M., Whittington, R.J., Griffin, D.A. and Bax, N.J. (1997). *Australasian Pilchard Mortalities*. World Journal of Microbiology and Biotechnology, 13 (4). pp. 383-392.

Jones K.E., Patel N.G., Levy M.A., Storeygard A., Balk D., Gittleman J.L., and Daskak P. (2008). *Global Trends in Emerging Infectious Diseases*. Nature 451 pp. 990-993.

Joshi Y.V. and Musalem A. (2021). *Lockdowns Lose One Third of Their Impact on Mobility in a Month*. Nature Scientific Reports 11 Article 22658.

Jost J.T., Glaser J., Kruglanski A. W., and Sulloway F.J. (2003). *Political Conservatism as Motivated Social Cognition*. Psychological Bulletin 129 pp. 339-375.

Jost J.T., Federico C.M., and Napier J.L. (2009). *Political Ideology: its Structure, Functions, and Elective Affinities*. Annual Review of Psychology *60* pp. 307-337.

Joy R. (2012). *Fiskville: Understanding the Past to Inform the Future*. Report of the Independent Fiskville Investigation, June 2012. Accessed at: https://apo.org.au/sites/default/files/resource-files/2012-07/apo-nid30192.pdf.

Juanola M.P. and Morgan C. (2022). *Ambulance Victoria Says Non-Urgent COVID Care Requests, Isolating Staff Prompted 'Code Red'*. The Age, 5 January 2022. Accessed at: https://www.theage.com.au/national/victoria/covid-s-strain-on-health-system-prompts-ambulance-victoria-code-red-call-20220105-p59lxm.html.

Jurkiewicz C.L. (2017). *Ethics and Crisis Management*. In: Global Encyclopedia of Public Administration, Public Policy, and Governance, (Editor: A. Farazmand). Springer International Publishing, Champs, Switzerland.

Judd B. (2017). *Internal Documents Reveal 'Toxic', 'Fearful' Culture at Victorian Hospital*. ABC News, 19 December 2017. Accessed at: https://www.abc.net.au/news/2017-12-19/toxic-culture-revealed-at-south-west-healthcare/9271182.

Juliano C., Castrucci B., Fraser M.R. (2021). *COVID-19 and Public Health: Looking Back, Moving Forward*. Journal of Public Health Management and Practice 27(1 Supp) PP. S1-S4.

LaRiviere J., Kling D., Sanchirico J.N., Sims C., and Springborn M. (2018). *The Treatment of Uncertainty and Learning in the Economics of Natural Resource and Environmental Management*. Review of Environmental Economics and Policy 12(1) pp. 92–112.

Lurie N., Wasserman J., and Nelson C. (2006). *Public Health Preparedness: Evolution or Revolution?* Health Affairs 25 4. Accessed at: http://www.healthaffairs.org/doi/10.1377/hlthaff.25.4.935

Kadam A. (2003). *Secure View: Because Business Must Go On*. Network Magazine August 2003. Accessed at: http://www.networkmagazineindia.com/200308/security2.shtml.

Kak V. (2015). Infections on Cruise Ships. Microbiology Spectrum 3(4) DOI: https://doi.org/10.1128/microbiolspec.IOL5-0007-2015.

Kan B., Wang M., Jing H., Xu H., Jian X., et al. (2005). *Molecular Evolution Analysis and Geographic Investigation of Severe Acute Respiratory Syndrome Coronavirus-Like Virus in Palm Civets at an Animal Market and on Farms*. Journal of Virology 79(18) pp. 11892-11900.

Kaina B. (2021). *On the Origin of SARS-CoV-2: Did Cell Culture Experiments Lead to Increased Virulence of the Progenitor Virus for Humans?* In Vivo 35 pp.1313-1326.

Kalra N., Hallegatte S., Lempert R., Brown C., Fozzard A., Gill S., and Shah A. (2014). *Agreeing on Robust Decisions New Processes for Decision Making Under Deep Uncertainty*. Policy Research Working Paper 6906. The World Bank, Climate Change Group Office of the Chief Economist June 2014. Accessed at: https://openknowledge.worldbank.org/bitstream/handle/10986/18772/WPS6906.pdf

Kamradt-Scott A. (2018). *What Went Wrong? The World Health Organisation from Swine Flu to Ebola*. In: Political Mistakes and Policy Failures in International Relations pp. 193-215, (Editors: A. Kruck, K. Oppermann, and A. Spencer). Palgrave Macmillan, Cham.

Kaplan R.S. and Mikes A. (2012). *Managing Risk: A New Framework*. Harvard Business Review June 2012.

Karpin J. (2020). *Government Has Failed Victoria and Victoria Has Failed Government*. Spectator Australia 6 August 2020. Accessed at:
https://www.spectator.com.au/2020/08/government-has-failed-victoria-and-victoria-has-failed-government/.

Kapucu N. and Garayev V. (2011) *Collaborative Decision-Making in Emergency and Disaster Management*. International Journal of Public Administration 34 pp. 366-375.

Kapucu N. and Ustun Y. (2018). *Collaborative Crisis Management and Leadership in the Public Sector*. International Journal of Public Administration 41(7) pp. 548-561.

Kahneman D., 2011. Thinking, Fast and Slow. Macmillan, Basingstoke, UK.

Kamradtt-Scott A. and Roper K. (2020). *Coronavirus Pandemic Shows it's time for an Australian Centre for Disease Control in Darwin*. The Conversation, accessed at:
https://theconversation.com/coronavirus-pandemic-shows-its-time-for-an-australian-centre-for-disease-control-in-darwin-138724.

Karelaia N. and Van der Heyden L. (2020). *Leading in Wicked Times: A Shift to Inquiry, Humility, Fairness*. Working paper 2020/55/DSC/TOM, Insead. Accessed at:
https://sites.insead.edu/facultyresearch/research/doc.cfm?c=1789&did=67197&disciplines=36&field_cs_publication_date%5Bmax%5D=&field_cs_publication_date%5Bmin%5D=&op=&search=Blue%20Ocean%20Strategy

Karpin J. (2020). *Government has Failed Victoria – and Victoria Has Failed Government*. The Spectator, 6 August 2020. Accessed at:
https://www.spectator.com.au/2020/08/government-has-failed-victoria-and-victoria-has-failed-government/

Katz R., Attal-Juncqua A., and Fischer J.E. (2017). *Funding Public Health Emergency Preparedness in the United States*. AJPH Policy 107(Suppl 2) pp. S148-S152.

Kahneman D. and Sibony O. (2021). *Noise: A Flaw in Human Judgement*. Hatchett Book Group.

Kaufmann D. (2020). *What the Pandemic Reveals About Governance, State Capture and Natural Resources*. Brookings Institution, 10 July 2020. Accessed at:
https://www.brookings.edu/blog/future-development/2020/07/10/what-the-pandemic-reveals-about-governance-state-capture-and-natural-resources/.

Kaul V., Shah V.H., and El-Serag H. (2020). *Leadership During Crisis: Lessons and Applications from the COVID-19 Pandemic*. Gastroenterology 159 pp. 809-812.

Kavanagh K. (2022a). *Evidence Shows Students Need to Wear Masks in Schools Despite Misinformation*. Infection Control Today, 15 March 2022. Accessed at:
https://www.infectioncontroltoday.com/view/evidence-shows-students-need-wear-masks-schools-despite-disinformation.

Kavanagh K. (2022b). *Viewpoint: Those Who Underestimate Omicron Aren't Doing the Math*. Infection Control Today, 5 January 2022. Accessed at:
https://www.infectioncontroltoday.com/view/viewpoint-those-who-underestimate-omicron-aren-t-doing-the-math.

Kealy E. (2022). *Questions Silenced as Victorian Labor Side-steps Allegations of Bullying, Toxic Treatment of Women*. Nationals for Regional Victoria. 9 March 2022. Accessed at:
https://vic.nationals.org.au/media-releases/questions-silenced-as-victorian-labor-side-steps-allegations-of-bullying-toxic-treatment-of-women/.

Keen P.K., Gilkey R., and Baker E.L. (2020). *Crisis Leadership—From the Haiti Earthquake to the COVID Pandemic*. Journal of Public Health Management Practice 26(5) pp. 503-505.

Kemp D. (2020). Australia's Greatest Governance Fail. Australian Financial Review, 6 August 2020. Accessed at: https://www.afr.com/policy/economy/australia-s-greatest-governance-fail-20200806-p55j0j.
Kemp S. and Dwyer L. (2001). *An Examination of Organisational Culture – The Regent Hotel, Sydney*. Hospitality Management 20 pp. 77-93.
Kernebone E. (2020). *Bendigo Ambulance Victoria Former Manager Voices Harassment Experience*. Canberra Times, 6 November 2020. Accessed at:
https://www.canberratimes.com.au/story/7001063/bullying-drove-her-out-of-ambulance-victoria-now-she-wants-others-to-speak-up/.
Kerrisey M.J. and Edmondson A.C. (2020). *What Good Leadership Looks Like During This Pandemic*. Harvard Business Review 13 April 2020.
Khalid A.F., Lavis J.N., El-Jardali F., and Vanstone M. (2020). *Supporting the Use of Research Evidence in*
Decision-making in Crisis Zones in Low- and Middle-income Countries: A Critical Interpretive Synthesis. Health Research Policy and Systems 18 Article 21.
Khan Y., O'Sullivan T., Brown A., Tracey S., Gibson J., Généreux M., Henry B., and Schwartz B. (2018). *Public Health Emergency Preparedness: A Framework to Promote Resilience.* BMC Public Health 18 Article 1344.
Khan Y., Brown A.D., Gagliardi A.R., O'Sullivan T., Lacarte S., Henry B., and Schwartz B. (2019) Are We Prepared? The Development of Performance Indicators for Public Health Emergency Preparedness Using a Modified Delphi Approach. PLoS ONE 14(12) Article e0226489.
Kharroubi S. and Saleh F. (2020). *Are Lockdown Measures Effective Against COVID-19?* Frontiers in Public Health doi.org/10.3389/fpubh.2020.549692.
Kiehl K. (2018). *The Psychopath Whisperer: Inside the Minds of Those Without Conscience*. Oneworld Publications, London UK.
Kilbourne E.D. *Influenza Pandemics of the 20th Century*. Emerging Infectious Diseases 12(1) pp. 9-14.
Kiley D. (2017). *VW Shareholders Demand Transparency That is Not Coming*. Forbes, 11 May 2017.
Killey I.D. (2017). *Police and the Executive. Thesis*. Victoria University, Melbourne, Australia.
Kim K.H., Tandi T.E., Choi J.W., Moon J.M., and Kim M.S. (2017). *Middle East Respiratory Syndrome Coronavirus (MERS-CoV) Outbreak in South Korea, 2015: Epidemiology, Characteristics and Public Health Implications*. The Journal of Hospital Infection 95(2) pp. 207-213.
Kim Y., Ku M., and Soo Oh S. (2020). *Public Health Emergency Response Coordination: Putting the Plan into Practice*. Journal of Risk Research, 23(7-8) pp. 928-944.
Kitayama S., Varnum M.E.W., and Salavador C.E. (2019). *Cultural Neuroscience.*
In: Handbook of Cultural Psychology (Editors: D. Cohen and S. Kitayama) pp. 79–118. The Guilford Press.
Klarskov Jeppesen K and Leder C. (2016). *Auditors' Experience with Corporate Psychopaths*. Journal of Financial Crime 23(4) pp. 870-881.
Kleczkowski A. (2022). *Did the COVID Lockdowns Work? Here's What We Know Two Years On*. The Conversation, 24 March 2022. Accessed at:
https://theconversation.com/did-the-covid-lockdowns-work-heres-what-we-know-two-years-on-176623.
Klein G. (1998). *Sources of Power: How People Make Decisions.*: MIT Press, Cambridge, MA.
Kline R. (2019). *Leadership in the NHS.* BMJ Leader 3(4) pp. 129-132.
Klippenstein M. and Pardy B. (2019). *How Social Justice Ideologues Hijacked a Legal Regulator*. Quillette, 11 February 2019. Accessed at:

https://quillette.com/2019/02/11/how-social-justice-ideologues-hijacked-a-legal-regulator/.
Knapton S. (2022). *Scientists Believed That COVID Leaked From Wuhan Lab – but Feared Debate Could Hurt 'International Harmony'.* The Telegraph, 11 January 2022. Accessed at: https://www.telegraph.co.uk/news/2022/01/11/scientists-believed-covid-leaked-wuhan-lab-feared-debate-could/.
Knauss C. (2019). *Murdoch University Sues Whistleblower After Comments on International Students*. The Guardian, 11 October 2019. Accessed at: https://www.theguardian.com/australia-news/2019/oct/11/murdoch-university-sues-whistleblower-after-comments-on-international-students.
Knibbs J. (2017). *Are Sonic and Primary Sitting on Digital Health Progress?* Medical Republic, 21 April 2017. Accessed at: https://medicalrepublic.com.au/sonic-primary-sitting-digital-health-progress/8562.
Knudson W.A. (2008). *The Environment, Energy, and the Tinbergen Rule*. Bulletin of Science, Technology and Society 29(4) pp. 308-312.
Koehn N. (2020). *Real Leaders are Forged in Crisis*. Harvard Business Review, 3 April 2020.
Kolovos B. (2020a). *Treat Andrews Claims with Caution: Mikakos*. The Canberra Times 9 October 2020. Accessed at: https://www.canberratimes.com.au/story/6961317/treat-andrews-claims-with-caution-mikakos/.
Kolovos B. (2020b*). Vic CHO Wanted Review of Hotel Quarantine*. The Canberra Times, 16 September 2020. Accessed at: https://www.canberratimes.com.au/story/6926948/vic-cho-wanted-review-of-hotel-quarantine/.
Kolovos C. (2020c). *Uncertainty Over Who Ran Vic Quarantine*. Australian Associated Press 11 September 2020. Accessed at : https://www.wellingtontimes.com.au/story/6920247/uncertainty-over-who-ran-vic-quarantine/.
Kolovos B. (2020d). *Vic Premier Says He Couldn't Stop Protests*. The Canberra Times, 9 June 2020. Accessed at: https://www.canberratimes.com.au/story/6786602/vic-premier-says-he-couldnt-stop-protests/.
Kolovos B. (2020e). *Coronavirus Victoria: Melbourne Public Housing Tower Residents Claim Food Shortage in Lockdown*. Perth Now, 7 July 2020. Accessed at: https://www.perthnow.com.au/news/vic/coronavirus-victoria-melbourne-public-housing-tower-residents-claim-food-shortage-in-lockdown-ng-b881601282z.
Kolovos B. and McGowan M. (2022). *QR Code Check-ins 'Useless' in Australia's Omicron Wave but Experts Urge for Them to Stay*. The Guardian, 27 January 2022. Accessed at: https://www.theguardian.com/australia-news/2022/jan/27/qr-code-check-ins-useless-in-australias-omicron-wave-but-experts-urge-for-them-to-stay.
Kolovos B. (2023). *Victorian Government Hired Lawyers Weeks Before Commonwealth Games Cancellation*. The Guardian, 4th October 2023. Accessed at: https://www.theguardian.com/australia-news/2023/oct/04/commonwealth-games-cancellation-2026-victoria-government-hired-lawyers#:~:text=Victorian%20government%20hired%20lawyers%20weeks%20before%20Commonwealth%20Games%20cancellation,-Law%20firm%20was&text=The%20Victorian%20premier%2C%20Jacinta%20Allan,the%20event%20would%20go%20ahead.
Kontovas C.A. and Psaraftis H.N. (2009). *Formal Safety Assessment: A Critical Review*. Marine Technology 46 pp. 45–59.

Koob S.F. (2020). *Police Stand by Arrest of Pregnant Mum but Handcuffing Stokes Debate*. The Age, 3 September 2020. Accessed at: https://www.theage.com.au/national/victoria/pregnant-ballarat-mum-blames-bimbo-moment-for-lockdown-protest-20200903-p55rz1.html.

Korać S. (2016). *Police Organisational Culture: "Cloud" Over Good Ethical Decision Making?* In: Thematic Conference Proceedings of International Significance, Volume II, pp. 173-183. Academy of Criminalistic and Police Studies, Belgrade.

Körner M., Wirtz M.A., Bengel J., and Göritz A. (2015). *Relationship of Organizational Culture, Teamwork and Job Satisfaction in Interprofessional Teams*. BMC Health Services Research. 14 Article 243.

Kornilova T. and Krasavtseva Y. (2017). *Role of the Dark Triad Traits and Attitude Towards Uncertainty in Decision-Making Strategies in Managers*. Social Sciences 6(6) pp. 187-195.

Kosonen P. (2014). *Corporate Psychopaths Talk Their Way Up*. The Glasgow Insight into Science and Technology. Accessed at: https://the-gist.org/2014/10/corporate-psychopaths-talk-their-way-up/#easy-footnote-bottom-2-4964.

Kozasa E.H., Lacerda S.S., Polissici M.A., da Silva Coelho R., da Silva Farias G., Chaves P., and Leão E.R. (2020). *An Intervention to Increase Situational Awareness and the Culture of Mutual Care (Foco) and Its Effects During COVID-19 Pandemic: A Randomized Controlled Trial and Qualitative Analysis*. Frontiers in Psychology 11 Article 570786.

Kovács G., Moshtari M., Kachali H., and Polsa P. (2019). *Research Methods in Humanitarian Logistics*. Journal of Humanitarian Logistics and Supply Chain Management 9 pp. 325–331.

Koskinen-Kannisto A. (2013). *Situational Awareness Concept in a Multinational Collaboration Environment*. Department of Military Technology, National Defense University, Helsinki, Finland.

Kryola M. (2021). *Do Lockdowns Make a Difference in a Pandemic?* C2C Journal, 20 March, 2021. Accessed at: https://c2cjournal.ca/2021/03/do-lockdowns-make-a-difference-in-a-pandemic/.

Kuchipudi S.V. (2020). *Why So Many Epidemics Originate in Asia and Africa*. US News 4 March 2020. Accessed at: https://www.usnews.com/news/best-countries/articles/2020-03-04/why-so-many-epidemics-originate-in-asia-and-africa.

Kurtz R.S. (2020). *Piper Alpha and Deepwater Horizon – Coincidence of Causation or Failure of Lessons Learned.* Accessed at: https://www.researchgate.net/publication/343167589_Piper_Alpha_and_Deepwater_Horizon_-Coincidence_of_Causation_or_Failure_of_Lessons_Learned.

Kwan C. (2020). *Victoria was not Fit to deal with COVID-19 and 'Misguided' in Choosing IBM Health Tracing*. ZDNet, 14 December 2020. Accessed at: https://www.zdnet.com/article/victoria-was-not-fit-to-deal-with-covid-19-and-misguided-in-choosing-ibm-health-tracing/.

Lackey B. and Parsons L. (2021). *Snarky Dan Andrews Refuses to Answer Questions About Nebuliser Which Sparked New Covid Cluster and Passes the Buck to his Quarantine Boss Instead - Leaving Her to be Grilled Over the Debacle*. Daily Mail Australia 13 February 2021. Accessed at: https://www.dailymail.co.uk/news/article-9256207/Dan-Andrews-REFUSES-answer-questions-man-ICU-accused-starting-outbreak.html.

Lane S. (2018). *Our Politicians Are Using Royal Commissions to Handball Big Issues They Can't Solve*. ABC, 18 September 2018. Accessed at: https://www.abc.net.au/news/2018-09-18/analysis-politicians-handballing-big-issues-to-royal-commissions/10262988.

Lapinski M.K. and Rimal R.N. (2005). *An Explication of Social Norms*. Communication Theory 15(2) pp. 127-147.

Lathouris O. (2021). *Returned Traveller Blamed for Melbourne Virus Outbreak Feels 'Like a Criminal' After Being Allowed to Use Nebuliser in Quarantine Hotel.* 9 News, 13 February 2021. Accessed at: https://www.9news.com.au/national/coronavirus-melbourne-return-traveller-blamed-for-holiday-inn-cluster-feels-like-criminal-after-using-nebuliser/6a8657c5-4442-4c6b-ada3-64658ff535bc.

Lauder M. (2018). *It Should Never Happen Again: The Failure of Inquiries and Commissions to Enhance Risk Governance*. Gower Publishing, Farnham UK.

Laur C.V., Agarwal P., Mukerji G., Goulbourne E., Baranek H., Pus L., Bhatia R.S., Martin D., and Bhattacharyya O. (2021). *Building Health Services in a Rapidly Changing Landscape: Lessons in Adaptive Leadership and Pivots in a COVID-19 Remote Monitoring Program*. Journal of Medical Internet Research 23(1) Article e25507.

Lee A.C.K. (2015). *Developing Evidence-Based Practice in Emergency Planning and Management*. PhD Thesis, University of Sheffield, UK.

Lee V.K. and Harris L.T. *How Social Cognition Can Inform Social Decision-making*. Frontiers in Neuroscience 7 Article 259.

Le Grand C. (2020a). *Victoria Abandoned Pandemic Plan by Failing to Put Sutton in Key Role*. The Sydney Morning Herald, 14 August 2020. Accessed at: https://www.smh.com.au/national/victoria-abandoned-pandemic-plan-by-failing-to-put-sutton-in-key-role-20200814-p55lxf.html.

Le Grand C. (2020b). *'He Did Not Even Glance at Him': The Day that Brett Sutton Felt the Inside of the Premier's 'Freezer'*. The Age, 11 December 2020. Accessed at: https://www.theage.com.au/national/victoria/how-we-beat-covid-part-one-the-way-in-20201210-p56mdr.html.

Le Grand C. and Cooper A. (2019). *Very Dark Corners': Former Top Cop Makes Dramatic Claims About Police. The Age 13 December 2019*. Accessed at: https://www.theage.com.au/national/victoria/very-dark-corners-former-top-cop-makes-dramatic-claims-about-police-20191213-p53jvo.html.

Le Grand C. and Sakkal P. (2021). *The Chosen Few: How Victoria is Really Governed*. The Age, 14 August 2021. Accessed at: https://www.theage.com.au/politics/victoria/the-chosen-few-how-victoria-is-really-governed-20210803-p58fk4.html.

Le Grand C., Houston C., and Sakkal P. (2021). *Running with Foxes: Daniel's Dining and Dealings with 'go-to billionaire'*. The Age, 27 February 2021. Accessed at: https://www.theage.com.au/politics/victoria/running-with-foxes-daniel-s-dining-and-dealings-with-go-to-billionaire-20210225-p575yu.html.

Leigh A. (2016). *Ethical Fading: Is it Happening Right Under Your Nose*. Ethical Leadership. Accessed at: https://www.ethical-leadership.co.uk/ethical-fading/.

Leigh M. (2016). *Critical Thinking in Crisis Management*. Emergency Planning College Occasional Papers New Series Number 15, August 2016.

Leland F. (2009). *Critical Decision Making Under Pressure*. The Homeland Security Review 3(1) pp. 43-72.

Le May R. (2011a). *Vic Government IT in Flames: $1.4 Billion Over Budget, All Projects Late or Failed*. Delimiter. 23 November 2011. Accessed at: http://delimiter.com.au/2011/11/23/vic-government-it-in-flames-1-4-billion-over-budget-all-projects-late-or-failed/.

LeMay R. (2011b). *Breaking Victoria's IT Fail Cycle: What Not to Do*. Delimiter, 28 November 2011. Accessed at: https://delimiter.com.au/2011/11/28/breaking-victorias-it-fail-cycle-what-not-to-do/.

Leppänen I., Hämäläinen R.P., ·Saarinen E., and Viinikainen M. (2018). *Intrapersonal Emotional Responses to the Inquiry and Advocacy Modes of Interaction: A Psychophysiological Study.* Group Decision and Negotiation 27 pp. 933-948.

Lewis A. (2021). *Good Leadership? It All Starts with Trust.* Harvard Business Publishing, 4 March, 2021. Accessed at: https://www.harvardbusiness.org/good-leadership-it-all-starts-with-trust/.

Lewis C. (2019). *Appointment of Assistant Commissioner is Just Plain Wrong.* The Age, 4 December 2019. Accessed at: https://www.theage.com.au/politics/victoria/appointment-of-assistant-commissioner-is-just-plain-wrong-20191203-p53ggp.html.

Lewis H. (2020a). *How Capitalism Drives Cancel Culture.* The Atlantic, 14 July 2020. Accessed at: https://www.theatlantic.com/international/archive/2020/07/cancel-culture-and-problem-woke-capitalism/614086/.

Lewis J. **(**2020b). *New Police Powers After 'State of Disaster' Declaration.* Star Observer, 4 August 2020. Accessed at: https://www.starobserver.com.au/news/new-police-powers-after-state-of-disaster-declaration/197020.

Leslie L. (2014). *Ebola – The Classic Creeping Crisis.* Disaster Recovery Journal Blogs. Accessed on 8 July 2017 at: https://www.drj.com/myblog/ebola-the-classic-creeping-crisis.html.

Li F. (2016). *Structure, Function, Evolution of Coronavirus Spike Proteins.* Annual Review of Virology 3 pp. 237-261.

Li N., Huang J., Feng Y., Huang K., and Cheng G. (2020). *A Review of Naturalistic Decision-making and its Applications to the Future Military.* IEEE Access 8 pp. 38276- 38284.

Liddell B. (2018). *Culture May Affect the Way Your Brain Processes Everything. Here's Why That's Important.* ABC Science, 17 August 2018. Accessed at: https://www.abc.net.au/news/science/2018-08-17/culture-may-affect-the-way-your-brain-processes-everything/10120068.

Light P.C. (2008). *Predicting Organizational Crisis Readiness: Perspectives and Practices Toward a Pathway to Preparedness.* NYU Center for Catastrophe and Preparedness and Response and the Public Entity Research Institute, New York, NY.

Lin L.C. and Telzer E.H. (2017). *An Introduction to Cultural Neuroscience.* In: The Handbook of Culture and Biology pp. 1-29, (Editors: J.M Causadias, E.H. Telzer, and Gonzales N.A). John Wiley and Sons Inc.

Lindeberg M.F. and Krasnici V. (2020). *Strategic Thinking in Crisis Management: A Study into How Organisations Use Strategic Thinking to Overcome Unusually Demanding Situations.* School of Business, Economics, and Statistics, Umeå University, Sweden.

Liotta M. (2020). *Tower Lockdown 'Confusion and Distress' could have been Prevented: GP.* News GP, Royal Australian College of General Practitioners. Accessed at: https://www1.racgp.org.au/newsgp/clinical/tower-lockdown-confusion-and-distress-could-have-b.

Lipman-Blumen J. (2005). *The Allure of Toxic Leaders: Why Followers Rarely Escape Their Clutches.* Ivey Business Journal January/ February 2005.

Liu B.F., Iles I.A., and Herovic E. (2020). *Leadership Under Fire: How Governments Manage Crisis Communication.* Communication Studies, 71(1) pp. 128-147.

Liu M. (2017). *Is China Ground Zero for a Future Pandemic?* Smithsonian Magazine, November 2017. Accessed at: https://www.smithsonianmag.com/science-nature/china-ground-zero-future-pandemic-180965213/.

LGiU (2015). *Care and Continuity: Contingency Planning for Provider Failure*. A Guide for Local Authorities. Local Government Information Unit, London.

Longbottom J. (2021). *Victorian Contact Tracing Still Plagued by 'Infuriating' Data Errors, Contractors Say*. ABC News, 25 February 2021. Accessed at: https://www.abc.net.au/news/2021-02-25/victoria-coronavirus-contact-tracers-concerns-cake-shop/13186678.

Lathouris O. (2020). *'Absolutely Devastating': Daniel Andrew Slammed Over 'Crippling' Coronavirus Restrictions*. Nine News, 20 October 2020. Accessed at: https://www.9news.com.au/national/coronavirus-liberals-slam-daniel-andrews-crippling-small-businesses-covid19-lockdown-restrictions/4ddbf575-1ece-454d-ba15-bd15f0ad0f42.

Li Q, Guan X., Wu P., Wang X., Zhou L., Tong Y, Ren R., Leung K.S.M, Lau E.H.Y., Wong J.Y., Xing X., Xiang N., Wu Y., Li C., Chen Q., Li D., Liu T., Zhao J. Liu M., Tu W., Chen C., Jin L., Yang R., WangQ., Zhou S., Wang R., Liu H., Luo Y., Liu Y., Shao G., Li H., Tao Z., Yang Y., Deng Z., Liu B., Ma Z., Zhang Y. , Shi G., Lam T.T.Y., Wu J.T., Gao G.F., Cowling B.J., Yang B., Leung G.M., and Feng Z. (2020). *Early Transmission Dynamics in Wuhan, China, of Novel Coronavirus-infected Pneumonia*. New England Journal of Medicine 382(13) pp.1199–1207.

Lipman-Blumen J. (2005). *Toxic leadership*. In: Political and Civic Leadership, Part VIII, The Psychology of Political and Civic Leadership pp. 652-660, (Edited by: R.A. Couto). Sage Publishing.

Lucas C. (2020). *St Basil's and Epping Gardens Review 'Not Independent', Say Experts, Families*. The Age, 1 January 2021, Accessed at: https://www.theage.com.au/politics/victoria/st-basil-s-and-epping-gardens-review-not-independent-say-experts-families-20201230-p56qsp.html.

Lucas C. and Clune R. (2020). Report *into St Basil's and Epping Gardens COVID-19 Outbreaks Highlights Failures*. The Sydney Morning Herald, 21 December 2020. Accessed at: https://www.smh.com.au/politics/federal/report-into-st-basil-s-and-epping-gardens-covid-19-outbreaks-highlights-failures-20201221-p56pcw.html.

Lucas F. *The Ripple Effect of Toxic Leadership in Education Settings: New Analysis from USyd*. The Sector13 September 2019. Accessed at: https://thesector.com.au/2019/09/13/the-ripple-effect-of-toxic-leadership-in-education-settings-new-analysis-from-usyd/.

Lucas H.C. and Goh J.M. (2009). *Disruptive Technology: How Kodak Missed the Digital Photography Revolution*. Journal of Strategic Information Systems 18 pp. 46-55.

Lucas C. and Kline T. (2008). *Understandıng the Influence of Organizational Culture and Group Dynamics on Organizational Change and Learning*. The Learning Organisation 15(3) pp. 277-287.

Lundberg J., Rollenhagen C., Hollnagel E., and Rankin A., (2012). *Strategies for Dealing with Resistance to Recommendations from Accident Investigations*. Accident Analysis and Prevention 45 pp. 455–467.

Luscombe B. (2020). *A Year After Christchurch, Jacinda Ardern has the World's Attention. How Will She Use It?* Time Magazine, 20 February 2020.

Ma J. (2020). *China's First Confirmed Covid-19 Case Traced Back to November 17*. South China Morning
Post, 13 March 2020. Accessed at: www.scmp.com/news/china/society/article/3074991/coronavirus-chinas-first-confirmed-covid-19-case-traced-back.

McCall G. (2021). *How Toxic Cultures Impact Organisations*. TJ, Training Journal, 26 November 2021. Accessed at:

https://www.trainingjournal.com/articles/features/how-toxic-working-cultures-impact-organisations.

McCallum J. (2019). *Where Next for Royal Commissions? Try Social Issues.* In The Black, 1 October 2019. Accessed at: https://www.intheblack.com/articles/2019/10/01/where-to-next-for-royal-commissions.

McCalla-Chen D. (2000). *Towards an Understanding of the Concept of Non-Decision Making and its Manifestation in the Schools Sector.* Educational Management and Administration 28(1) pp. 33-46.

McCaul M.T. (2020). *The Origins of the Covid-19 Global Pandemic, including the Roles of the Chinese Communist Party and The World Health Organization.* House Foreign Affairs Committee Minority Staff Report. Final Report. 116 Congress. Washington DC.

McCauley D. (2020). *'Failure of Leadership': Health Workers Denied Access to PPE.* The Sydney Morning Herald 21 September 2020. Accessed at: https://www.smh.com.au/politics/federal/failure-of-leadership-health-workers-denied-proper-gear-20200918-p55x10.html.

McCulloch D. (2020). *Andrews Pledges Exit Plan After Pressure.* The Canberra Times, 31 August 2020. Accessed at: https://www.canberratimes.com.au/story/6902056/andrews-pledges-exit-plan-after-pressure/.

McGubbing G. (2021). *Vic Treasurer Says Lockdown Cost Unknown.* 7 News, 27 May 2021. Accessed at: https://7news.com.au/lifestyle/health-wellbeing/tim-pallas-weathers-lockdown-grilling-c-2944031.

McQuire G. (2020). Modelling Victoria's Second Wave of COVID 19 Cases. Taylor Fry, 24 September 2020. Accessed at: https://taylorfry.com.au/articles/covid-19-in-victoria-modelling-the-second-wave/.

Macdonald D. (2021). *The Wet Market Sources of Covid-19: Bats and Pangolins Have an Alibi.* Oxfrod University News Blog. Oxford UK. Accessed at: https://www.ox.ac.uk/news/science-blog/wet-market-sources-covid-19-bats-and-pangolins-have-alibi.

MacLean J.P., Campbell G., and Seals S. (2004). *Analysis of the Columbia Shuttle Disaster—Anatomy of a Flawed Investigation in a Pathological Organization.* Journal of Scientific Exploration 18(2) pp. 187–215.

Mclellan P., Coate J., Atkinson B., Fitgerald R., Milroy H., Murray A. (2017) *Our Inquiry: Final Report. Royal Commission into Institutional Response to Child Sexual Abuse.* Commonwealth of Australia, Canberra, Australia.

McConnell A. and Stark A. (2002). *Foot-and-Mouth 2001: The Politics of Crisis Management.* Parliamentary Affairs 55 pp.664-781, Hansard Society for Parliamentary Government.

McCracken J. and Ahmed A. (2020). *Sick Politics at the Heart of Public Health England Closure.* The Guardian 21 August 2020.

McGhee A. (2020). *Public Housing Tenants Caught Out by Victoria's Sudden COVID-19 Lockdown of Tower Blocks.* https://www.abc.net.au/news/2020-07-07/covid-19-lockdown-catches-tower-public-tenants-by-surprise/12426804.

McGinn D. (2015). *What Companies can Learn from Military Teams.* Harvard Business Review 6 August 2015. Accessed at: https://hbr.org/2015/08/what-companies-can-learn-from-military-teams on 30 June 2018.

McGinn C. (2019a). *Vic Launches Review into Private Security.* Canberra Times 10 June 2019. Accessed at: https://www.canberratimes.com.au/story/6208002/vic-launches-review-into-private-security/.

McGinn C. (2019b). *MFB Top Firefighter Pulls Pin on Vic Job*. Canberra Times, 12 July 2019. Accessed at: https://www.canberratimes.com.au/story/6271942/mfb-top-firefighter-pulls-pin-on-vic-job/.

McGuinness J. 2020. *4 COVID-19 Leadership Lessons*. Chief Executive 12 May. Accessed at: https://chief executive.net/4-covid-19-leadership-lessons/.

McHugh F. (2021). *'I Don't Care': Berejiklian Defends Delayed Lockdown Amid Growing Criticism*. News.com.au, 27 June, 201. Accessed at: https://www.news.com.au/national/nsw-act/politics/barilaro-defends-berejiklian-after-premier-said-there-would-be-no-further-lockdowns/news-story/f4a188069c2c560fa05513616bcb74d1.

McIntyre C.R. (2011). *Public Health and Heath Reform in Australia.* Medical Journal of Australia. 194(1) pp.38-40 p.487.

McKenzie N. and Sakkal P. (2022). *Warrant Reveals IBAC Probing 'Suspected Corrupt Conduct' Between Andrews Government and Firefighters' Union*. The Age 23 February 2022. Accessed at: https://www.theage.com.au/politics/victoria/warrant-reveals-ibac-probing-suspected-corrupt-conduct-between-andrews-government-and-firefighters-union-20220221-p59ycd.html.

McKenzie N. Ilanbey S., and Sakkal P. (2021). *IBAC Scrutiny on Andrews Over Firefighters' Union Deal*. The Age, 6 October 2021. Accessed at: https://www.theage.com.au/politics/victoria/ibac-scrutiny-on-andrews-over-firefighters-union-deal-20211005-p58xhm.html.

McKeever A. (2022). *Do Masks Really harm Kids? Here's What the Science Says*. National Geographic, 18 February 2022. Accessed at: https://www.nationalgeographic.com/science/article/do-masks-really-harm-kids-heres-what-the-science-says.

McPhee E. and Coe C. (2021). *Traveller Accused of Sparking Melbourne's Hotel Quarantine Outbreak that led to a Five-day Lockdown by Using a Nebuliser Breaks His Silence as Secret Reports Suggests it was Not His Fault*. Daily Mail Australia 5 May 2021. Accessed at: https://www.dailymail.co.uk/news/article-9544597/Man-accused-sparking-Melbournes-five-day-lockdown-quarantine-breaks-silence.html.

Mahoney J. (2022). *Former Labor MP Emma Husar Slams Kristina Keneally's Treatment Saying She 'ostracised' and 'froze me out'*. Sky News, 21 March 2022. Accessed at: https://www.skynews.com.au/australia-news/politics/former-labor-mp-emma-husar-slams-kristina-keneallys-treatment-saying-she-ostracised-and-froze-me-out/news-story/9b8c40ded030c590abfc6f19b793d15b.

Maiden S. (2020). *Tapes Solve the Mystery of Victoria's COVID Hotel Whodunit. News.com.au, 27 September 2020*. Accessed at: https://www.news.com.au/world/coronavirus/australia/tapes-solve-the-mystery-of-victorias-covid-hotel-whodunit/news-story/68067f4af991a8dc15a962c5173a8283.

MALS (2020). *Statement of Concern: Police Use of Projectile Weapons*. Melbourne Activist Legal Support. Accessed at: https://melbactivistlegal.org.au/2021/08/22/statement-of-concern-police-use-of-projectile-weapons/.

Mallapaty S. (2022). *Where did Omicron Come From? Three Key Theories*. Nature, 28 January 2022.

Manadvilli A. (2003). *SARS Epidemic Unmasks Age-old Quarantine Conundrum.* Nature Medicine 9(5)

Manko R. (2021). *Judicial Decision-Making, Ideology and the Political: Towards an Agonistic Theory of Adjudication*. Law and Critique. Accessed at: https://doi.org/10.1007/s10978-021-09288-w.

Mannix L. (2021). *Victoria's QE Codes Badly Made, Developers Say*. The Age, 18 June 2021. Accessed at: https://www.theage.com.au/national/victoria/victoria-s-qr-codes-badly-made-developers-say-20210617-p581r6.html.

Mannix L. and Ilanbey S. (2020). *'Just Makes Logical Sense': Top Adviser Joins Calls to Move COVID-19 Quarantine Out of Big Cities*. The Sydney Morning Herald, 23 November 2020. Accessed at: https://www.smh.com.au/national/just-makes-logical-sense-top-adviser-joins-calls-to-move-covid-quarantine-out-of-big-cities-20201122-p56gun.html.

Markel H. (2020). *Will the Largest Quarantine in History Just Make Things Worse*? The New York Times, 27 January 2020. Access at: https://www.nytimes.com/2020/01/27/opinion/china-wuhan-virus-quarantine.html.

Marks R. (2021). Mutation in Highly Infectious Alpha Variant May Help Coronavirus Evade Immune System. University of California San Francisco, 17 June 2021. Accessed at: https://www.ucsf.edu/news/2021/06/420826/mutation-highly-infectious-alpha-variant-may-help-coronavirus-evade-immune.

Markson S. (2021a). *Wuhan Live Bat Video Contradicts WHO Investigation*. The Australian, 14 June 2021. Accessed at: https://www.theaustralian.com.au/nation/wuhan-live-bat-video-contradicts-who-investigation/news-story/3c9445445f7cd1e1ad0229665660b1df.

Markson S. (2021b). *Shocking Scale of China's Cover-up Exposed: What Really Happened in Wuhan*. News.com.au, 27 September 2021. Accessed at: https://www.news.com.au/entertainment/books-magazines/books/doctors-courage-and-official-coverup-exposed-in-exclusive-extract-from-what-really-happened-in-wuhan/news-story/45679ce050df46cc7c7112036c966bb2.

Markson S. (2021c). *WHO Wuhan Covid-19 probe's 'clear' Conflicts of Interest*. The Australian, 28 September 2021. Accessed at: https://www.theaustralian.com.au/world/who-wuhan-covid19-probes-clear-conflicts-of-interest/news-story/7e9f195aa4ac5ef08e9dc0b9af5c9328.

Markson S. and Mendes L. (2021). *Fauci led Push for Research at Wuhan Institute of Virology*. The Weekend Australian 5 September 2021. Accessed at: https://www.theaustralian.com.au/world/fauci-led-push-for-research-at-wuhan-institute-of-virology/news-story/31024790d0a83bb6398f40b9dc712b18.

Martin S. (2022). *Australian Government was Warned About Covid Testing Overburden Almost a Year Ago*. 7 January 2022. Accessed at: https://www.theguardian.com/australia-news/2022/jan/07/australian-government-was-warned-about-covid-testing-overburden-almost-a-year-ago.

Martins E.C. and Terblanche F. (2003). *Building Organisational Culture that Stimulates Creativity and Innovation*. European Journal of Innovation Management 6(1) pp. 64-74.

Martin G. (2021). *Protest, Policing and Law During COVID-19: On the Legality of Mass Gatherings in a Health Crisis*. Alternative Law Journal. https://doi.org/10.1177/1037969X211029963.

Mattera P. (2020). *Boeing: Corporate Rap Sheet*. Corporate Research Project. Accessed at: https://www.corp-research.org/boeing.

Maunder R., Hunter J., Vincent L., Bennett J., Peladeau N., Leszcz J., Dadavoy J., Verhaeghe L.M., Setinberg R., Mazzulli T. (2003). *The Immediate Psychological and Occupational*

Impact of the 2003 SARS Outbreak in a Teaching Hospital. Canadian Medical Association Journal 168(10) pp. 1245-1251.

Maurens D.M. and Fauci A.S. (2020). *Emerging Pandemic Diseases: How We Got COVID-19*. Cell 182(5) pp. 1077-1092.

Meadowcraft J. (2008). *Patients, Politics, and Power: Government Failure and the Politicization of UK Health Care*. Journal of Medicine and Philosophy 33(5) pp. 427-44.

Meehan M. (2022). *Vic CHO Not Asked About Third Dose Mandate*. Canberra Times, 1 February 2022. Accessed at: https://www.canberratimes.com.au/story/7601997/vic-cho-not-asked-about-third-dose-mandate/.

Mégarbane B., Bourasset F., and Schermann J.-M. (2020). *Is Lockdown Effective in Limiting SARS-CoV-2 Epidemic Progression?—a Cross-Country Comparative Evaluation Using Epidemiokinetic Tools*. Journal of General Internal Medicine 36(3) pp.746-752.

Meixner S. (2020). *Australia's Outbound Travel Ban is One of the Strictest Coronavirus Public Health Responses in the World*. ABC News 31 August 2020. Accessed at: https://www.abc.net.au/news/2020-08-31/coronavirus-covid-outbound-international-travel-ban-morrison/12605404.

Menachery V.D., Yount B.L., Debbink K., Agnihothram S., Gralinski L.E., Plante J.A., Graham R.L., Scobey T., Ge X.Y., Donaldson E.F., Randell S.H., Lanzavecchia A., Marasco W.A., Shi Z.L. and Baric R.S. (2015). *A SARS-like Cluster of Circulating Bat Coronaviruses Shows Potential for Human Emergence*. Nature Medicine 21(12) pp. 1508-1513.

Meng B., Ferreira I.A.T.M,, Abdullahi A., Goonawardane N., Saito A.,, Kimura I., Yamasoba D., Gerba P.P, Fatihi S., Rathore S. , Zepeda S.K., Papa G., Kemp S.A, Ikeda T., Toyoda M., Tan T.S, Kuramochi J., Mitsunaga S., Ueno T., Shirakawa K., Takaori-Kondo A., Brevini T., Mallery D.L., Charles O.J., CITIID-NIHR BioResource COVID-19 Collaboration, The Genotype to Phenotype Japan (G2P-Japan) Consortium, Ecuador-COVID19 Consortium, Bowen J.E., Joshi A., Walls A.C., Jackson L., Cele S., Martin D.,. Smith K.G.C., Bradley J., Briggs J.A.G., Choi J., Madissoon E., Meyer K., Mlcochova P., Ceron-Gutierrez L., Doffinger R., Teichmann S., Pizzuto M., de Marco A., Corti D., Sigal A., James L., Veesler D., Hosmillo M., Lee J.H., Sampaziotis F., Goodfellow I.G., Matheson N.J., Thukral L., Sato K., and Gupta R.K. (2022). *SARS-CoV-2 Omicron Spike Mediated Immune Escape and Tropism Shift*. BiRxiv preprint, 13 January 2022. https://doi.org/10.1101/2021.12.17.473248.

Mendez-Brito A., El Bcheraoui C., and Pozo-Martin F. (2021). *Systematic Review of Empirical Studies Comparing the Effectiveness of Non-pharmaceutical Interventions Against COVID-19*. Journal of Infection 83(3) pp. P281-293.

Menon K.U. and Goh K.T. *Transparency and Trust: Risk Communications and the Singapore Experience in Managing SARS*. Journal of Communication Management 9 pp. 375-83.

Michelle D S., Maier R., and Jardine C. (2018). *Damned If You Do, and Damned If You Don't: Communicating about Uncertainty and Evolving Science During the H1N1 Influenza Pandemic*. Journal of Risk Research.
DOI: 10.1080/13669877.2018.1459793.

Miller H.E. (2018). *Intuition and Decision Making for Crisis Situations*. In: The Routledge Companion to Risk, Crisis and Security in Business (Editor: K.J. Engemann). Routledge.

Millon D. (2003). *Who 'Caused' the Enron Debacle*. Washington and Lee Law Review 601 (1) pp. 310-329.

Mills T., Ward M., and Houston C. (2022). *Doubts Over Usefulness of QR Codes as Cases Spread, Close Contact Rules Change*. Accessed at: https://www.theage.com.au/politics/victoria/doubts-over-usefulness-of-qr-codes-as-cases-spread-close-contact-rules-change-20220102-p59lch.html.

Milne P. (2007). *Motivation, Incentives and Organisational Culture*. Journal of Knowledge Management 11(6) pp. 28-38.

Milsom P., Smith R., Baker P., and Walls H. (2020). *Corporate Power and the International Trade Regime Preventing Progressive Policy Action on Non-communicable Diseases: A Realist Review*. Health Policy and Planning 2020 pp. 1-16.

Mimis S. (2022) *State Governments Warned Six Months Ago About Rapid Antigen Test Shortages*. A Current Affair, 12 January 2022. Accessed at: https://9now.nine.com.au/a-current-affair/coronavirus-aussie-emergency-physician-ian-norton-says-rapid-antigen-test-shortage-could-have-been-avoided/502bcfe9-39dc-48d4-a83b-b8a883c45bb8.

Minear T. (2018). *Police Investigation into Labor's Rorts-for-Votes Schemes "Set Up to Fail"*. AMP News, 22 November 2018. Accessed at: https://amp.news.com.au/police-investigation-into-labors-rorts-for-votes-set-up-to-fail/news-story/6e02439f26c66d15dffe15de768fed3a.

Ministry of Health (2020). *Fifth Case of COVID-19 Fits Pattern of Previous Case*. Media Release, 5 March 2020, Ministry of Health. Accessed at: https://www.health.govt.nz/news-media/media-releases/fifth-case-covid-19-fits-pattern-previous-case.

Minooee A. and Rickman L.S. (1999). *Infectious Diseases on Cruise Ships*. Clinical Infectious Diseases 29 pp. 737-44.

Minsky S. *The Wells Fargo Scandal is a Failure in Risk Management*. Accessed at: https://www.logicmanager.com/erm-software/2016/09/20/wells-fargo-scandal-risk-management/.

Mintron M., O'Neill D., and O'Connor R. (2021). *We Have Studied 50 Years of Royal Commissions – Here's How They Make a Difference*. The Conversation, 21 April 2021. Accessed at: https://theconversation.com/we-studied-50-years-of-royal-commissions-heres-how-they-make-a-difference-159231.

Mintz A. and Wayne C. (2014). *Group Decision Making in Conflict: From Groupthink to Polythink in the War in Iraq*. In: The Handbook of Conflict Resolution: Theory and Practice pp. 331–352. (Editors: P. T. Coleman, M. Deutsch, and E. C. Marcus). Jossey-Bass/Wiley.

Mintz A. and Barr K. (2021). *Rethinking Group Dynamics: The Cuban Missile Crisis Revisited*. In: The Cambridge Handbook of Pollical Psychology, (Editors: D. Osborne and C. Sibley), Cambridge University Press, Cambridge, UK.

Mirage (2021a). *Man Killed in Farming Accident*. Live WorkSafe Victoria News, 15 December 2021. Accessed at: https://www.miragenews.com/tag/worksafe-victoria/.

Mirage (2021b). *Operator Charged After Car Wash Fatality*. Live WorkSafe Victoria News, 2 December 2021. Accessed at: https://www.miragenews.com/operator-charged-after-car-wash-fatality-685371/.

Mirage (2021c). *Truck Driver Killed by Falling Road Barrier*. Live WorkSafe Victoria News, 29 November 2021. Accessed at: https://www.miragenews.com/truck-driver-killed-by-falling-road-barrier-682635/.

Mirage (2021d). *Driver Killed in Rollover Incident*. Live WorkSafe Victoria News, 25 November 2021. Accessed at: https://www.miragenews.com/driver-killed-in-rollover-incident-680991/.

Mirage (2021e). *WorkSafe Investigates Rollover Death*. Live WorkSafe Victoria News, 19 November 2021. Accessed at: https://www.miragenews.com/worksafe-investigates-rollover-death-677031/.

Mirage (2021f). *WorkSafe Investigates Road Worker Death*. Live WorkSafe Victoria News, 10 November 2021. Accessed at: https://www.miragenews.com/worksafe-investigates-road-worker-death-670181/.

Mitchel E. and O'Brian N.A. (2020*). Social Groups and Ideological Belief Systems. Fresh Evidence on an Old Theory*. Princeton University. Accessed at: https://csdp.princeton.edu/sites/csdp/files/media/mitchell_obrian_socialgroups_sept2020 .pdf.

Mitchell N. (2021). *'Vilified' Man with Nebuliser Speaks Out After Damning Report Reveals Hotel Quarantine Failings*. 3aw Radio, News Talk, 5 May 2021. Accessed at: https://www.3aw.com.au/vilified-man-with-nebuliser-speaks-out-after-damning-report-reveals-hotel-quarantine-failings/.

Mitchell T., Yu S., Liu X., Peel M. (2020). *China and Covid-19: What Went Wrong in Wuhan?* Financial Times. 18 October 2020. Accessed at: https://www.ft.com/content/82574e3d-1633-48ad-8afb-71ebb3fe3dee.

Mohelska H. and Sokolova M. (2015). *Organisational Culture and Leadership – Joint Vessels?* Procedia – Social and Behavioral Sciences 171 pp. 1011-1016.

Mohr D.C., Young G.J., and Burgess J.F. (2011). *Employee Turnover and Operational Performance: The Moderating Effect of Group-oriented Organisational Culture*. Human Resource Management Journal 22(2) pp. 216-233.

MOHW (2016). *2015 MERS White Paper*. Korea Institute for Health and Social Affairs, Ministry of Health and Welfare. Seoul, South Korea.

Moloney J. (2014). *Error Modelling in Anaesthesia: Slices of Swiss Cheese or Shavings of Parmesan*. British Journal of Anaesthesia 113(6) pp. 905–906.

Monat J.P. and Doremus S. (2018). *Deficiencies in and Alternatives to Heat Map Risk Matrices for Project Risk Prioritization.* The Journal of Modern Project Management 6(1) Article 11.

Montefiori D., Mohanan M., and Udayakumar K. (2021). *Failed Leadership, Late Assistance Behind India's COVID Crisis, Experts Say.* Campus News, Duke University. Accessed at: https://today.duke.edu/2021/05/failed-leadership-late-assistance-behind-india's-covid-crisis-experts-say.

Moore C. (2021). *Is Victoria Going 'Woke and Broke'? Inside Dan Andrews' Extraordinary Assault on Business as He's Accused of an 'Aggressive Tax Attack' That's Driven by an 'Envy of Success and Aspiration'*. Daily Mail Australia, 21 May 2021. Accessed at: https://www.dailymail.co.uk/news/article-9603273/Inside-Dan-Andrews-extraordinary-assault-business.html.

Moore G. (2021*). 'Toxic' Workplace Culture at Vic Prison*. 7 News, 21 May 2021. Accessed at: https://7news.com.au/news/crime/toxic-workplace-culture-at-vic-prison-c-2899549.

Mooren L., Grzebieta R.H., and Williamson A. (2009). *Lessons from Occupational Safety for Work Related Road Safety*. Road Safety Research, Policing and Education Conference, 10-13 November 2009, Sydney, New South Wales, Australia.

More H.W and More T.L. (2012). *Teams-Groups-Task Forces in Law Enforcement*: The Wave of the Future. Charles C. Thomas Publisher Ltd., Springfield, IL.

Morecombe J.D. (2018). *"They Day" Mayday*. Spectator, 6 August 2018. Accessed at: https://www.spectator.com.au/2018/08/they-day-mayday/.

Morgan C. (2021). *Second Ambulance 'Code Red' in a Week as Victoria Records 37,994 New COVID Cases, 13 Deaths*. The Age 11 January 2022. Accessed at: https://www.theage.com.au/national/victoria/second-ambulance-code-red-in-a-week-as-victoria-records-37-994-new-covid-cases-13-deaths-20220111-p59n9u.html.

Morgan P.B.C., Fletcher D. and Sarkar M., (2015). *Understanding Team Resilience in the World's Best Athletes: A Case of a Rugby Union World Cup Winning Team.* Psychology of Sport and Exercise 16 (1) pp. 91-100.

Morriss P. (1987) *Power: A Philosophical Analysis*. Manchester University Press, Manchester, UK.

Moynihan D.P. (2008). *The Network Governance of Crisis Response: Case Studies of Incident Command Systems*. a Follette School Working Paper No. 2008-020

MSAV (2018). *Public Hospitals and Private Pathology Providers*. Medical Scientists Association of Victoria, 18 January 2018. Accessed at: http://msav.org.au/news/public-hospitals-private-pathology/.

Mulholland E. (2017). *Pedestrian Signals, Pedestrian Thinking*. Institute of Public Affairs. 7 March 2017. Accessed at: https://ipa.org.au/publications-ipa/opinion/pedestrian-signals-pedestrian-thinking.

Mullane P. (2017). *What the Cuban Missile Crisis can Teach us about Decision-making*. Harvard Business Review Online 15 August 2017. Accessed at: https://online.hbs.edu/blog/post/what-the-cuban-missile-crisis-can-teach-us-about-decision-making.

Mumley W.E. (2019). *Organizational Culture and Ethical Decision-Making During Major Crises*. The Journal of Values-Based Leadership 12(2) Article 9.

Munro P. (2011). *Call to Take Politics Out of Top Police Appointments*. The Age, 8 May 2011. Accessed at: https://www.theage.com.au/national/victoria/call-to-take-politics-out-of-top-police-appointments-20110507-1edje.html.

Murray P. (2021). *Daniel Andrews 'banged on' about Gold Standard Days After Improvement Notices*. Herald Sun, 17 February 2021. Accessed at: https://www.heraldsun.com.au/news/national/daniel-andrews-banged-on-about-gold-standard-days-after-improvement-notices/video/146cc2611168d22c9af4f46ed8d84be1.

Murray S.K. and Cowden J.A. (1999). *The Role of "Enemy Images" and Ideology in Elite Belief Systems*. International Studies Quarterly 43(3) pp. 455-481.

Murray A. and Meyer D. (2020). *On the COVID-19 front, the US Has Had a Massive Leadership Failure*. Fortune, CEO Daily, 13 July 2020. Accessed at: https://fortune.com/2020/07/13/us-health-care-leadership-failure-covid-19-ceo-daily/.

Murray-Atfield Y. (2021a). *Victoria Moves to Single QR Code COVID-19 Check-in System Amid Concerns About Compliance*. ABC NEWS, 7 May 2021. Accessed at: https://www.abc.net.au/news/2021-05-07/victoria-moves-to-single-qr-code-system-compliance-concerns/100121552.

Murray-Atfield Y. (2021b*). Details of Previously Secret Battle Over Victorian COVID Contact Tracing Information Made Public*. ABC News, 29 December 2021. Accessed at: https://www.abc.net.au/news/2021-12-28/victorian-government-covid-contact-tracing-legal-fight/100728412.

Murray-Atfield Y. (2022). *Victorian Government MPs Defend Labor Party Culture in Wake of Kaushaliya Vaghela Bullying Allegations*. ABC, 12 February 2022. Accessed at: https://www.abc.net.au/news/2022-02-12/victorian-labor-mps-defend-party-andrews-vaghela-bullying-claims/100825634

Nai A. and Toros E. (2019). *The Peculiar Personality of Strongmen: Comparing the Big Five and Dark Triad Traits of Autocrats and Non-autocrats*. Political Research Exchange. 2(2) Article 1707697.

Nakazawa E., Ino H., and Akabayashi A. (2020). *Chronology of COVID-19 Cases on the Diamond Princess Cruise Ship and Ethical Considerations: A Report from Japan*. Disaster Medicine and Public Health Preparedness Mar 24 pp. 1-8.

Nam H.H., Jost J.T., and Van Bavel J.J. (2013). *"Not for All the Tea in China!" Political Ideology and the Avoidance of Dissonance-Arousing Situations*. PLoS One 8(4) Article: e59837.

NARI (2021). *What Worked Well? Lessons Learnt from the Second Wave of COVID-19 Outbreaks in Victorian Aged Care Services: Mapping Activity*. National Ageing Research Institute. Report for DHVic May 2021. Accessed at:

https://www.nari.net.au/Handlers/Download.ashx?IDMF=51cd2eef-eb47-432b-a662-c162d1cfe24a.

National Commission (2011a). *Deep Water: The Gulf Oil Disaster and the Future for Offshore Drilling*. Report to the President. National Commission on the BP Deepwater Horizon Oil Spill and Offshore Drilling, January 2011.

National Commission (2011b). *Macondo: The Gulf Oil Disaster. Chief Counsels' Report. National Commission on the BP Deepwater Horizon Oil Spill and Offshore Drilling.*

Neilson N. (2020). *'Dream Job to Nightmare"" Investigation into Senior Lawyers Suicide Reveals Toxic Culture at Victoria's Coroners Court.* Lawyers Weekly, 9 November 2020. Accessed at:
https://www.lawyersweekly.com.au/biglaw/29934-dream-job-to-nightmare-investigation-into-senior-lawyer-s-suicide-reveals-toxic-culture-at-victoria-s-coroners-court.

Neiva F.W. and Borges M.R.S. (2019). *Sharing Gut Feelings to Support Collaborative Decision Making.* In: WiPe Paper – Intelligent and Semantic Web Systems Proceedings of the 16th ISCRAM Conference (Editors Z. Franco, J.J. González, and J.H. Canós) May 2019, València, Spain.

Nescolarde-Selva J.A Usó-Doménech J-L., and Gash H. (2017). What are Ideological Systems? Systems 6(1) 21.

Newell D. and Matti S. (2017). *Values, Beliefs and Elite Decision-making: The Case of the Markbygden Wind Power Development*. Environmental Policy and Governance. Accessed at: http://www.diva-portal.org/smash/get/diva2:1143956/FULLTEXT01.pdf.

News.com (2022). *Daniel Andrews' Secret Data System Monitoring Victorians*. News.com.au, 5 June 2022. Accessed at:
https://www.news.com.au/technology/online/daniel-andrews-secret-data-system-monitoring-victorians/news-story/42cf74edcebebac6944ca4a8d3d1521a#share-tools.

Neyman G. and Dalsey W. (2020). *Black Lives Matter Protests and COVID-19 Cases: Relationship in Two Databases*. Journal of Public Health, doi:10.1093/pubmed/fdaa212.

Nguyen T., Lim C.P., Nguyen N.D., Gordon-Brown L., Nahavandi S. (2019). *A Review of Situation Awareness Assessment Approaches in Aviation Environments.* IEEE Systems Journal DOI: 10.1109/JSYST.2019.2918283

NHMRC (2019). *Australian Guidelines for the Prevention and Control of Infection in Healthcare*. Australian Government, National Health and Medical Research Council, Australian Commission on Safety and Quality in Health Care. Accessed at:
https://www.nhmrc.gov.au/sites/default/files/documents/Infection-control-guidelines-feb2020.pdf.

NIC (20210). *Updated Assessment on COVID-19 Origins*. National Intelligence Council, Office of the Director of National Intelligence, Washington DC.

Nicola M., Sohrabi C., Mathew G., Kerwan A., Al-Jabir A., Griffin M., Agha M., and Agha R. (2020). *Health Policy and Leadership Models During the COVID-19 Pandemic: A Review.* International Journal of Surgery 81 pp. 122-129.

Nine News (2022). *Worrying Account of 'Chaos' Inside Victoria COVID-19 Ward*. Nine News, 21 January 2022. Accessed at: https://www.youtube.com/watch?v=fb5DVyzcYHs.

NNDSS (2010). *Australia's Notifiable Disease Status, 2016*: Annual Report of the National Notifiable Diseases Surveillance System NNDSS Annual Report Working Group. Communicable Diseases Intelligence 45 pp. 62-63.

Noah L. (2021). *'Lack of Transparency' the 'Most Concerning Thing' About Victoria's Hotel Quarantine System.* Times News Express, May 2021. Accessed at:
https://timesnewsexpress.com/news/world/australia/lack-of-transparency-the-most-concerning-thing-about-victorias-hotel-quarantine-system/.

Nofi A.A. (2000). *Defining and Measuring Shared Situational Awareness.* Center for Naval Analysis, Alexandria VA.

Nojoumi A.R., Givehchi S., and Mahmood Zadeh A. (2015). *Crisis Management Arising from Technological Risks and its Models in South Pars: A Systematic Review*. Journal of Materials and Environmental Science 6(7) pp. 1965-1974.

Normile D. *The Metropole, Superspreaders, and Other Mysteries*. Science 339 pp. 1272-1273.

NSW Health (2015). *Planning and Preparedness Resources.* NSW Government, Sydney. Accessed at: https://www.health.nsw.gov.au/emergency_preparedness/planning/Pages/default.aspx.

NSW Health (2019). *Public Health Emergency Response Preparedness Minimum Standards.* NSW Government, Sydney. Accessed at: https://www1.health.nsw.gov.au/pds/ActivePDSDocuments/PD2019_007.pdf.

Nuwer R. (2012). *Research Suggests Politicians are More Likely to Be Psychopaths.* Smithsonian Magazine, 1 August 212. Accessed at: https://www.smithsonianmag.com/smart-news/research-suggests-politicians-are-more-likely-to-be-psychopaths-11364143/.

Nwachukwu S.L.S. and Vitell S.J. (1997). *The Influence of Corporate Culture on Managerial Judgments*. Journal of Business Ethics 16 pp. 757-776.

Nye J.S. (2020). *An Abysmal Failure of Leadership*. Project Syndicate 7 May 2020. https://www.project-syndicate.org/commentary/trump-xi-leadership-failures-covid19-pandemic-by-joseph-s-nye-2020-05

Nyenswah T., Engineer C.Y., and Peters D.H. (2016). *Leadership in Times of Crisis: The Example of Ebola Virus Disease in Liberia*. Health Systems and Reform 2(3) pp. 194-207.

Obrenovic B., Du J., Godinic D., Tsoy D., Khan M.A., Jakhongirov I. (2020). *Sustaining Enterprise Operations and Productivity during the COVID-19 Pandemic: "Enterprise Effectiveness and Sustainability Model*. Sustainability 12 Article 5981.

O'Brien M. (2021a). *Hospitals Exposed as Premier Fails to Deliver on Promise*. Media Release, Michael O'Brien MP, 3 September 2021. Accessed at : https://www.michaelobrien.com.au/hospitals-exposed-as-premier-fails-to-deliver-on-promise/.

O'Brien M. (2021b). *More Hypocrisy from the Andrews Labor Government Surrounding Hotel Quarantine*. Media Release, Michael O'Brien MP, 12 May 2021. Accessed at: https://www.michaelobrien.com.au/more-hypocrisy-from-the-andrews-labor-government-surrounding-hotel-quarantine/.

OECD (2021). *Making Better Policies for Food Systems*. OECD Publishing, Paris, France.

Oeij P.R.A., Dhondt S., Gaspersz J.B.R., and van Vuuren T. (2017). *Innovation Resilience Behavior and Critical Incidents: Validating the Innovation Resilience Behavior-Scale with Qualitative Data*. Project Management Journal 48(5) pp. 49-63.

Offer K. (2021). *Lack of Strategy Behind Vic Build Blowouts*. Canberra Times 19 August 2021. Accessed at: https://www.canberratimes.com.au/story/7393430/lack-of-strategy-behind-vic-build-blowouts/.

Ohlheiser A. (2013). *The Bizarre PR Disaster of the Quebec Train Explosion*. The Atlantic, 11 July 2011. Accessed at: https://www.theatlantic.com/international/archive/2013/07/bizarre-pr-disaster-quebec-train-explosion/313404/.

Okoli J. and Watt J. (2018). *Crisis Decision-making: The Overlap Between Intuitive and Analytical Strategies*. Management Decision, 56 (5). pp. 1122-1134.

Om J. (2020). *Coronavirus Hard Lockdown of Melbourne Public Housing Towers Left Residents Feeling Like 'Criminals', Inquiry Hears*. ABC News, 25 August 2020. Accessed at: https://www.abc.net.au/news/2020-08-25/coronavirus-melbourne-public-housing-tower-shutdown-inquiry/12589372.

Omar A.T., Robinson S. and Dudau A. (2017). *Leaders Behaving Badly: Constructing a Toxic leadership for Public University Leaders.* International Journal of Management and Applied Science 3(6) pp.75-80.

O'Malley P., Rainford J., and Thompson A. (2009). *Transparency During Public Health Emergencies: From Rhetoric to Reality*. Bulletin of the World Health Organisation B7 pp. 614-618.

Ombudsman (2020*). Investigation into the Detention and Treatment of Public Housing Residents Arising from a COVID-19 'Hard Lockdown' in July 2020.* Victorian Ombudsman, December 2020. Accessed at: https://assets.ombudsman.vic.gov.au/assets/Reports/Parliamentary-Reports/Public-housing-tower-lockdown/Victorian-Ombudsman-report-Investigation-into-the-detention-and-treatment-of-public-housing-residents-arising-from-a-COVID-19-hard-lockdown-in-July-2020.pdf.

Ombudsman (2021). *The Ombudsman for Human Rights*: A Casebook. Victorian Ombudsman, 4 August 2021. Accessed at: https://www.parliament.vic.gov.au/file_uploads/The_Ombudsman_for_Human_Rights_-_A_Casebook_mztsThT0.pdf.

OneSharedWorld.com (2020). *Declaring COVID-19 the Ultimate Failure of Leadership, Citizens of 43 Countries and Territories Together Release "Declaration of Interdependence".* Cision PR Newswire, 12 May 2020. Accessed at: https://www.prnewswire.com/news-releases/declaring-covid-19-the-ultimate-failure-of-leadership-citizens-of-43-countries-and-territories-together-release-declaration-of-interdependence-301057812.html.

Op Ed (2011). *New Police Chief Needs to Restore Confidence: The Government Must Remain at Arms Length*, Sydney Morning Herald 15 November 2011. Access at: https://www.smh.com.au/politics/federal/new-police-chief-needs-to-restore-confidence-20111114-1nfi6.html.

O'Reilly D., Leitch C.M., Harrison R.T. and Lamprou E. (2015). *Introduction: Leadership in a Crises-constructing World*. Leadership 11(4) pp. 387-395.

O'Sullivan M. (2020). *Protests Have Been Criminalised Under COVID. What is Incitement? How Is It Being Used in the Pandemic*. The Conversation, 3 September 2020. Accessed at: https://theconversation.com/protests-have-been-criminalised-under-covid-what-is-incitement-how-is-it-being-used-in-the-pandemic-145538.

Oraby T., Tyshenko M.G., Maldonado J.C., Vatcheva K., Elassdany S., Alali W.Q., Longenecker J.C., and Al-Zoughool M. (2021). *Modeling the Effect of Lockdown Timing as a COVID-19 Control Measure in Countries with Differing Social Contacts*. Scientific Reports 11 Article 3354.

Oullier O. (2013). *Behavioural Insights Are Vital to Policy-making*. Nature 501 pp. 463.

Oxford J.S., and Gill D. (2018). *Unanswered Questions about the 1918 Influenza Pandemic: Origin, Pathology, and the Virus Itself*. The Lancet Infectious Diseases 18(11) pp. E248-E354.

Padgett D.R.G., Cheng S.S., and Parekh V. (2013). *The Quest for Transparency and Accountability: Communicating Responsibly to Stakeholders in Crises*. Asian Social Science; 9(9) pp. 31-44.

Padilla A., Hogan R., and Kaiser R.B. (2007). *The Toxic Triangle: Destructive Leaders, Susceptible Followers, and Conducive Environments*. The Leadership Quarterly 18 pp. 176-194.

PAEC (2020). *Inquiry into the Victorian Government's Response to the COVID-19 Pandemic*. Transcript of Hearing held on Tuesday 12 May 2020. Public Accounts and Estimates Committee, p. 12. Accessed at:
https://www.parliament.vic.gov.au/images/stories/committees/paec/COVID-19_Inquiry/Transcripts/DPC_12_May_verified_transcript.pdf.

PAEC (2021). *Inquiry into the Victorian Government's Response to the COVID-19 Pandemic*. Report, p. 8, Public Accounts and Estimates Committee. February 2021 PP No 203, Session 2018-201.

Pak A., Adegboye O.A., and McBryde E.S. (2021). *Are We Better Off? The Benefit and Costs of Australian COVID-19 Lockdown*. Frontiers in Public Health 9 Article Number:798478.

Parker A.M., Nelson C., Shelton S.R., Dausey D.J., Lewis M.W., Pomeroy A., and Luschner K.J. (2009). *Measuring Crisis Decision Making for Public Health Emergencies*. Rand Corporation, Santa Monica, CA.

Parkhurst J.O. (2016). *Appeals to Evidence for the Resolution of Wicked Problems: The Origins and Mechanisms of Evidentiary Bias*. Policy Science 49 pp. 373-393.

Parliament of Victoria (2020). *Inquiry into the Victorian Government's COVID-19 Contact Tracing System and Testing Regime*. Parliament of Victoria Legislative Council and Social Issues Committee, December 2020. Melbourne Australia.

Parks Victoria (2021). *Quarantine Station, Nepean National Park*. Accessed at:
https://www.parks.vic.gov.au/places-to-see/parks/point-nepean-national-park/attractions/quarantine-station.

Parnell J.A. and Crandall W.R. (2020). *The Contribution of Behavioral Economics to Crisis Management Decision-making*. Journal of Management and Organization 26(4) pp. 585-600.

Parnell J.A., Spillan J.E., and Crandall W. (2013). *The Underlying Role of Ethics in Crisis Management*. In: Crisis Management: Leading in the New Strategy Landscape. Sage Publishing, Thousand Oaks, CA.

Parsons L. (2021). *How Dan Andrews' Ran Secret 'virus surveys' to Monitor his Political Popularity with Victorians – Despite Always Insisting Lockdown Decisions Were Made on 'health advice'*. Daily Mail Australia, 13 July 2021. Accessed at:
https://www.dailymail.co.uk/news/article-9780691/Dan-Andrews-virus-surveys-used-monitor-popular-Victoria-Covid-lockdown.html.

Pascault J. (2021). *WHO COVID-19 Investigation Is Tainted by Conflict of Interest, Says AHF*. AIDS Health, 1 February 2021. Accessed at:
https://www.aidshealth.org/2021/02/who-covid-19-investigation-is-tainted-by-conflict-of-interest-says-ahf/.

Paulhus D.L. (2014). *Toward a Taxonomy of Dark Personalities*. Current Directions in Psychological Science 23(6) pp. 421-426.

Paulhus D. L. and Williams K. (2002). *The Dark Triad of Personality: Narcissism, Machiavellianism, and Psychopathy*. Journal of Research in Personality 36 pp. 556-568.

Paull S.H., Song S., McClure K.M., Sackett L.C., Kilpatrick A.M., and Johnson P.T.J. (2012). *From Superspreaders to Disease Hotspots: Linking Transmission Across Hosts and Space*. Frontiers in Ecology and Environment 10(2) pp. 75-82.

Paynter J. (2021a). *Victorian Government Admits Contact Tracing 'Fell Down' as Wrong Woolworths Store Listed*. NCA Newswire 25 May 2021. Accessed at:

https://www.news.com.au/national/victoria/news/victorian-government-admits-contact-tracing-fell-down-as-wrong-woolworths-store-listed/news-story/b4749a281e9d072eace9c12e4005238.

Paynter J. (2021). *Victoria Records 867 new Local Covid Cases, Surpasses daily NSW Figure.* New.com.au, 29 September 2021. Accessed at: https://www.news.com.au/national/victoria/news/victoria-records-867-new-local-covid-cases-melburnians-to-get-extra-freedoms-on-wednesday/news-story/a64d00d58d61fbbba916112f93fb45af.

Penta S., Marlowe V.G., Gill K., and Kendra J. (2017). *Of Earthquakes and Epidemics: Examining the Applicability of the All-Hazards Approach in Public Health Emergencies.* Risk Hazards and Crisis in Public Policy 8(1) pp. 48-67.

Pentland A. *The New Science of Building Great Teams.* Harvard Business Review April 2012.

Phillips K. (2021). *The Rule of Law is Cracking in Victoria – and so is the Labor Establishment.* Spectator Australia, 22 September 2021. Accessed at: https://www.spectator.com.au/2021/09/the-rule-of-law-is-cracking-in-victoria-and-so-is-the-labor-establishment/.

Peplow S. (2017). *Why People Have Long Questioned the Point of Public Inquiries.* The Conversation, 9 November, 2019. Accessed at: https://theconversation.com/why-people-have-long-questioned-the-point-of-public-inquiries-86648.

Perrin P.C., McCabe L., Everly G.S., and Links J.M. (2009). *Preparing for an Influenza Pandemic: Mental Health Considerations.* Prehospital and Disaster Medicine 24(3) pp. 223-230.

Persson T., Parker C.F., and Widmalm S. (2017). *Social Trust, Impartial Administration and Public Confidence in Eu Crisis Management Institutions.* Public Administration 95(1) pp. 97-114.

Peters B.G. (2021). *Governing in a Time of Global Crises: The Good, The Bad, and The Merely Normal.* Global Public Policy and Governance 1 pp. 4-19.

Petersen D.C. (1978). *Techniques of Safety Management.* Second Edition, McGraw-Hill, New York.

Pezenik S. (2021). *Criticism of WHO Wuhan Report Exposes Limits of Agency's Power and Influence.* ABC News, 31 March 2021. Accessed at: https://abcnews.go.com/Health/criticism-wuhan-report-exposes-limits-agencys-power-influence/story?id=76761378.

Phillips R. (2008). *Why Vietnam Matters: An Eyewitness Account of Lessons Not Learned.* Naval Institute Press, US Naval Institute, Annapolis, MD.

Phillips G. and Green J. (2015). *Working for the Public Health: Politics, Localism and Epistemologies of Practice.* Sociology of Health and Illness 37(4) pp. 491-505.

Philips K. (2021). *Is WorkSafe Grossly Incompetent – or is Something Else Going on?* Spectator Australia, 30 June 2021. Accessed at: https://www.spectator.com.au/2021/06/is-worksafe-victoria-grossly-incompetent-or-is-something-else-going-on/.

PHO (2022). *Mask Wearing in Children and COVID-19... What We Know So Far.* Synthesis, Public Health Ontario, 17 February 2022. Accessed at: https://www.publichealthontario.ca/-/media/documents/ncov/covid-wwksf/2021/08/wwksf-wearing-masks-children.pdf?sc_lang=en.

Piovesan A. (2020). *Former Health Minister Jenny Mikakos Takes Aim at Daniel Andrews After Hotel Quarantine Inquiry Findings.* The Australian, 21 December 2020. Accessed at:

https://www.theaustralian.com.au/breaking-news/former-health-minister-jenny-mikakos-takes-aim-at-daniel-andrews-after-hotel-quarantine-inquiry-findings/news-story/051b32dc2b46b7cec58ded5c6f45ccb7.

Piovesan A. (2021a) *Victorian Opposition Call for New Law to Stop Police Accessing Contact Tracing Data*. News.com.au, 23 June 2021. Accessed at: https://www.news.com.au/technology/gadgets/mobile-phones/victorian-opposition-call-for-new-law-to-stop-police-accessing-contact-tracing-data/news-story/f2cf5888fb891392a84cc77ea21ee560.

Piovesan A. (2021b). *WorkSafe Victoria Investigates 24 Companies Over Potential COVID-19 Breaches*. News.com.au, 7 January 2021. Accessed at: https://www.news.com.au/finance/work/at-work/worksafe-victoria-investigates-24-companies-over-potential-covid19-breaches/news-story/2fd386532aee61d891620caa99038af9.

Piovesan A. (2021c). *Victorians Lodging Formal Complaints About Human Rights in 'Record' Numbers, Victorian Ombudsman Finds*. News.com.au, 28 October 2021. Accessed at: https://www.news.com.au/national/victoria/news/victorians-lodging-formal-complaints-about-human-rights-in-record-numbers-victorian-ombudsman-finds/news-story/e802c9efe3501c742bcf7608c6e1fbe9.

Piovesan A. (2021d). *Andrews Government Ordered to Reveal Secret Documents that Justify Victorian Lockdown*. News.com.au, 20 October 2021. Accessed at: https://www.news.com.au/national/victoria/politics/andrews-government-ordered-to-reveal-secret-documents-that-justify-victorian-lockdown/news-story/4954176823fbf13b4e3e2c6ae1d56d98.

Piovesan A. (2022). *Jim's Mowing Franchisee Steve Thompson to Fight Victorian Government for Loss of Income During Lockdown*. The Australian, 24 May 2022. Accessed at: https://www.theaustralian.com.au/breaking-news/jims-mowing-franchisee-steve-thompson-to-fight-victorian-government-for-loss-of-income-during-lockdown/news-story/3380bd0bb23f4c1d9d975988ab9a767c.

Plotkin B. (2007). *Human Rights and Other Provisions in the Revised International Health Regulations (2005)*. Journal of the Royal Institute of Human Health 121 pp. 840-845.

Pockett D. (2020). *Our Lives Matter – Melbourne Public Housing Residents Talk About Why Covid 19 Hits Them Hard.* The Conversation, 24 July 2020. Accessed at: https://theconversation.com/our-lives-matter-melbourne-public-housing-residents-talk-about-why-covid-19-hits-them-hard-142901.

Popoli P. (2017). *Organisational Culture as a Driver of Outsourcing Choices: A Conceptual Model.* African Journal of Business Management 11(18) pp. 524-536.

Porter R. (1997). *The Greatest Benefit to Mankind: A Medical History of Humanity from Antiquity to the Present*. Harper Collins Publishing, London, UK.

PoV (2016). *Inquiry into the CFA Training College at Fiskville: Final Report*. Environment, Natural Resources and Regional Development Committee, Parliament of Victoria. Accessed at: https://www.parliament.vic.gov.au/images/stories/committees/enrc/Fiskville_training_college/Final_report/ENRRDC_58-03_Text_WEB.pdf.

Powell M. (2023). *Toxic Legacy*. Spectator Australia. 9 October 2023/ Accessed at: https://www.spectator.com.au/2023/10/toxic-legacy/

Prasser S. (2020). *How Royal Commissions Can Both Help and Hinder*. Financial Review 14 January 2020. Accessed at: https://www.afr.com/politics/federal/how-royal-commissions-can-both-help-and-hinder-20200113-p53r20.

Preston O.C. and Anestis J.C. (2017). *Psychopathic Traits and Politics: Examining Affiliation, Support of Political Issues, and the Role of Empathy*. Personality and Individual Differences 131 pp. 142-148.
Price D., Shearer F.M., Meehan M.T., McBryde E., Moss., Golding N., Conway E.J., Dawson P., Cromer D., Wood J., Abbott S., McVernon J., and McCaw J.M. (2020). *Early Analysis of the Australian COVID-19 Epidemic*. eLife 9 Article: e58785.
Probyn A. (2020). *Ruby Princess Passengers Infected Others with COVID-19 on Qantas Flight, Research Suggests*. ABC News, 30 September 2020. Accessed at: https://www.abc.net.au/news/2020-09-30/covid19-ruby-princess-passengers-infected-qantas-coronavirus/12718748.
Pronin E. (2007). *Perception and Misperception of Bias in Human Judgement*. Trends in Cognitive Sciences 11(1) pp. 37-43.
Public Health Ontario (2020). *Public Health Emergency Preparedness Framework and Indicators: A Workbook to Support Public Health Practice*. Ontario Agency for Health Protection and Promotion, Toronto ON.
Public Pathology Australia (2020a). *Public Pathology: Value and Opportunities*. Public Pathology Australia, 9 June 2020. Accessed at: https://publicpathology.org.au/wp-content/uploads/2020/06/Public-Pathology-Values-and-Opportunities-Paper.pdf.
Public Pathology Australia (2020b). *Submission: Inquiry into the Victorian Government's Response to COVID-19 Pandemic*. Submission no. 225. Accessed at: https://www.parliament.vic.gov.au/images/stories/committees/paec/COVID-19_Inquiry/Submissions/224._Public_Pathology_Australia.pdf.
Puchan H. (2001). *The Mercedes-Benz A Class Crisis*. Corporate Communications: An International Journal 6(1) pp. 43-46.
Pupulidy I. and Vesel C. (2017). *The Learning Review: Adding to the Accident Investigation Toolbox*. Proceedings of the 53rd ESReDA Seminar, 14 – 15 November 2017, Ispra, Italy.
QStation (2018). Investigate Infectious Disease at Q Station. Accessed at: https://www.qstation.com.au/blog/infectious-diseases-at-q-station.
Quinlan M. (2014). *Ten Pathways to Death and Disaster: Learning from Fatal Incidents in Mines and Other High Hazard Workplaces*. The Federation Press, Leichardt, NSW, Australia.
Rainie L. and Perrin A. (2019). *Key Findings About Americans' Declining Trust in Government and Each Other*. Pew Research Centre, 22 July 2019. Accessed at: https://www.pewresearch.org/fact-tank/2019/07/22/key-findings-about-americans-declining-trust-in-government-and-each-other/.
Ramaswamy V. (2021). Woke, Inc.: Inside Corporate America's Social Justice Scam. Center Street, Hachette Book Group.
Rasmussen H.B., Drupsteen L., and Dyreborg J. (2013). *Near Miss Reporting in the Danish Oil & Gas Industry*. Safety Science Monitor 17 (2) pp. 1-12.
Rauch J. (2018). *The Constitution of Knowledge*. National Affairs 48, Fall 2018. Accessed at: https://www.nationalaffairs.com/publications/detail/the-constitution-of-knowledge.
Reardon S. (2021). The Most Worrying Mutations in Five Emerging Coronavirus Variants. Scientific American, 29 January 2021. Accessed at: https://www.scientificamerican.com/article/the-most-worrying-mutations-in-five-emerging-coronavirus-variants/.
Reis B. (2020). *CFA in Disarray as Chief Quits on Eve of Fire Service Restructure*. The Age, 26 June 2020. Accessed at: https://www.theage.com.au/national/victoria/cfa-in-disarray-as-chief-quits-on-eve-of-fire-service-restructure-20200626-p556ko.html.

Rego L. and Garu R. (2007). *Stepping into the Void*. Reflections and Insights from a Forum on Crisis Leadership Convened at the Center for Creative Leadership, 13–15 March 2007. Center for Creative Leadership.
Riley W., Davis S., Miller K., and McCullough M. (2010). *A Model for Developing High-reliability Teams*. Journal of Nursing Management 18(5) pp. 556–563.
Riley W., Lownik E., Parrotta C., Miller K., and Davis S. (2011). *Creating High Reliability Teams in Healthcare Through in situ Simulation Training*. Administrative Sciences 1 pp. 14-31.
Roach K. (2017). *Police Government Relations and Police Independence*. Accessed at: https://www.cepcsj.gouv.qc.ca/fileadmin/documents_client/recherche/Quebec_Police_Independence_pour_depot.pdf.
Roach K. (2018). *Balancing Police Independence and Political Responsibility for the Police: Some Recent Developments in Australia, Canada, and the UK*. Policing: A Journal of Policy and Practice Article pay055.
Roper W. (2020). *Science, Politics, and Public Health*. Science 370(6515) pp. 385.
Roberts R. (2020). *COVID-19, Leadership and Lessons from Physics*. Australian Journal of Rural Health 28 pp. 232-235.
Robin M. (2020). *Victorian Government Doesn't Stint on Legal Representation*. Financial Review, 27 September 2020.
Robinson B. (2022). *Toxic Workplace Culture 10 Times More Likely to Drive Employees Away, Study Shows*. Forbes, 3 February 2022. Accessed at: https://www.forbes.com/sites/bryanrobinson/2022/02/03/toxic-workplace-culture-10-times-more-likely-to-drive-employees-away-study-shows/?sh=532d3f141386.
Rodger J.J. (1985). *Natural Justice and the Big Public Inquiry: A Sociological Perspective*. The Sociological Review 33(3) pp. 409-429.
Roe E. and Schulman P. (2008). *High Reliability Management: Operating on the Edge*. Stanford University Press, Stanford, CA.
Rogers W.P. (1986). *Report to the President by the Presidential Commission on the Space Shuttle Challenger Accident*. June 6th 1986, Washington DC.
Rollason B. (2021). *Victorian Parliament Decriminalises Public Drunkenness in a Victory for the Family of Tanya Day*. ABC News, 19 February 2021. Accessed at: https://www.abc.net.au/news/2021-02-19/victorian-parliament-decriminalises-public-drunkenness-tanya-day/13172136
Rollason B. (2021). *COVID-19 Quarantine Victoria Infection Control Manager Stood Down After Allegedly Breaching Protocols*. ABC News, 5 May 2021. Accessed at: https://www.abc.net.au/news/2021-05-05/victoria-covid-hotel-quarantine-infection-manager-stood-down/100116928.
Rollason B. and Wong L. (2023). *When and How Victoria's Plans for the 2026 Commonwealth Games Went Awry*. ABC News 17 September 2023. Accessed at: https://www.abc.net.au/news/2023-09-17/vic-commonwealth-games-cancellation-timeline/102862566.
Ronnie L. (2017). *Toxic Leaders Affect Companies, and Governments. How to Deal with Them*. The Conversation 29 May 2017. Accessed at: https://theconversation.com/toxic-leaders-affect-companies-and-governments-how-to-deal-with-them-78265.
Ronson J. (2011). *The Psychopath Test: A Journey Through the Madness Industry*. Picador, London, UK.
Rosa W.E., Schlak A.E., and Rushton C.H. (2020). *A Blueprint for Leadership During COVID-19*. Nursing management August 202 pp. 29-34.
Rose R. and Davies P.L. (1994*) Inheritance in Public Policy: Chang without Choice in Britain*.

Yale University Press, New Haven, CT.

Rosenthal U., Boin R.A., and Comfort L. (2001). *Managing Crises: Threats, Dilemmas, Opportunities*. Charles C. Thomas Publisher, Springfield, Illinois.

Rosenthal U., 't Hart P., and Charles M.T. (1989). *The World of Crises and Crisis Management*. In: Coping with Crises: The Management of Disasters, Riots and Terrorism (Editors: U. Rosenthal, M.T. Charles, and P. Hart) Charles C. Thomas, Springfield, Illinois.

Roskam J. (2020a). Beautiful One Day, Police State the Next. Institute of Public Affairs, 3 April 2020. Accessed at: https://ipa.org.au/publications-ipa/beautiful-one-day-police-state-the-next.

Roskam J. (2020b). *Why I was Right About Victoria's Police State*. Financial Review 24 September 2020. Accessed at: https://www.afr.com/politics/why-i-was-right-about-victoria-s-police-state-20200923-p55yky.

Ross D. (2021a). *Banned Security Boss David Millward 'Never Left'*. The Australian 14 April 2021. Accessed at:
https://www.theaustralian.com.au/nation/politics/banned-security-boss-david-millward-never-left/news-story/80d1faed7824a1617669591a1473e679.

Ross D. (2021b). *Unified Security Shadow Directors Pulled $20m from Sinking Business*. The Australian 30 August 2021. Accessed at:
https://www.theaustralian.com.au/nation/unified-security-shadow-directors-pulled-20m-from-sinking-business/news-story/73473da4889a12a7503513020c9c1e25.

Rossheim J. (2019). *The Cost of Toxic Cultures*. Workhuman, 30 October 2019. Accessed at: https://www.workhuman.com/resources/globoforce-blog/the-cost-of-toxic-cultures.

Rothstein M.A., Alcalde M.G., Elster N.R., Majumder M.A. Plamer L.I., Stone T.H., and Hoffman R.E. (2003). *Quarantine and Isolation: Lessons Learned from SARS. A Report to the Centers for Disease Control and Prevention*. Institute for Bioethics, Health Policy and Law University of Louisville School of Medicine. Accessed at:
https://biotech.law.lsu.edu/blaw/cdc/SARS_REPORT.pdf.

Roulet T.J. and Pichler R. (2020). *Blame Game Theory: Scapegoating, Whistleblowing and Discursive Struggles following Accusations of Organizational Misconduct*. Organization Theory 1 pp. 1-30.

Rowland D., Casimir S., and Pivcevic P. (2020). *Covid-19 Pandemic: Now id the Time for Emergent Leadership*. LSE Business Review, 30th April 2020. London School of Economics and Political Science.

Rowley D. (2008). *The Fires that Created an Incident Management System*. In Uninets.net - Dale Rowley, January 1. Accessed at:
http://www.uninets.net/~dsrowley/The%20Fires%20that%20Created%20an%20IMS.pdf.

Rostis A. (2007). *Make no Mistake: the Effectiveness of the Lessons-learned Approach to Emergency Management in Canada*. International Journal of Emergency Management 4(2) pp. 197-210.

Rulli M.C., D'Odorico P., Galli N., and Hayman D.T.S. (2021). *Land-use Change and the Livestock Revolution Increase the Risk of Zoonotic Coronavirus Transmission from Rhinolophid Bats*. Nature Food 2 pp. 409-416.

Rutledge P.E. (2020). *Trump, COVID-19, and the War on Expertise*. American Review of Public Administration 50 pp.505-511.

Ryan L. (2010). *Ten Unmistakable Signs of a Toxic Culture*. Forbes 19 October 2016. Accessed at:
https://www.forbes.com/sites/lizryan/2016/10/19/ten-unmistakable-signs-of-a-toxic-culture/?sh=6285137a115f.

Sanford S., Schwartz B., and Khan Y. (2020). *The Role of Tacit Knowledge in Communication and Decision-making During Emerging Public Health Incidents.* International Journal of Disaster Risk Reduction. 50 Article 101681.

SA Health (2015). *Public Health Emergency Management Plan.* Government of South Australia, Adelaide.

Sadiq A-A., Kapucu N., and Hu Q. (2021). *Crisis Leadership During COVID-19; The Role of Governor in the Unites States.* International Journal of Public Leadership 17(1) pp. 65-80.

Sadler D. (2021). *Victoria Won't Prevent Police Accessing QR Code Check-in Data.* Innovation Australia, 22 June 2021. Accessed at: https://www.innovationaus.com/victoria-wont-prevent-police-accessing-qr-code-check-in-data/.

SAGO (2022). *Preliminary Report of the SAGO.* 9 June 2022. Scientific Advisory Group for the Origins of Novel Pathogens (SAGO). World Health Organisation.

Salas E. and Rosen M.A. (2013). *Building High Reliability Teams: Progress and Some Reflections on Teamwork Training.* Quality and Safety in Health Care22 pp. 369–373.

Sakkal P. (2020). *'Disaster': Calls for External Audit of Health Department after Scathing Hotel Quarantine Assessment.* The Age, 21 December 2021. The Age, 24 March, 2021. Accessed at: https://www.theage.com.au/national/victoria/disaster-calls-for-external-audit-of-health-department-after-scathing-hotel-quarantine-assessment-20201221-p56pcu.html.

Sakkal P. (2020a). *'Coverup' Claims After Man Avoided Hotel Quarantine, Drove to Toorak.* The Age, 16 December 2020. Accessed at: https://www.theage.com.au/politics/victoria/coverup-claims-after-man-avoided-hotel-quarantine-drove-to-toorak-20201215-p56nor.html.

Sakkal P. (2020b). *Hotel Infection Data Kept Secret as Opposition Calls for Ministers to be Dumped.* The Age, 14 July 2020. Accessed at: https://www.theage.com.au/national/victoria/hotel-infection-data-kept-secret-as-opposition-calls-for-ministers-to-be-dumped-20200714-p55by9.html.

Sakkal P. (2021a). *'They Don't Care About Our Safety ': Quarantine Workers Move Between Hotels, Offices.* The Age, 16 February 2021. Accessed at : https://www.theage.com.au/national/victoria/they-don-t-care-about-safety-quarantine-workers-move-between-hotels-offices-20210216-p572w8.html.

Sakkal P. (2021b). *Probe Into Hotel Quarantine Security Contracts.* The Age 8 March 2021. Accessed at: https://www.theage.com.au/national/victoria/probe-into-hotel-quarantine-security-contracts-20210307-p578jn.html.

Sakkal P. (2022). *Second IBAC probe into Victorian Firefighter Union Revealed.* 8 April 2022. Accessed at: https://www.theage.com.au/politics/victoria/second-ibac-probe-into-victorian-firefighter-pay-deal-revealed-20220407-p5abq0.html

Sakkal P. and Ilanbey S. (2021a). *Quarantine Hotel Doctors Working at More Than One Site.* WA Today, 7 April 2021. Accessed at: https://www.watoday.com.au/national/victoria/quarantine-hotel-doctors-working-at-more-than-one-site-20210407-p57has.html?ref=rss&utm_medium=rss&utm_source=rss_feed.

Sakkal P. and Ilanbey S. (2021b). *International Flights, Revamped Hotel Quarantine Program in Victoria Set to Restart in Next Fortnight.* The Age, 24 March 2021. Accessed at: https://www.theage.com.au/national/victoria/international-flights-revamped-hotel-quarantine-program-in-victoria-set-to-restart-in-next-fortnight-20210324-p57dt9.html.

Sakkal P. and Rooney K. (2023). *Andrews Skips Commonwealth Games Inquiry but Pakula to be Grilled.* The Sydney Morning Herald, 24 August, 2023. Accessed at:

https://www.smh.com.au/politics/federal/andrews-skips-commonwealth-games-inquiry-but-pakula-to-be-grilled-20230824-p5dz4t.html.

Salin D. (2008). *The Prevention of Workplace Bullying as a Question of Human Resource Management: Measures adopted and Underlying Organisational Factors.* Scandinavian Journal of Management 24 pp. 221-231.

Sanne J.M. (2008). *Incident Reporting or Storytelling? Competing Schemes in a Safety-Critical and Hazardous*
Work Setting. Safety Science 46(8) pp. 1205–1222.

Sapat A. and Esnard A. (2016). *Learning from Transboundary Crises and Disasters: The 2010 Haiti Earthquake.* In: Global Cases in Best and Worst Practice in Crisis and Emergency Management pp. 237-258, (Editor: A Farazmand) CRC Press, Boca Raton, FL.

Saposnik G., Redelmeier D., Ruff C.C., and Tobler P.N. (2016). *Cognitive Biases Associated with Medical Decisions: A Systematic Review.* BMC Medical Informatics and Decision Making 16 Article 138.

Satell G. and Windschitl C. (2021). *High-Performing Teams Start with a Culture of Shared Values.* Harvard Business Review 11 May 2021.

Savage A. (2015). *Cancer Cluster at CFA Fiskville Training Centre Confirmed by Study: Premier.* ABC News, 21 January 2015. Accessed at:
https://www.abc.net.au/news/2015-01-21/fiskville-cfa-health-study-daniel-andrews/6030020.

Sayegh L., Anthony W.P., Perrewé P.L. (2004). *Managerial Decision-making Under Crisis: The Role of Emotion in an Intuitive Decision Process.* Human Resource Management Review 14 pp.179-199.

SBS (2017). *Andrews Government Splits CFA in Two.* 18 May 2017.

SBS (2020). *Worried About Coronavirus, Daniel Andrews Urges Victorians to Avoid Black Lives Matter Rally.* SBS News, 4 June 2020. Accessed at:
https://www.sbs.com.au/news/article/worried-about-coronavirus-daniel-andrews-urges-victorians-to-avoid-black-lives-matter-rally/3l33hood1.

Schaefer P.V. and Willardsen K. (2020). *A Note of the Tinbergen Rule.* Working Paper. Accessed at:
https://www.petervschaeffer.com/uploads/7/4/3/3/74334295/a_note_on_the_relevance_of_tinbergen.pdf.

Schakel J.K. and Wolbers J. (2021). *To the Edge and Beyond: How Fast- Response Organizations Adapt in Rapidly Changing Crisis Situations.* Human Relations 74(3) pp. 405-436.

Sharov K.S. (2020). *Creating and Applying SIR Modified Compartmental Model for Calculation of COVID-19 Lockdown Efficiency.* Chaos, Solitons & Fractals 141 Article 110295.

Schein E.H. (2010). *Organizational Culture and Leadership* 4th Edition. Jossey-Bass Publishers, San Francisco, CA.

Schelle C. (2021). *Pregnant Ballarat Mum Zoe Buhler to Argue Police Search Wasn't Legal.* The Australian, 27 March 2021. Accessed at:
https://www.theaustralian.com.au/breaking-news/pregnant-ballarat-mum-zoe-buhler-to-argue-police-search-wasnt-legal/news-story/0ff35793350adc2a8b319a5a48605d09.

Schiltz N.K. (2012). *Quarantine and Isolation.* In: Mental Health Practitioner's Guide to HIV/AIDS, pp. 339-343 (Editor S. Loue). Springer Science and Business Media, New York.

Schippers M.C. and Rus D.C. (2021). *Optimizing Decision-Making Processes in Times of COVID-19: Using Reflexivity to Counteract Information-Processing Failures.* Frontiers in Psychology 12 Article 650525.

Schmitt L. (2018). *Go Fast and Break Things: The Difference Between Reversible and Irreversible Decisions.* Inovo. Accessed at: https://www.theinovogroup.com/reversible-irreversible/.

Schraagen J.M. and van de Ven J.G.M. (2008). *Improving Decision Making in Crisis Response Through Critical Thinking Support*. Journal of Cognitive Engineering and Decision Making 2(4) pp. 311-327.

Schultz J.M., Baingana F., and Neria Y. (2015). *The 2014 Ebola Outbreak and Mental Health: Current Status and Recommended Response.* JAMA 313(6) pp. 567-568.

Schubert S. and Miles D. (2021). *COVID Contact Tracing, Health Department 'Shambles' for These Victorians Amid Reopening*. ABC News, 26 November 2021. Accessed at: https://www.abc.net.au/news/2021-11-26/regional-victorians-concerned-about-contact-tracing-delays/100649988.

Schwabe L. and Wolf O.Y. (2013). *Stress and Multiple Memory Systems: From 'Thinking' to 'Doing'*. Trends in Cognitive Sciences 17 pp. 60-68.

Schyns B. (2015) *Dark Personality in the Workplace: Introduction to the Special Issue*. Applied Psychology: An International Review 64(1) pp. 1-14.

SEA (2021a). *The Case for the Prosecution: Victorian Quarantine Hotel Work Safety Breaches. The Evidence Requiring Prosecution of the Victorian Government.* Self Employed Australia. Accessed at: https://selfemployedaustralia.com.au/Downloads/NATL/SEA-Prosecution-Case-Victorian-Government-Quarantine-August-2021.pdf.

SEA (2021b). *Is WorkSafe Victoria Grossly Incompetent or is Something Else Going On?* Self Employed Australia, 29 June 2021. Accessed at: https://selfemployedaustralia.com.au/is-worksafe-victoria-grossly-incompetent-or-is-something-else-going-on/.

Seeger M.W, Pechta L.E., Price S.M., Lubell K.M., Rose D.A., Sapru S., Chansky M.C., and Smith B.J. (2018). *A Conceptual Model for Evaluating Emergency Risk Communication in Public Health*. Health Security 16(3) pp. 193-203.

Seerval S. and Shah S. (2021). *India's Failure of Leadership Collapses Health System in COVID-19 Surge*. Improving Health Care Quality, The Commonwealth Fund. Accessed at: https://www.commonwealthfund.org/blog/2021/indias-failure-leadership-collapses-health-system-covid-19-surge.

Setiawan M.A. (2019). *In the Making of Effective Decision-making in Public Health Domain with Business Intelligence Dashboard.* IOP Conference Series Material Science and Engineering 482 Article 012029.

Seyfort S. (2022a). *Almost 100,000 Victorians Told They Will Not Get Their PCR Test Results.* 9 News, 15 January 2020. Accessed at: https://www.9news.com.au/national/around-100000-victorians-told-they-will-not-get-their-pcr-test-results-from-melbourne-pathology-and-australian-clinical-labs/88ca51aa-478b-4afe-a517-ea5d37275df9.

Seyfort S. (2022b). *Up to 1000 Patients May Have Been Harmed by Victoria's Triple Zero Delays*. 9 News, 16 August 2022. Accessed at: https://www.9news.com.au/national/ambulance-crisis-victoria-1000-patients-may-have-been-harmed-by-victorias-triple-zero-delays/c642b7a0-2a28-452d-b8f3-848b62fd9db7.

Shanahan A. (2021). *Lockdowns, Right or Wrong, Must be Learned From*. The Australian, 12 June 2021. Accessed at: https://www.theaustralian.com.au/inquirer/lockdowns-right-or-wrong-must-be-learned-from/news-story/f1ef99b77b0f6223fa0d31f92617c8c6.

Sharkansky I. and Friedberg A. (2002). *Toward a Typology of Non-decisions: Three Israeli Cases*. International Journal of Organization Theory and Behavior 5(1&2) pp. 145-158.

Sharma M. (2017). *Securing Critical Information Infrastructure: Global Perspectives and Practices*. IDSA Monograph Series No. 60, April 2017.

Sheehan M.C. and Fox M.A. (2020). *Early Warnings: The Lessons of COVID-19 for Public Health Climate Preparedness*. International Journal of Health Services 50(3) pp. 264–270.

Shell R. (2021). *Tackling a Toxic Work Culture*. Human Resources Professional Association, 12 May 2021. Accessed at: https://www.hrpa.ca/hr-insights/tackling-a-toxic-work-culture/.

Shepheard M. (2019). *Royal Commissions Are Outdate and Will Not Deliver Real Change*. Institute for Government. Accessed at: https://www.instituteforgovernment.org.uk/blog/labours-manifesto-fails-recognise-royal-commissions-are-past-their-sell-date.

Shepherd K. (2021). *Rick Perry says Texans Would Accept Even Longer Power Outages 'to Keep the Federal Government out of their Business'*. The Washington Post 18 February 2021. Accessed at: https://www.washingtonpost.com/nation/2021/02/17/texas-abbott-wind-turbines-outages/.

Sheridan G. (2020). *While Daniel Andrews was Rooting out Sexism in Fairy Tales, Victoria's Health Team was Overlooked*. The Australian, 10 September 2020. Accessed at: https://www.theaustralian.com.au/commentary/while-daniel-andrews-was-rooting-out-sexism-in-fairy-tales-victorias-health-team-was-overlooked/news-story/c36281af2bf955096a78142ba46fc384.

Shi Z-L. (2021). *Origins of SARS-CoV-2: Focusing on Science*. Editorial, Infectious Diseases and Immunity 1(1) pp.3-5.

Sikora K. (2020). *COVID-19 Kills – But so do Lockdowns*. The Spectator, 19 October 2020. Accessed at: https://www.spectator.co.uk/article/covid-19-kills-but-so-does-lockdown.

Silver J. (2012). *The Startling Accuracy of Referring to Politicians as 'Psychopaths'*. The Atlantic 31 July 2012. Accessed at: https://www.theatlantic.com/health/archive/2012/07/the-startling-accuracy-of-referring-to-politicians-as-psychopaths/260517/.

Sim G. (2016). *Individual Disrupters and Economic Gamechangers: Netflix, New Media, and Neoliberalism*. In: The Netflix Effect: Technology and Entertainment in the 21st Century (Editors: K. McDonald and D. Smith Rowsey), Bloomsbury Academic and Professional, London UK.

Simons M. (2020a). *Victoria Hotel Quarantine Inquiry: Systemic Issues More Urgent Than Individual Blame*. The Guardian 29 September 2020. Accessed at: https://www.theguardian.com/australia-news/2020/sep/29/victoria-hotel-quarantine-inquiry-systemic-issues-more-urgent-than-individual-blame.

Simons M. (2020b). *Melbourne Towers Sudden Hard Lockdown Caught Police, Health Workers and Residents Off-guard*. The Guardian 5 July 2020. Accessed at: https://www.theguardian.com/australia-news/2020/jul/05/melbourne-towers-sudden-hard-lockdown-caught-police-health-workers-and-residents-off-guard.

Simons M. (2020c). *'It Was Paternalism': How Government Support for Melbourne's Locked Down Public Housing Blocks Fell Short*. The Guardian, 11 July 2020. Accessed at: https://www.dailymail.co.uk/news/article-8517311/Victorian-authorities-knew-housing-commission-tower-infected-TWO-MONTHS-covid-outbreak.html.

Simpson J. (2020a). *Woke and Broke: What's Honorable About Victoria?* The Spectator 18 December 2020. Accessed at:

https://www.spectator.com.au/2020/12/woke-and-broke-whats-honourable-about-victoria/.

Simpson J. (2020). *Daniel Andrews: "You Can Now Get a Haircut. Aren't You Going to Thank Me?"* Spectator Australia, 19 October 2020. Accessed at: https://www.spectator.com.au/2020/10/daniel-andrews-you-can-now-get-a-haircut-arent-you-going-to-thank-me/.

Simpson J. (2021). *The New COVID Crisis Shows Victoria's Public Health Administration is in Deadly Decline*. Spectator Australia, 4 January 2021. Accessed at: https://www.spectator.com.au/2021/01/the-new-covid-crisis-shows-victorias-public-health-administration-is-in-deadly-decline/.

Sisemore J.D. (1991). *The Russo-Japanese War, Lessons not Learned*. Thesis, M.S. Southwest Missouri State University, Springfield, MO.

Skatssoon J. (2020). *Victorian ICT Provider Failing, Auditor Finds*. Government News 23 October 2019. Accessed at: https://www.governmentnews.com.au/victorian-ict-provider-failing-audit-finds/.

Skatssoon J. (2020). *DHHS Slammed for Bungling Homelessness Plan*. Government News, 21 September 2020. Accessed at: https://www.governmentnews.com.au/dhhs-slammed-for-bungling-homelessness-plan/.

Skatssoon J. (2021). *Victoria Falling Short on Infrastructure Planning*. Government News, 23 August 2021. Accessed at: https://www.governmentnews.com.au/victoria-falling-short-on-infrastructure-planning/.

Sky News (2020a). *Victoria's Second Wave Lockdown Costing $300-$400 Million Each Day*. Sky News, 30 August 2020. Accessed at: https://www.skynews.com.au/australia-news/victorias-second-wave-lockdown-costing-300400-million-each-day/video/06fcf9aff7d2f6d77d8c8d2944799e4d

Sky News (2020b). *Leaked Video Shows Bureaucrats Congratulating Themselves for Botched Hotel Quarantine System*. Sky News Australia 10 August 2020. Accessed at: https://www.youtube.com/watch?v=gq51zvmN7j4.

Sky News (2020c). *Daniel Andrews is a 'one man band' just as culpable as his bureaucrats*. The Kenny Report, Sky News Australia, 29 September 2020.

Sky News (2021a). *Reports Hotel Quarantine Company Unified Security in Liquidation*. 21 May 2021. Accessed at: https://www.skynews.com.au/australia-news/reports-hotel-quarantine-company-unified-security-in-liquidation/video/f928a497dbca0570390e9e4239736749.

Sky News (2021b). *'Craven Spin' by Daniel Andrews is the 'Tip of the iceberg': Credlin*. Sky News 15 February 2021. Accessed at: https://www.youtube.com/watch?v=3zNZqKvEKdk.

Sky News (2021c). *Victorian Government's QR Code Problem Led to the 'Most Crippling Lockdown' Yet*. Sky News 5 June 2021. Accessed at: https://www.skynews.com.au/australia-news/victorian-governments-qr-code-problem-led-to-the-most-crippling-lockdown-yet/video/932bce6939e8d1188ac1f529c5440ed3.

Slattery C. (2009). *The Dark Side of Leadership: Troubling Times at the Top*. Seaman and Slattery, November 2009. Sydney Australia.

Sloan J. (2021). *Politicians Flout Tinbergen Rule, to the Nation's Peril*. The Australian 27 July 2021. Accessed at: https://www.theaustralian.com.au/commentary/politicians-flout-tinbergen-rule-tothe-nations-peril/news-story/e067be6192aea092180f801787d524e7.

Smethurst A. (2021a). *'Seriously worried': Whistleblower Reveals Hotel Quarantine 'Breaches'*. The Age 6 March 2021.

Smethurst A. (2021b). *Culture of Cover-up Puts Victorians at Risk*. The Age, 7 May 2021. Accessed at: https://www.theage.com.au/national/victoria/culture-of-cover-up-puts-victorians-at-risk-20210506-p57pl5.html.

Smethurst A. and Sakkal P. (2021). *Contact Tracing Faltered as 'Hyper-Infectious' COVID Strain Pushes State into Lockdown*. The Age 13 February 2021. Accessed at: https://www.theage.com.au/national/victoria/contact-tracing-faltered-as-hyper-infectious-covid-strain-pushes-state-into-lockdown-20210212-p5723f.html.

Smith C. (2020). *Premier Andrews Buckling Under 'Police Union Pressure to Refuse ADF Aid': Kroger*. Sky News, 25 June 2020. Accessed at: https://www.adelaidenow.com.au/news/national/premier-andrews-buckling-under-police-union-pressure-to-refuse-adf-aid-kroger/video/544c883618d85888b3b4c2277d3bac50.

Smith E.D., Siefert W.T., and Drain D. (2009). *Risk Matrix Input Data Biases. Systems Engineering* 12 (4) pp. 344–360.

Smith F. (2020). *'Woke' Companies: Do They Really Mean What They Say?* The Ethics Centre, The Ethics Alliance. Accessed at: https://ethics.org.au/woke-companies-do-they-really-mean-what-they-say/.

Smith K.M., Machalaba C.C., Seifman R., Feferholtz Y., and Karesh W.B. (2019). *Infectious Disease and Economics: The Case for Considering Multi-sectoral Impacts*. One Health 7 Article 100080.

Smith M. (2016). *What's Happened to the Victoria Police AWU Fraud Investigation Since Dan Andrews Became Premier?* Michael Smith News, 15 March 2016. Accessed at: https://www.michaelsmithnews.com/2016/03/whats-happened-to-victoria-polices-awu-fraud-investigation-since-dan-andrews-became-premier.html.

Smith M. (2018). *Victoria Police Told to Go Easy on Labor MPs in Fraud Investigation*. Michael Smith News, 16 October 2018.Accessed at: https://www.michaelsmithnews.com/2018/10/victoria-police-told-to-go-easy-on-labor-mps-in-fraud-investigation.html.

Smith R. (2021). *Covid-19 back in Aged Care, Rule banning Staff at Multiple Sites Lifted*. News.com.au. 1st June 2021. Accessed at: https://www.news.com.au/national/politics/covid19-back-in-aged-care-rule-banning-staff-at-multiple-sites-lifted/news-story/875eef78b219af19dcd1876b67836e5b.

Smith S.F., Watts A.L., and Lilienfeld S.O. (2014). *On the Trail of the Elusive Successful Psychopath*. The Psychologist 27(7) pp. 506-510.

Smith T. (2021). *Toxic Culture Still Running Through Victoria's Fire Service*. Accessed at: https://vic.liberal.org.au/media-releases/2021-02-20-toxic-culture-still-running-through-victorias-fire-service

Smits M., Groenewegen P.P., Timmermans D.R.M., van der Wal G. and Wagner C. (2009). *The Nature and Causes of Unintended Events Reported at Ten Emergency Departments*. BMC Emergency Medicine 9 Article 16.

Smollen R.K. (2014). *Organisational Culture, Organisational Change and Emotions: A Qualitative Study*. ANZAM, 2008. Auckland, New Zealand.

Snijders V., Burd H., Prestt J., Judah G., Huf S., and Halpern D. (2016). *Applying Behavioral Insights: Simple Ways to Improve Health Outcomes*. World Innovation Summit for Health, 2016. Doha, Qatar. Accessed at: https://www.bi.team/wp-content/uploads/2016/11/WISH-2016_Behavioral_Insights_Report.pdf

Snow D. (2018). *Siege: The Powerful and Uncompromising Story of What Happened Inside the Lindt Cafe and Why the Police Response Went so Tragically Wrong*. Allen and Unwin, Crows Nest. NSW Australia.

Snow F.M. (2020). *Epidemics and Society: From the Black Death to the Present*. Yale University Press, New Haven and London.

Song H-D., Tu C-C., Zhang G-W., Wang S-Y., Zheng K., et al. (2005). *Cross-host Evolution of Severe Acute Respiratory Syndrome Coronavirus in Palm Civet and Human*. PNAS 102 pp. 2430-2435.

Spalluto L.B., Planz V.B., Stokes L.S., Pierce R., Aronoff D.M., McPheeters M.L., and Omary R.A. (2020). *Transparency and Trust During the Coronavirus Disease 2019 (COVID-19) Pandemic*. Journal of the American College of Radiology 17(7) pp. 909-912.

Sparrow A. (2021). *The Chinese Government's Cover-up Killed Health Care Workers Worldwide*. Foreign Policy, Special Reports, 18 March 2021. Accessed at: https://foreignpolicy.com/2021/03/18/china-covid-19-killed-health-care-workers-worldwide/.

Spiliopoulos L. (2022). *On the Effectiveness of COVID-19 Restrictions and Lockdowns: Pan Metron Ariston. BMC Public Health* 22, Article 1842.

Staley L. (2021). *Andrews Labor Government Continues to Hide Public Health Advice*. Media release, 21 July 2021. Accessed at: https://www.louisestaley.com.au/media-releases/2021-07-21-crozier-andrews-labor-government-continues-to-hide-public-health-advice.

Standards Australia (2018). *AS ISO 31000:2018 Risk management – Guidelines*. Standards Australia, Sydney, Australia.

Starcke K, and Brand M. (2012). *Decision Making Under Stress: A Selective Review*. Neuroscience and Behavioral Reviews 36(4) pp. 1228-1248.

State Services Authority (2013). *Organisational Culture*. State Services Authority, Government of Victoria, Melbourne, Australia.

Stenning P. (2016). *The Idea of Political 'Independence' of the Police: International Interpretations and Experiences*. In Police and Government Relations pp. 183-256. University of Toronto Press.

Stenning P.C. (2011). *Governance the Police: Independence, Accountability and Interference*. Ray Whitrod Memorial Lecture, 6 October 2011, TAFE SA, Adelaide, Australia.

Sterman J.D. (2006). *Learning from Evidence in a Complex World*. American Journal of Public Health. 96(3) pp. 505-514.

Stern E. (2013). *Preparing: The Sixth Task of Crisis Leadership*. Journal of Leadership Studies 7(3) pp. 51-56.

Stern E., 't Hart P., and McConnell A. (2020). *Leading in a Crisis: How to Avoid Common Pitfalls and Build a High Performing Team*. ANSOG. Accessed at: https://www.anzsog.edu.au/resource-library/research/how-to-avoid-common-pitfalls-and-build-a-high-performing-team

Stewart C. (2021). *Locked-down and Out in Daniel Andrews' Penal Pandemic Paradise*. The Weekend Australian 22 September 2021. Accessed at: https://www.theaustralian.com.au/commentary/lockeddown-and-out-in-daniel-andrews-penal-pandemic-paradise/news-story/1ba7dd9395b26505b83f578f06b12f5a.

Stewart G. (2020). *Will Boris go for Woke?* The Critic, 22 November 2020. Accessed at: https://thecritic.co.uk/will-boris-go-for-woke/.

Stout S., Zallman L., and Arsenault L. (2017). *Developing High-Functioning Teams: Factors Associated with Operating as a "Real Team" and Implications for Patient-centered Medical Home Development*. Inquiry: The Journal of Health Care Organization, Provision, and Financing 54, 12 June 2017.

Strassheim H. (2019). *Behavioural Mechanisms and Public Policy Design: Preventing Failures in Behavioural Public Policy*. Public Policy and Administration 36(2) pp. 187-204.

Steibel L. (2021). *Update on Emergency Incident*. Victorian Big Battery 2 August 2021. Accessed at: https://victorianbigbattery.com.au/incident-at-vbb/.

Sumpton J. (2020). *Covid Measures will be seen as 'Monument of Collective Hysteria and Folly' Says Ex-judge*. The Guardian (Australian edition) 28 October 2021. Accessed at: https://www.theguardian.com/law/2020/oct/27/covid-measures-will-be-seen-as-monument-of-collective-hysteria-and-folly-says-ex-judge.

Sundin J. (2019). *Public Health of Politics*. Interchange 50 pp. 129-136.

Supreme Court of Victoria (2022). *Independent Contractors of Australia Inc (Trading as Self-Employed Australia) vs Victorian WorkCover Authority (Trading as WorkSafe Victoria)*. S ECI 2022 00427.

Sunraysia (2022). Labor Fighting to Keep Victoria in the Dark. Sunraysia Daily, 3 June 2022. Accessed at: https://www.sunraysiadaily.com.au/letters/5967723/labor-fighting-to-keep-victoria-in-the-dark-on-covid-survey.

Surraweera A. and Ofner B. (2020). *The Voice of Reason or Just More Noise: Understanding the Significance of the Royal Commission*. Sydney University Law Society, 11 October 2020. Accessed at: https://www.suls.org.au/law-in-society-2019-content/2020/10/11/the-voice-of-reason-or-just-more-noise-understanding-the-significance-of-the-royal-commission.

Sutton B. (2020). *Transcript of Day 18 Hearing, P-1491*. COVID-19 Hotel Quarantine Inquiry, 16 September 2020. Accessed at: https://www.quarantineinquiry.vic.gov.au/hearings-transcripts.

Swainston J., Chapman B., Grunfeld E.A. and Derakshan N. (2020). *COVID-19 Lockdown and Its Adverse Impact on Psychological Health in Breast Cancer*. Frontiers in Psychology 11 Article 2033.

Sweeney R.J. (2003). *Self-Denial in Federalizing Power in the European Union: Lessons from the Causes of the American Revolution.* LEFIC Working Paper 2003-10. Centre for Law, Economics and Financial Institutions, Copenhagen Business School, Frederiksberg, Denmark.

Tabesh P. and Vera D.M. (2020). *Top Managers' Improvisational Decision-making in Crisis: A Paradox Perspective*. Management Decision 58(10) pp. 2235-2256.

Tahir Q. (2021). *The Second Ambulance, Code Red, in a Week as Victoria Recorded 37,994 New COVID Cases and 13 Deaths*. Sydney News Today, 11 January 2022. Accessed at: https://sydneynewstoday.com/the-second-ambulance-code-red-in-a-week-as-victoria-recorded-37994-new-covid-cases-and-13-deaths/494337/.

Talbot J. (2021). *Victoria Premier Daniel Andrews Grilled Over IBAC Investigation Knowledge*. Sky News, 7 October 2021. Accessed at: https://www.skynews.com.au/australia-news/politics/victoria-premier-daniel-andrews-grilled-over-ibac-investigation-knowledge/news-story/c6755ad48dd1c7df2fe88ca394794d56.

Talbot T. (2022). *Victorian Premier Daniel Andrews Private Office Under Workplace Watchdog Investigation After MP Alleges Bullying.* Sky News, 20 February 2022. Accessed at: https://www.skynews.com.au/australia-news/politics/victorian-premier-daniel-andrews-office-under-workplace-watchdog-investigation-after-mp-alleges-bullying/news-story/2e2a6cf9fd62f7112525e2f044ff13d8#share-tools.

Talevski J. (2021). *How Poor Advice and Planning Led Victoria's Department of Justice to Complete Project Failure*. ARN 6 May 2021. Accessed at: https://www.arnnet.com.au/article/688195/how-poor-advice-planning-led-victoria-department-justice-complete-project-failure/.

Tang W. (2021a). *Coronavirus: It's too Early to Rule out Lab Leak, says WHO Chief*. The Times, 16 July 2021. Accessed at:

https://www.theaustralian.com.au/world/the-times/coronavirus-its-too-early-to-rule-out-lab-leak-says-who-chief/news-story/b69549fa8f192224796a6d0648d84489.

Tang D. (2021b). *Coronavirus: China Fakes Swiss Expert for Wuhan Laboratory Leak Propaganda*. The Australian 12 August 2021. Accessed at: https://www.theaustralian.com.au/world/the-times/coronavirus-china-fakes-swiss-expert-for-wuhan-laboratory-leak-propaganda/news-story/fc1fcc62cc8de03b13ed2d11ccd6b367.

Tang J. (2022). *Expert Reaction to 'Evidence Summary: Coronavirus (COVID-19) and the Use of face Coverings in Education Settings'*. Science Media Centre 6 January 2022. Accessed at: https://www.sciencemediacentre.org/expert-reaction-to-evidence-summary-coronavirus-covid-19-and-the-use-of-face-coverings-in-education-settings/.

Tardivel K., White S.B., and Duong K.K. (2020). *Cruise Ship Travel.* In: Travelers' Health, CDC Yellow Book, Chapter 8: Travel by Air, Sea & Land. Centers for Disease Control and Prevention. Accessed at: https://wwwnc.cdc.gov/travel/yellowbook/2020/travel-by-air-land-sea/cruise-ship-travel.

Tarakji G. (1992). *Lessons not Learned From 1998 Loma Prieta Earthquake*. Journal of Professional issues in Engineering Education and Practice 118(2) 132.

Taştan S.B. and Türker M.V. (2014). *A Study of the Relationship between Organizational Culture and Job Involvement: The Moderating Role of Psychological Conditions of Meaningfulness and Safety*. Procedia – Social and Behavioral Sciences 149 pp. 943-947.

Taylor J. (2020a). *Hotel Quarantine Linked to 99% of Victoria's COVID Cases, Inquiry Told*. The Guardian 18 August 2020.

Taylor J. (2020b). *Victoria's Hotel Quarantine Inquiry No Excuse to Dodge Questions, Judge Says*. The Guardian 5 August 2020. Accessed at: https://www.theguardian.com/australia-news/2020/aug/05/victorias-hotel-quarantine-inquiry-granted-a-six-week-extension.

Taylor S. (2021). *How to Stop Psychopaths and Narcissists from Winning Positions of Power*. The Conversation 8 April 2021. Accessed at: https://theconversation.com/how-to-stop-psychopaths-and-narcissists-from-winning-positions-of-power-158183.

Teague B., Catford J., and Petering S. (2014). *Hazelwood Mine Fire Inquiry Report*. Hazelwood Mine Fire Inquiry. Government of Victoria, Melbourne, Victoria.

Teague B., McLeod R., Pascoe S. (2010). *Final Report, 2009 Victorian Bushfires Royal Commission*. Government of Victoria, Melbourne, Victoria.

Tenbrunsel A.E., Diekmann K.A., Wade-Benzoni K.A., and Bazerman M.H. (2009). *The Ethical Mirage: A Temporal Explanation as to Why We Aren't as Ethical as We Think We Are*. Harvard Business School, Working Paper 08-012. Accessed at: https://www.hbs.edu/faculty/Publication%20Files/08-012.pdf.

Tenbrunsel A.E. and Messick D.M. (2004). *Ethical Fading: The Role of Self-Deception in Unethical Behavior*. Social Justice Research 17 pp. 223-236.

Terrill M. (2021). *Billion Dollar Blowouts in Major Projects Predictable - and Avoidable*. The Age, 11 August 2021. Accessed at: https://www.theage.com.au/national/victoria/billion-dollar-blowouts-in-major-projects-predictable-and-avoidable-20210811-p58hsa.html.

Thacker P.D. (2021a). *The Covid-19 Lab Leak Hypothesis: Did the Media Fall Victim to a Misinformation Campaign?* British Medical Journal 7, Article: n1656.

Thacker P.D. (2021b). *Covid-19: Lancet Investigation into Origin of Pandemic Shuts Down Over Bias Risk*. British Medical Journal 375 Article: n2414.

't Hart P., and Boin A. (2001). *Between Crisis and Normalcy: The Long Shadow of Post-politics*. In: Managing crises: Threats, Dilemmas and Opportunities, (Editors: C.C. Thomas. U. Rosenthal, A. Boin, and L.K. Comfort (Eds.), Springfield.

Thawley M, and Comley B. (2015). *Martin Place Siege, Joint Commonwealth-New South Wales Review*. January 2015.

The Australian (2020). *Leaked Video Celebrates Melbourne Hotel Quarantine Program's Success*. The Australian, 11 August 2020. Accessed at: https://www.theaustralian.com.au/breaking-news/leaked-video-celebrates-melbourne-hotel-quarantine-programs-success/news-story/4648daf87eaac3ec512768b3c5e2d7bb.

The Editors (2020). *Dying in a Leadership Vacuum*. New England Journal of Medicine 283 pp. 1479-1480.

Thiessen T. (2020). *Ruby Princess Inquiry Slams Health Officials Over Covid-19 Cruise: Australia US Deaths*. Forbes 14 August 2020. Accessed at: https://www.forbes.com/sites/tamarathiessen/2020/08/14/ruby-princess-inquiry-health-covid-australia-us/?sh=58b4a15c3809.

Thorne L. (2020). *Victoria's Coronavirus Quarantine Program to Get a 'Reset' After Breaches*. ABC News 1 July, 2020. Accessed at: https://www.abc.net.au/news/2020-07-01/victoria-coronavirus-hotel-quarantine-how-did-we-get-here/12408256.

Tichy M. (2014). *Analogies in Entity Risk Mechanics*. Journal of Risk Analysis and Crisis Response 4(2) pp. 96-107.

Tinbergen J. (1952). *On the Theory of Economic Policy*. North-Holland Publishing Company, Amsterdam, The Netherlands.

Tsirtsakis A. (2022). *GPs Step up to Avoid 'Absolute Collapse' of Health System*. News GP, 2 February 2022. Royal Australian College of General Practitioners. Accessed at: https://www1.racgp.org.au/newsgp/professional/gps-step-up-to-avoid-absolute-collapse-of-health-s.

Tognotti E. (2013). *Lessons from the History of Quarantine, From Plague to Influenza A*. Emerging Infectious Diseases 19(2) pp. 254-9.

Tomazin F. (2019). *Anti-corruption Chiefs Warn of Political Interference, Call for Independent Funding*. The Sydney Morning Herald, 1 November 2019.

Tomazin F., Dow A., and Cunningham M. (2021). *System Overload: Why Victoria's Health Network is on its Knees*. The Age, 4 September 2021. Accessed at: https://www.theage.com.au/national/victoria/system-overload-why-victoria-s-health-network-is-on-its-knees-20210901-p58nry.html.

Torossian R. (2019). *Boeing's Ongoing PR Nightmare*. Accessed at: https://www.odwyerpr.com/story/public/13356/2019-11-11/boeings-ongoing-pr-nightmare.html.

Towell N. (2021). *Latest Cost Victoria $2.8 Billion and Counting*. The Age, 16 November 2021. Accessed at: https://www.theage.com.au/national/victoria/latest-lockdowns-cost-2-8-billion-and-counting-20211116-p59985.html.

Towell N. and Crock L. (2021). *State Consultant Bill Blows Out by 300 per cent*. The Age, 3 December 2021. Accessed at: https://www.theage.com.au/national/victoria/state-consultant-bill-blows-out-by-300-per-cent-20211130-p59dbw.html.

Tran K., Cimon K., Severn M., Pessoa-Silva C.L., Conly J. (2012). *Aerosol Generating Procedures and Risk of Transmission of Acute Respiratory Infections to Healthcare Workers: A Systematic Review*. PLoS One 7(4) Article e35797.

Treurniet W and Wolbers J. (2021). *Codifying a Crisis: Progression from Information Sharing to Distributed Decision-making*. Journal of Contingencies and Crisis Management 29 pp. 23-35.

Trioli V. (2021). *'It's not Working Properly': Infectious Disease Expert Calls for Pause of Victoria's Hotel Quarantine Program*. ABC Radio Melbourne. 17 February 2021. Accessed at: https://www.abc.net.au/melbourne/programs/mornings/lindsay-grayson-hotel-quarantine/13163066.

Trioli V. (2021). Look*ing at Victoria's Fourth COVID Lockdown from Behind is Maddening*. ABC News, 29 May 2021. Accessed at: https://www.abc.net.au/news/2021-05-29/victoria-fourth-covid-lockdown-behind-solutions-staring-face/100173884

Triple M (2020). *The Hot Breakfast Explains the Issues with Victoria's Contact Tracing: "A Farce"*. Triple M Newsroom, 17 October 2020. Accessed at: https://www.triplem.com.au/story/the-hot-breakfast-explains-the-issues-with-victoria-s-contact-tracing-168049.

Tsai Y. (2011). *Relationship between Organizational Culture, Leadership Behavior and Job Satisfaction*. BMC Health Services Research 11 Article 98.

Tuffield R. (2021a). *Ombudsman Details Shocking Human Rights Complaints in New Report*. News.com.au, 4 August 2021. Accessed at: https://www.news.com.au/national/victoria/politics/ombudsman-details-shocking-human-rights-complaints-in-new-report/news-story/9023aeb1c8b49fe0b9549b3784798dcd.

Tuffield R. (2021b). *Woman $180 Out of Pocket in Body Corporate Fees for QR Code*. News.com.au, 14 May 2021. Accessed at: https://www.news.com.au/national/victoria/politics/woman-180-out-of-pocket-in-body-corporate-fees-for-qr-code/news-story/2e25053d8c5c2c4be2cf2733b67bf1f1.

Tuffield R. (2021c). *Victorian Government Orders Senior Bureaucrat Matiu Bush to Stand Aside Following Hotel Quarantine Breaches*. News.com, 5 May 2021. Accessed at: https://www.news.com.au/travel/travel-updates/victorian-government-orders-senior-bureaucrat-matiu-bush-to-stand-aside-following-hotel-quarantine-breaches/news-story/848c7932e957f6c70a8c0eade045611a.

Tuffield R. (2021d). *'Secret' Curfew Documents May Soon be Revealed*. The Australian, 13 October 2021. Accessed at: https://www.theaustralian.com.au/news/latest-news/secret-curfew-documents-may-soon-be-revealed/news-story/5d603b1eac08f8213bbb1c452ce9436f.

Tuffield R, (2021e). *Victorian Opposition Slams Daniel Andrews Government Over 'corrupt' Taxpayer Spend*. News.com.au, 4 August 2021. Accessed at: https://www.news.com.au/national/victoria/politics/victorian-opposition-slams-daniel-andrews-government-over-corrupt-taxpayer-spend/news-story/45fa662b6fe887071b6fbc8978b8991a.

Tuffield R. and Piovesan A. (2021). *Victorian Opposition Leader Matthew Guy Calls for Daniel Andrews to Resign Amid IBAC Investigation*. News.com.au, 6 October 2021. Accessed at: https://www.news.com.au/national/victoria/news/victorian-opposition-leader-matthew-guy-calls-for-daniel-andrews-to-resign-amid-ibac-investigation/news-story/2df563e21ca751185caf3a61aa6f3389.

Tuohy W. (2020). *Ambulance Victoria Chief Vows to Shine a Light into the Rotten Corners of our Culture*. The Age, 28 October 2020. Accessed at: https://www.theage.com.au/national/victoria/call-for-worksafe-to-investigate-dangers-to-mental-health-of-ambulance-victoria-staff-20201028-p569ep.html.

Turner B.A. (1976). *The Organizational and Interorganizational Development of Disasters*. Administrative Science Quarterly 21(3) pp. 378–397.
Turner-Cohen A (2021). *Relatives of COVID Victims During Victoria's Second Wave Warn 'History is Repeating' As the State's Aged Care Crisis Deepens*. 7 News, 1 June 2021. Accessed at:
https://7news.com.au/lifestyle/health-wellbeing/relatives-of-covid-victims-during-victorias-second-wave-warn-history-is-repeating-as-the-states-aged-care-crisis-deepens-c-2982309.
Uitdewilligen S. and Waller M.J. (2018). *Information Sharing and Decision-making in Multidisciplinary Crisis Management Teams*. Journal of Organizational Behaviour 39(6) pp. 731-748.
UN/DESA (2020). UN/DESA Policy Brief #74: *Resilient Institutions in Times of Crisis: Transparency, Accountability and Participation at the National Level Key to Effective Response to COVID-19*. United Nations, Department of Economic and Social Affairs. Accessed at:
https://www.un.org/development/desa/dpad/publication/un-desa-policy-brief-74-resilient-institutions-in-times-of-crisis-transparency-accountability-and-participation-at-the-national-level-key-to-effective-response-to-covid-19/.
UNDRR (2019). *Accountability in the Context of Disaster Risk Governance*. Un Office for Disaster Recovery. Accessed at:
https://reliefweb.int/sites/reliefweb.int/files/resources/Accountability%20in%20the%20context%20of%20disaster%20risk%20governance.pdf.
Urban R. (2018). *Bureaucrats Told: Use Gender-Neutral Speech*. The Australian, 2 August 2018. Accessed at:
https://www.theaustralian.com.au/nation/politics/bureaucrats-told-use-genderneutral-speech/news-story/9cb64690112ae646369010490e60ca7e.
USAID (2021). *Emerging Pandemic Threats*. Emerging Pandemic Threats Program. Accessed at:
https://www.usaid.gov/news-information/fact-sheets/emerging-pandemic-threats-program.
US Army (2015). *Leader's Guide to Team Building: Building Adaptive High-performance Teams*. Handbook No 14-02. Center for Army Lessons Learned, Washington, DC.
US-Canada PSOTF (2003). Final Report on the August 14, 2003 Blackout in the United States and Canada. US-Canada Power System Outage Task Force.
US DHSS (2007). *Public Health Emergency Response: A Guide for Leaders and Responders*. US Department of Health and Human Services, Washington DC.
VAGO (2008). *Biosecurity Incidents: Planning and Risk Management for Livestock Diseases*. Victorian Auditor General's Report, November 2008. Accessed at:
https://www.parliament.vic.gov.au/papers/govpub/VPARL2006-10No153.pdf.
VAGO (2016a). *Bullying and Harassment in the Health Sector*. Victorian Auditor-General's Report, March 2016, 2015-16:28. Accessed at:
https://www.audit.vic.gov.au/sites/default/files/20160323-Bullying.pdf.
VAGO (2016b). *Digital Dashboard: Status Review of ICT Projects and Initiatives – Phase 2*. Victorian Auditor General's Office, 9 March 2016. Accessed at:
https://www.audit.vic.gov.au/report/digital-dashboard-status-review-ict-projects-and-initiatives-phase-2.
VAGO (2021a). *Major Projects Performance, September 2021, Independent Assurance Report to Parliament 2021-22:05*. Victorian Auditor-General's Office. Accessed at:
https://www.audit.vic.gov.au/sites/default/files/2021-09/20210922-Major-Projects_1.pdf.

VAGO (2021b). *Major Infrastructure Program Delivery Capability, August 2021. Independent Assurance Report to Parliament 2021-22:2*. Victorian Auditor-General's Office. Accessed at: https://www.audit.vic.gov.au/sites/default/files/2021-08/20210818-Major-Infrastructure.pdf.

VAGO (2021c). *Clinical Governance: Department of Health September 2021*. Independent Assurance Report to Parliament 2021-22: 03. Victorian Auditor-General's Office. Accessed at: https://www.audit.vic.gov.au/sites/default/files/2021-08/20210901-Clinical-Governance.pdf.

VAGO (2021d). *Managing Conflicts of Interest in Procurement*. Independent Assurance Report to Parliament 2021–22: 04, September 2021. Victorian Auditor-General's Office. Accessed at:

VAGO (2021e). *Measuring and Reporting on Service Delivery May 2021. Independent Assurance Report to Parliament 2020-21:19*. Victorian Auditor-General's Office. Accessed at: https://www.audit.vic.gov.au/sites/default/files/2021-05/20210526-Service-Delivery-report.pdf.

VAGO (2021f). *Service Victoria —Digital Delivery of Government Services March 2021. Independent Assurance Report to Parliament 2020–21:16*. Victorian Auditor-General's Office. Accessed at:
https://www.audit.vic.gov.au/sites/default/files/2021-03/20210318-Service-Victoria-report.pdf.

VAGO (2021g). *Grants to the Migrant Workers Centre February 2021. Independent assurance report to Parliament 2020–21:12*. Victorian Auditor General's Office. Accessed at: https://www.audit.vic.gov.au/sites/default/files/2021-02/20210217-Grants-to-MWC.pdf.

VAGO (2021h). *Victoria's Homelessness Response September 2020. Independent Assurance Report to Parliament 2020–21: 3*. Victorian Auditor General's Office. Accessed at: https://www.audit.vic.gov.au/sites/default/files/2020-09/20200917-Homelessness-Response-report_2.pdf.

VAGO (2021i). *Implementing a New Infringements Management System*. VAGO, 5 May 2021. Accessed at: https://www.audit.vic.gov.au/report/implementing-a-new-infringements-management-system.

VALS (2020). *Increased Police Powers Must Not be Free Kick for Discrimination*. Victorian Aboriginal Legal Service. 11 August 2020. Accessed at: https://www.vals.org.au/increased-police-powers-must-not-be-free-kick-for-discrimination/.

Van Beusekorn M. (2020). *Scientists: 'Exactly Zero' Evidence COVID-19 Came from a Lab*. Center for Infectious Disease Research and Policy, 12 May 2020. Accessed at: https://www.cidrap.umn.edu/news-perspective/2020/05/scientists-exactly-zero-evidence-covid-19-came-lab.

Van Diemen A. (2020). *Transcript of Day 18 Hearing, P-1536*. COVID-19 Hotel Quarantine Inquiry, 16 September 2020. Accessed at:
https://www.quarantineinquiry.vic.gov.au/hearings-transcripts.

Van Onselen L. (2021). *Dan's Wasteland: Victorian Project Costs Blowout by $6bn*. Unconventional Economist, Macrobusiness, 23 September 2021. Accessed at:
https://www.macrobusiness.com.au/2021/09/victorian-project-costs-blowout-by-6b/.

Van Onselen L. (2022). *Victoria has Nation's Unhealthiest Hospital System*. Accessed at: https://www.macrobusiness.com.au/2022/02/victoria-has-nations-unhealthiest-hospital-system/.

Van de Walle B., Brugghemans B., and Come T. (2016). *Improving Situation Awareness in Crisis Response Teams: an Experimental Analysis of Enriched Information and Centralized Coordination*. International Journal of Human Computer Studies 95 pp. 66-79.

Van Winsen R., Henriqson E., Schuler B., and Dekker S.W.A. (2015). *Situation Awareness: Some Conditions of Possibility*. Theoretical Issues in Ergonomics Science 16 (1) pp. 53-68.

Varga R. (2019). *Sir Ken Jones Slams Toxic Loyalty over Law in Victoria Police*. The Australian 13 December 2019. Accessed at: https://www.theaustralian.com.au/nation/sir-ken-jones-slams-toxic-loyalty-over-law-in-victoria-police/news-story/6aa501049c70a36ab5f2ff299f4f2ef4.

Varga R. (2020). *Coronavirus: Victorian CHO Brett Sutton 'Should Lead Response, not Bureaucrats'*. The Weekend Australian 29 September 2020. Accessed at: https://www.theaustralian.com.au/nation/politics/coronavirus-victorian-cho-brett-sutton-should-lead-response-not-bureaucrats/news-story/57ebd3181c86293a8471f13ef1c07d5d.

Varga R. (2021a). *Victoria's Hotel Quarantine Legal Bill Soars to $12.3 million*. The Australian, 3 May 2021. Accessed at: https://www.theaustralian.com.au/nation/politics/victorias-hotel-quarantine-legal-bill-soars-to-123-million/news-story/9c04f53a7752389f3b4aefed595af3b8.

Varga R. (2021b). *Hotel Quarantine: Nebuliser Man Vindicated After 'Cover Up*. The Australian 6 July 2021. Accessed at: https://www.theaustralian.com.au/nation/hotel-quarantine-nebuliser-man-vindicated-after-cover-up/news-story/ca09931ca5c765a3d101d8bbeaf1eb9a.

Varga R. (2021c). *Coronavirus: Hundreds Wait for Beds Amid Victorian Hotel Quarantine*. The Australian 15 September 2021. Accessed at: https://www.theaustralian.com.au/nation/politics/coronavirus-hundreds-wait-for-beds-amid-victorian-hotel-quarantine-chaos/news-story/820ddf2b6fe84a8302259c91ef491e84

Varga R. (2021d). *IBAC Inquiry: Faction Mates 'played racism cover-up card'*. The Australian, 19 October 2021. Accessed at: https://www.theaustralian.com.au/nation/ibac-inquiry-banyule-mayor-rick-garotti-admits-factional-aim-over-grant/news-story/5d5ea1721a9b522f577ac9e004a0ca30.

Varga R. (2020). *Coronavirus: Brett Sutton was Blocked from Leading Response, Inquiry Told*. The Australian 11 September 2020. Accessed at: https://www.theaustralian.com.au/nation/hotel-quarantine-inquiry-five-calls-before-body-found-at-pan-pacific/news-story/0647d938eb1ef74c7b9bb9500fc7918d.

Varga R. and Snowden A. (2020). *Coronavirus Australia Live News: Botched Victorian Hotel Quarantine Program Cost $195m*. The Australian, 6 November 2020. Accessed at: https://www.theaustralian.com.au/nation/coronavirus-australia-live-news-mealticket-plan-to-get-economy-cooking/news-story/0f4f245cbfcf91814320775d7e075dcd#U702940738355iED.

Vaughan D. (2016). *The Challenger Launch Decision: Risky Technology, Culture, and Deviance at NASA*. University of Chicago Press, Chicago, IL.

Vinall F. (2020). *'I Don't agree': Daniel Andrews Contradicted in Court by Top Health Bureaucrat*. News.com.au, 1 October 2020. Accessed at: https://www.news.com.au/lifestyle/health/health-problems/seeing-the-premier-gives-me-anxiety-says-woman-suing-victorian-government/news-story/da1d3648d42a1ba9dfe2bab107b9cc27.

Vinall F. (2021). *Hotel Quarantine Company Unified Security Goes into Liquidation as Lawsuit Looms*. The Australian, 4 June 2021. Accessed at: https://www.theaustralian.com.au/breaking-news/hotel-quarantine-company-unified-security-goes-into-liquidation-as-lawsuit-looms/news-story/e43fd10f26ce74276d75ac7466480cbe.

Veil S. R. (2020). *Revisiting the Best Practices in Risk and Crisis Communication: A Multi-case Analysis*. In The Handbook of Applied Communication Research, edited by H. Dan O'Hair, 377–396. John Wiley & Sons, New York NY.
VEOHRC (2020). *Policing and Emergency Powers in the COVID-19 Recovery. Victorian Equal Opportunity and Human Rights Commission*. Accessed at: https://www.humanrights.vic.gov.au/legal-and-policy/covid-19-and-human-rights/centring-human-rights-in-the-covid-19-recovery/policing-and-emergency-powers-in-the-covid-19-recovery/.
Vergano D. (2014). *1918 Flu Pandemic That Killed 50 Million Originated in China, Historians Say*. National Geographic 25 January 2014. Accessed at: https://www.nationalgeographic.com/adventure/article/140123-spanish-flu-1918-china-origins-pandemic-science-health.
Vic Health (2017). *State Health Emergency Response Plan* Edition 4. Health.Vic, Victoria's hub for health services & businesses. Accessed at https://www2.health.vic.gov.au/emergencies/shera.
Victorian Government (2018). *Guide for Security Arrangements to Prevent and Manage Occupational Violence and Aggression: Guiding Principles.* Department of Health and Humans Services. Accessed at: https://www.health.vic.gov.au/publications/guide-for-security-arrangements-to-prevent-and-manage-occupational-violence-and.
Victorian Government (2019). *Victorian Public Health and Wellbeing Plan 2019-2023*. Victoria State Government, Melbourne.
Victorian Government (2020). *Victoria's Private Security Industry: Issues Paper for Consultation Police Policy and Strategy*. Justice and Community Safety, Melbourne, Victoria.
Victorian Government (2020). *Victorian Government Response to the Hotel Quarantine Inquiry*. Accessed at: https://www.vic.gov.au/hotel-quarantine-inquiry-victorian-government-response
Victorian Multicultural Commission (2020). *Submission 27, Inquiry into the Victorian Government's COVID–19 Contact Tracing System and Testing Regime*. Parliament of Victoria: Legislative Council Legal and Social Issues Committee. Accessed at: https://www.parliament.vic.gov.au/images/stories/committees/SCLSI/Inquiry_into_the_Victorian_Governments_COVID19_Contact_Tracing_System_and_Testing_Regime_/report/LCLSIC_59-05_Vic_Gov_COVID-19_contact_tracing_testing.pdf.
VOA News (2021). *New COVID-19 Outbreak Sends Australia's Victoria State into 4th Lockdown*. VOA News, 27 May 2021. Accessed at: https://www.voanews.com/covid-19-pandemic/new-covid-19-outbreak-sends-australias-victoria-state-4th-lockdown.
VPSC (2020). *Employee Numbers*. Victorian Public Sector Commission. 18 December 2020. Accessed at: https://vpsc.vic.gov.au/data-and-research/data-facts-visuals-state-of-the-sector/employee-numbers/.
Wade N. (2021). *Fauci Email Bolsters Lab Leak Theory*. Wall Street Journal 4 June 2021. Accessed at: https://www.wsj.com/articles/fauci-email-bolsters-the-lab-leak-theory-11622830092.
Wahlquist C. (2018). *Andrews Government's Release of Unredacted Mathew Guy Documents Condemned*. The Guardian, 6 September 2018. Accessed at: https://www.theguardian.com/australia-news/2018/sep/06/andrews-governments-release-of-unredacted-matthew-guy-documents-condemned.
Wahlquist C. (2020). *Questioning Daniel Andrews: How Reporters Came Under Attack in Victoria*. The Guardian 3 October 2020. Accessed at:

https://www.theguardian.com/australia-news/2020/oct/03/questioning-daniel-andrews-how-reporters-came-under-attack-in-victoria.
Wahlquist C. (2021). *Victorians Who Test Positive for Covid Will Need to Notify Close Contacts Themselves*. The Guardian, 20 November 2021. Accessed at:
https://www.theguardian.com/world/2021/nov/20/victorians-who-test-positive-for-covid-will-need-to-notify-close-contacts-themselves.
Wakeling N. (2020). *Victoria's Emergency Services Suffers Another Resignation Due to War on CFA*. Shadow Minister for Emergency Services, Media Statement, 18 December 2020. Accessed at:
https://vic.liberal.org.au/News/2020-12-18/wakeling-victorias-emergency-services-suffers-another-resignation-due-to-war-o.
Walker B. (2020). *Special Commission of Inquiry into the Ruby Princess*, Government of NSW.
Walshe K. (2005). *Are Public Inquiries Losing Their Independence?* British Medical Journal 331 pp. 117.
Wan G.H., Tsai Y.H., Wu Y.K., Tsao K.C. (2004). *A Large-volume Nebulizer Would Not be an Infectious Source for Severe Acute Respiratory Syndrome*. Infection Control and Hospital Epidemiology 25(12) pp. 1113–1115.
Wan W. and Blake A. (2020). *Coronavirus Modelers Factor in New Public Health Risk: Accusations Their Work is a Hoax*. The Washington Post, 27 March, 2020.
https://www.washingtonpost.com/health/2020/03/27/coronavirus-models-politized-trump.
Wang M., Li M., Ren R, Li L., Chen E-Q., Li W., and Ying B. (2020a). International Expansion of a Novel SARS-CoV-2 Mutant. Journal of Virology 94(12) Doi:
https://doi.org/10.1128/JVI.00567-20.
Wang R., Chen J., Gao K., Hozumi Y., Yin C., and Wei G-W. (2020b). *Characterizing SARS-CoV-2 Mutations in the United States*. Research Square Preprint 11 August 2020.
Wang Y., Hao H., and Platt L.S. (2021). *Examining Risk and Crisis Communications of Government Agencies and Stakeholders During Early-stages of COVID-19 on Twitter*. Computers in Human Behaviour 114 Article 106568.
Wankmüller C. (2020). *European Disaster Management in Response to the COVID-19 Pandemic*. Mind and Society https://doi.org/10.1007/s11299-020-00252-2.
Ward M and Rabe T. (2020). NSW Police Taking Organisers of Sydney Black Lives Matter Protest to Supreme Court. Sydney Morning Herald 5 June 2020. Accessed at:
https://www.smh.com.au/national/nsw/nsw-police-taking-organisers-of-sydney-black-lives-matter-protest-to-supreme-court-20200605-p54zw8.html.
Waters C. (2022). *Calls to Abolish Mandatory QR Check-ins*. The Age, 4 February 2022. Accessed at: https://www.theage.com.au/national/victoria/calls-to-abolish-mandatory-qr-check-ins-20220203-p59tgb.html.
Watson C.R., Watson M., and Sell T.K. (2017). *Public Health Preparedness Funding: Key Programs and Trends From 2001 to 2017*. American Journal of Public Health 107(S2) pp. S165-S167.
Way B., Khan F., and Veitch B. (2014). *Marine Transportation Application of Risk-Based Decision Making*. Proceedings of the 15th Annual General Assembly of the International Association of Maritime Universities, pp. 224-232, IAMU AGA 2014, 27-30 October 2014, Launceston, Tasmania, Australia.
Weber E.U. and Hse C.K. (2000). *Culture and Individual Judgement and Decision Making*. Applied Psychology: An International Review 49(1) pp. 32-61.
Weekly Source (2020*). Inquiry into VIC Government's COVID-19 Contact Tracing System was "Overwhelmed" from the Outset*. 15 December 2020. Accessed at:

https://www.theweeklysource.com.au/inquiry-into-vic-governments-covid-19-contact-tracing-system-concludes-system-was-overwhelmed-from-outset/

Weeramanthri T.S., Robertson A.G., Dows G.K., Effler P.V., Leclerq M.G., Burtenshaw J.D., Oldham S.J., Smith D.W., Gatti K.J., and Gladstones H.M. (2010). *Response to Pandemic (H1N1) 2009 Influenza in Australia – Lessons from a State Health Department Perspective.* Australian Health Review 34 pp. 477-486.

Weick K. and Sutcliffe K. (2002). *Managing the Unexpected.* Jossey-Bass, San Francisco, CA.

Weeramanthri T. (2021a). Review of Western Australia's Hotel Quarantine Arrangements. Interim Advice #1, 4 February 2021. Government of Western Australia. Accessed at: https://www.wa.gov.au/sites/default/files/2021-04/Review-of-Hotel-Quarantine-Arrangements-in-Western-Australia-Interim-Advice-1.pdf.

Weeramanthri T. (2021). *Review of Western Australia's Hotel Quarantine Arrangements.* Interim Advice #2: *Governance and Related Issues, 11 March 2021.* Government of Western Australia. Accessed at: https://www.wa.gov.au/sites/default/files/2021-04/Review-of-Hotel-Quarantine-Arrangements-in-Western-Australia-Interim-Advice-2.pdf.

Weeramanthri T. (2021c). *Review of Western Australia's Hotel Quarantine Arrangements. Final Advice 12 March 2021.* Government of Western Australia. Accessed at: https://www.wa.gov.au/sites/default/files/2021-04/Review-of-Hotel-Quarantine-Arrangements-in-Western-Australia-Final-Advice.pdf

Weidmann J. (2021). *What Role Should Central Banks Play in Combating Climate Change?* ILF Online-Conference "Green Banking and Green Central Banking: What are the Right Concepts?", 25 January 2021. Deutsche Bundesbank, Goethe University Frankfurt, Germany.

Weinshall K., Sommer U., and Ritov Y. (2018). *Ideological Influences on Governance and Regulation: The Comparative Case of Supreme Courts.* Regulation and Governance 12 pp. 334-353.

Weir K. (2017). *Why We Believe Alternative Facts.* Monitor on Psychology 48(4). American Psychological Association. Accessed at: https://www.apa.org/monitor/2017/05/alternative-facts.

Wernau J. (2021). *Fauci Says He Didn't Play Down China Lab-Leak Theory of Covid-19 Origins.* The Wall Street Journal, 9 June 2021. Accessed at: https://www.wsj.com/articles/fauci-says-he-didnt-play-down-china-lab-leak-theory-of-covid-19-origins-11623275288.

Wesnser B.S. (2015). *An Analysis of Reliability and Resilience in High Reliability Teams.* Journal of Management and Marketing Research 18 pp. 1-20.

West O. (2021). *UK Policing is at Real Risk of Direct Political Interference – But Does Anyone Care?* Policing Insight 2n July 2021. Accessed at: https://policinginsight.com/features/opinion/uk-policing-is-at-real-risk-of-direct-political-interference-but-does-anyone-care/.

Westcott R., Ronan K., Bambrick H., and Taylor M. (2019). *Public Health and Natural Hazards: New Policies and Preparedness Initiatives Developed from An Australian Bushfire Case Study.* Australia and New Zealand Journal of Public Health 43(4) pp. 395-400.

Whittaker J. (2015). *Thanks for Your Service, Liars': Di Dan Andrews Go too Far?* The Mandarin 11 March 2015. Accessed at: https://www.themandarin.com.au/25632-thanks-service-liars-daniel-andrews-go-far/.

White K.R.G, Kinnery D., Danek R.H., Smith B., and Harben C. (2020). *The Resistance to Change-Beliefs Scale: Validation of a New Measure of Conservative Ideology.* Personality and Social Psychology Bulletin 46(1) pp.20-30.

WHO (2005). *Article 32: Treatment of Travellers, International Health Regulations (2005).* Third Edition. World Health Organisation. Accessed at:
https://www.who.int/health-topics/international-health-regulations#tab=tab_1.
WHO (2014). *The Case for Investing in Public Health: A Public Health Summary Report for EPHO 8*. World Health Organisation Regional Office for Europe.
WHO (2017). *Communicating Risk in Public Health Emergencies: A WHO Guideline for Emergency Risk Communication (ERC) Policy and Practice*. World Health Organization, Geneva, Switzerland.
WHO (2019). *Five-Year Regional Strategic Plan to Strengthen Public Health Preparedness and Response – 2019–2023.* World Health Organization, Regional Office for South East Asia.
WHO (2020). *Key Considerations for Repatriation and Quarantine of Travellers in Relation to the Outbreak of Novel Coronavirus 2019-nCoV*. World Health Organisation, COVID -19 Travel Advice, 11 February 2020. Accessed at:
https://www.who.int/news-room/articles-detail/key-considerations-for-repatriation-and-quarantine-of-travellers-in-relation-to-the-outbreak-of-novel-coronavirus-2019-ncov.
WHO (2021a). *WHO-convened Global Study of Origins of SARS-CoV-2: China Part*. Joint WHO-China Study 14 January-14 February 2021. Joint Report. Workd Health Organisation.
WHO (2021b). *Behavioural Insights*. World Health Organisation. Accessed at:
https://www.who.int/our-work/science-division/behavioural-insights.
Whyte J., Thompson S., Marin-Guzman D., and Pelly M. (2018). *King & Wood Mallesons' Worksafe Investigation Lifts Lid on a Can of Worms*. Financial Review, 26 October 2018. Accessed at:
https://www.afr.com/work-and-careers/workplace/king--wood-mallesons-worksafe-investigation-lifts-lid-on-a-can-of-worms-20181025-h172ud.
Wibulpolprasert S. and Chowdhury M. (2016). *World Health Organization: Overhaul or Dismantle?* American Journal of Public Health 106(11) pp1910-1911.
Wick W.D. (2022). *Stopping the SuperSpreader Epidemic: The Lessons from SARS (with, perhaps, applications to MERS)*. ARVIX: 1308.6534v1, 29 August 2013
Wijtvliet W. and Dyevre A. (2021). *Does Ideology Influence Decision-making by EU Judges. London School of Economics and Political Science*. Accessed at:
https://blogs.lse.ac.uk/europpblog/2021/01/11/does-ideology-influence-decision-making-by-eu-judges/.
Wilhelm O., Hildebrandt A., and Oberauer K. (2013). *What is Working Memory Capacity, and How Can We Measure it*? Frontiers in Psychology 4 Article 433.
Whitehead J.W. (2016). *From Democracy to Pathocracy: The Rise of the Political Psychopath*. The HuffPost 1 April 2017. Accessed at:
https://www.huffpost.com/entry/from-democracy-to-pathocr_b_9566896.
Williams K.R. (2019). *The Cost of Tolerating Toxic Behaviors in the Department of Defense Workplace*. Military Review July-August 2019.
Willingham R. (2021). *Victorian Premier Daniel Andrews Knocks Back Questions on IBAC Investigation into Firefighting Saga*. ABC News, 6 October 2021. Accessed at:
https://www.abc.net.au/news/2021-10-06/ibac-premier-daniel-andrews-cfa-volunteers-pay-dispute/100517280.
Wilkins P. and Phillimore J. (2019). *What are the Merits of Royal Commissions and Other Forms of Inquiry*. The Mandarin, 18 February 2019. Accessed at:
https://www.themandarin.com.au/104199-what-are-the-merits-of-royal-commissions-and-other-forms-of-inquiry/.
Willingham R. (2023). *Victorians are still waiting for answers to simple questions on the Commonwealth Games*. ABC News 5 August, 2023. Accessed at:

https://www.abc.net.au/news/2023-08-05/daniel-andrews-victoria-commonwealth-games-questions-remain/102687944.

Windsor L.C., Reinhardt G.Y., Windsor A.J., Ostergard R., Allen S., Burns C., Giger J., Wood R. (2020). *Gender in the Time of COVID-19: Evaluating National Leadership and Covid-19 Fatalities*. PLoS ONE 15(12 Article e0244531.

Wollbers J., Boersma K., and Groenewegen P. (2018). *Introducing a Fragmentation Perspective on Coordination in Crisis Management*. Organization Studies 39)11) pp. 1521-1546.

Wong G., Liu W., Zhou B., Bi Y., and Gao G.F. (2015). *MERS, SARS, and Ebola: The Role of Super-Spreaders in Infectious Disease*. Cell Host & Microbe 18(4) pp. 398-401.

Woodley M. (2020a). *Inquiry Funds GPs Sidelined During Pandemic*. GP News, 5 August 2020. Accessed at:
https://www1.racgp.org.au/newsgp/clinical/parliamentary-inquiry-finds-gps-sidelined-during-p.

Woodley M. (2020b). *Restrictions Ease, but 'Main Problem' with Vic Contact Tracing Remains*. News GP, 26 October 2020, Royal Australian College of General Practitioners. Accessed at: https://www1.racgp.org.au/newsgp/clinical/as-restrictions-ease-the-main-problem-with-victori.

Woods E. (2021). *'Do you want to win the election or not?' Dan Andrews is Dragged into Labor Branch Stacking Probe – as Former MP Claims He Refused to Listen to Concerns Before 'red shirts' Scandal*. Daily Mail Australia, 9 November 2021.

Woods E. *Call for Vic Parliament Bullying Review*. Canberra Times 22 March 2022. Accessed at: https://www.canberratimes.com.au/story/7668182/calls-for-vic-parliament-bullying-review/.

Wooten L., and E. James. (2008). *Linking Crisis Management and Leadership Competencies: The Role of Human Resource Development*. Advances in Developing Human Resources 10 (3): 352–379.

WorkSafe (2019). *DHHS Charged for Alleged Health and Safety Discrimination*. WorkSafe Victoria, 5 July 2019. Accessed at:
https://www.worksafe.vic.gov.au/news/2019-07/dhhs-charged-alleged-health-and-safety-discrimination.

WorkSafe Victoria (2021). *Charges Laid Over Hotel Quarantine*. 29 September 2021. Accessed at: https://www.worksafe.vic.gov.au/news/2021-09/charges-laid-over-hotel-quarantine.

WorkSafe Victoria (2022). St Basil's Charged After Deadly COVID-19 Outbreak. News Article, 4 July 2022. Accessed at:
https://www.worksafe.vic.gov.au/news/2022-07/st-basils-charged-after-deadly-covid-19-outbreak.

Worobey M., Han G-Z. Rambault A. (2014). *Genesis and Pathogenesis of the 1918 Pandemic H1N1 Influenza A Virus*. PNAS 111(22) pp. 8107-8112.

Worobey M. Cox J., and Gill D. (2019). *The Origins of the Great Pandemic*. Evolution Medicine and Public Health [2019] pp. 18–25 doi:10.1093/emph/eoz001.

Worthington B. and Snape J. (2020). *Australia Blocks Arrival of all Non-citizens, Non-residents in Expanded Coronavirus Travel Ban*. ABC News 20 March 2020. Accessed at:
https://www.abc.net.au/news/2020-03-19/coronavirus-non-resident-travel-ban-australia/12071640.

Wright L. and van der Schaaf T. (2004). *Accident Versus Near Miss Causation: A Critical Review of the Literature, an Empirical Test in the UK Railway Domain, and Their Implications for Other Sectors*. Journal of Hazardous Materials 111 pp. 105-110.

Wu D. (2022). *Daniel Andrews' Department Told to Release COVID-19 Pandemic Surveys in the 'strong interest' of the Victorian Public*. Sky News, 1 June 2022. Accessed at: https://www.skynews.com.au/australia-news/coronavirus/daniel-andrews-department-told-to-release-covid19-pandemic-surveys-in-the-strong-interest-of-the-victorian-public/news-story/860d61076ab38fe609e043ced697677f.

Wu Z. and McGoogan J.M. (2020). *Characteristics of and Important Lessons from the Coronavirus Disease 2019 (COVID-19) Outbreak in China: Summary of a Report of 72314 Cases from the Chinese Center for Disease Control and Prevention*. JAMA 323 pp. 1239–1242.

Yang W., Shaff J., Shaman J. (2020). *COVID-19 Transmission Dynamics and Effectiveness of Public Health Interventions in New York City during the 2020 Spring Pandemic Wave*. medRxiv, 9 September 2020. Accessed at: https://www.medrxiv.org/content/10.1101/2020.09.08.20190710v1.full.pdf.

Yanovskiy M. and Socol Y. (2022). *Are Lockdowns Effective in Managing Pandemics?* International Journal of Environmental Research and Public Health 19 Article 9295.

Yates J.F. and de Oliveira S. (2016). *Culture and Decision Making.* Organizational Behaviour and Human Decision Processes 136 pp. 106-118.

Yemini A. (2021). *Breaking: Police Forcibly Eject Journalist Avi Yemini from Dan Andrews Press Conference*. Rebel News 17 February 2021. Accessed at: https://www.rebelnews.com/breaking_police_forcibly_eject_journalist_avi_yemini_from_dan_andrews_press_conference.

Yerka B. (2013). *Study Finds Political Ideology Impacts Decision-making Regarding Energy-efficient Products.* Phys.org, 30 April 210. Accessed at: https://phys.org/news/2013-04-political-ideology-impacts-decision-making-energy-efficient.html.

Young T. (2019). *The Rise of the Woke Corporation*. The Spectator, 9 March 2019. Accessed at: https://www.spectator.co.uk/article/the-rise-of-the-woke-corporation.

Young T. (2017). *Don't Like Our Diversity Agenda*? You're Fired. 12 August 2017. The Spectator, 12 August 2017. Accessed at: https://www.spectator.co.uk/article/don-t-like-our-diversity-agenda-you-re-fired.

Yuan S. (2020). *Inside the Early Days of China's Coronavirus Cover-Up*. Wired, 1 May 2020. Accessed at: https://www.wired.com/story/inside-the-early-days-of-chinas-coronavirus-coverup/.

Yuan H. and Miller S.M. (2013). *Target Controllability, Time Consistency, and the Tinbergen Rule*. Available at: SSRN: https://ssrn.com/abstract=2334342 or http://dx.doi.org/10.2139/ssrn.2334342.

Yussuf A. (2021). *Victorian Government Urged to Reconsider Need for Apology Over COVID-19 Public Housing Tower Lockdown*. ABC News, 2 July 2021. Accessed at: https://www.abc.net.au/news/2021-07-02/residents-wait-for-apology-for-public-housing-lockdown/100261552.

Zagon C., Swain S., and Waters C. (2021). *Testing Commander 'Very Unhappy' COVID-positive Nurse Worked at Multiple Sites*. 9 News 17 June 2021. Accessed at: https://www.9news.com.au/national/coronavirus-victoria-june-17-zero-new-local-cases-covid19/c66fce07-03be-4374-a4b5-88e83cd232eb.

Zaza S. (2020). *Politicization of Public Health*. American College of Preventive Health. Accessed at: https://www.acpm.org/news-publications/news/2020/politicization-of-public-health/.

Zelditch M. and Walker H.A. (2000). *The Normative Regulation of Power*. In: Advances in Group Processes Vol. *17*. Emerald Group Publishing Limited, Bingley, pp. 155-178.

References

Zhang N., Ruosong M., Huang H., and Chang E.Y.Y. (2016). *Contact Infection of Infectious Disease on Board a Cruise Ship*. Scientific Reports 6 Article number 38790.

Zhou A. (2016). *Analysis of the Volkswagen Scandal Possible Solutions for Recovery*. School of Global Policy and Strategy. University of California at San Diego, CA.

Zorn C. and Barnes Bowie J. (2010). *Ideological Influences on Decision Making in the Federal Judicial Hierarchy: An Empirical Assessment.* The Journal of Politics 72(4) pp. 1222-1235.

Index

E

F

G

H

L

M

N

O

P

Q

R

S

T

U

V

W